RUMINATION-FOCUSED COGNITIVE-BEHAVIORAL THERAPY FOR DEPRESSION

Also by Edward R. Watkins

Handbook of Cognition and Emotion
Edited by Michael D. Robinson,
Edward R. Watkins, and Eddie Harmon-Jones

Rumination-Focused Cognitive-Behavioral Therapy *for* DEPRESSION

EDWARD R. WATKINS

THE GUILFORD PRESS
New York   London

Copyright © 2016 The Guilford Press
A Division of Guilford Publications, Inc.
370 Seventh Avenue, Suite 1200, New York, NY 10001
www.guilford.com

Paperback edition 2018

Printed in the United States of America

This book is printed on acid-free paper.

Last digit is print number: 9 8 7 6 5 4

The author has checked with sources believed to be reliable in his efforts to provide information that is complete and generally in accord with the standards of practice that are accepted at the time of publication. However, in view of the possibility of human error or changes in behavioral, mental health, or medical sciences, neither the author nor the publisher, nor any other party who has been involved in the preparation or publication of this work warrants that the information contained herein is in every respect accurate or complete, and they are not responsible for any errors or omissions or the results obtained from the use of such information. Readers are encouraged to confirm the information contained in this book with other sources.

Library of Congress Cataloging-in-Publication Data

Names: Watkins, Edward R., author.
Title: Rumination-focused cognitive-behavioral therapy for depression /
   Edward R. Watkins.
Description: New York : The Guilford Press, [2016] | Includes bibliographical
   references and index.
Identifiers: LCCN 2016000631 | ISBN 9781462525102 (hardback : acid-free paper) |
   ISBN 9781462536047 (paperback : acid-free paper)
Subjects: LCSH: Depression, Mental—Treatment. | Emotions and cognition. |
   BISAC: PSYCHOLOGY / Psychopathology / Depression. | MEDICAL / Psychiatry /
   General. | SOCIAL SCIENCE / Social Work.
Classification: LCC RC537 .W28 2016 | DDC 616.85/27—dc23
LC record available at *http://lccn.loc.gov/2016000631*

About the Author

Edward R. Watkins, PhD, CPsychol, is Professor of Experimental and Applied Clinical Psychology at the University of Exeter, United Kingdom, and Director of the Mood Disorders Centre and the Study of Maladaptive to Adaptive Repetitive Thought (SMART) Lab. Dr. Watkins has practiced as a cognitive-behavioral therapist for 20 years, specializing in depression. His research focuses on the experimental understanding of psychopathology in depression—with a particular focus on repetitive negative thoughts and rumination—and the development and evaluation of new psychological interventions for mood disorders, including randomized controlled trials of treatments targeting rumination in depression. Dr. Watkins is a recipient of the British Psychological Society's May Davidson Award for outstanding contributions to the development of clinical psychology within the first 10 years of his career.

Preface

This is a book written for clinicians who want to find better ways to grapple with the thorny problems of rumination and worry in their patients. It is intended to be relevant for practicing clinicians at every level, from trainee to cognitive therapy supervisor.

Over the last 20 years, rumination and repetitive negative thought have increasingly been identified as among the most important cognitive mechanisms in the onset and maintenance of depression and anxiety. Despite this, to date there have been only limited and often sketchy descriptions of how to tackle rumination. I wrote this book to fill this important gap by providing a detailed and comprehensive how-to guide for therapists. The goal of this book is thus to present the state-of-the-art principles and strategies that I have found to be effective in reducing rumination in patients.

The book is based on the original treatment manual I wrote for a rumination-focused cognitive-behavioral therapy (RFCBT) research trial, and it is thus an evidence-based manual, utilizing a treatment proven to be effective. This book evolved from and built on that manual so that it incorporates the clinical lessons and experience learned over the last 15 years of developing and implementing RFCBT. While my treatment research originally focused only on rumination in the context of residual depression, the ideas and techniques in this book are not limited to this use alone. In the 2011 trial, rumination was targeted as the only focus of therapy to provide a strong test of whether reducing rumination would reduce residual depression. However, excitingly, a recently completed trial has confirmed the additional benefits of RFCBT for depression relative to existing treatments: the RFCBT group significantly outperformed the standard cognitive-behavioral therapy (CBT) group in reducing symptoms of depression in 131 adult patients with major depression recruited in a psychiatric outpatient service

(Hvenegaard, Watkins, Gondan, Grafton, & Moeller, 2015). Other work has indicated the efficacy of RFCBT in preventing depression and anxiety in young adults, and in reducing rumination and depression in adolescents with remitted histories of depression. Further, there are good theoretical and empirical reasons to support applying this treatment more broadly.

The approaches and techniques outlined in this manual could be used as a stand-alone treatment for depression, incorporated as a module focused on rumination or worry within a course of CBT for depression or other disorders, or used as an adjunct to other interventions. For example, if you are working with a patient who is struggling to make progress because of severe rumination or worry, then the interventions in this book may help to break this impasse, regardless of his or her diagnosis. I believe that this manual will help therapists to treat worry and rumination in all disorders in which these pernicious symptoms present.

The genesis of this book came over 20 years ago when I was working as a cognitive-behavioral therapist in the specialist Affective Disorders Unit at the Institute of Psychiatry and Maudsley Hospital, London. In this role, I was regularly engaged in CBT with patients with depression, who were referred to this tertiary service because they experienced the most persistent and severe depression. Although we obtained good outcomes using Aaron Beck's classic CBT for depression, there was still a substantial proportion of patients who showed little or no improvement. As I began to more closely observe and engage with these patients, it become apparent that nearly all of them reported rumination as a major problem, but that it had not been previously asked about or addressed. From these observations, I began to try to better understand the phenomenology of rumination and to experiment with better ways to treat it.

Running parallel to my research, the research literature on rumination was also rapidly expanding, with more and more evidence of its importance as a vulnerability factor emerging, principally from the laboratory of Susan Nolen-Hoeksema. Her research focused primarily on the consequences of rumination, and my own experimental research, building on some fortuitous observations emerging from my PhD work, began to investigate the mechanisms underpinning rumination. This research is described in Chapter 2, which illustrates the links between clinical research and clinical practice and provides further details for researchers and clinicians interested in developing research.

RFCBT has since emerged as the integration of many years of clinical observation and piloting of treatment approaches with the translation of experimental findings into clinical techniques. This book is a summary and culmination of all that clinical and research work, with the intention of widely disseminating these ideas to the therapy community.

The treatment described in this manual emerges from the classical CBT approach for depression, primarily because this is the approach in which I was trained. The development of RFCBT has also been heavily influenced by the reemergence of behavioral approaches for treating depression over the last decade, and, in particular, the growing evidence for behavioral activation. This treatment shares with behavioral activation a focus on contextual approaches and functional analysis, as developed by Christopher Martell, Sonja Dimidjian, and colleagues. Indeed, in conjunction with my work, Martell and colleagues have been proposing how behavioral activation can tackle rumination. Reassuringly, their suggestions closely mirror those described in this book.

Because the development of RFCBT has also built on my experimental research work indicating the importance of shifting processing style as a means to move patients out of pathological rumination, the intervention has a number of experiential approaches intended to shift mode of processing. As such, RFCBT overlaps with a number of recent therapeutic interventions, sometimes labeled as "third-wave" interventions, such as mindfulness and compassion-focused therapy. In particular, RFCBT involves exercises devised to increase engagement in the present moment and to support self-compassion. The key differences from these other interventions is that in RFCBT, these interventions are all derived from a solid empirical experimental research base and are tightly grounded in a functional analytic framework. For example, the approaches to increasing compassion in this manual, while inspired by Paul Gilbert's seminal work indicating the importance of compassion, differ from his approach in that they are based on patients' identifying and imagining their own experiences of compassion.

At its heart, this book is focused on trying to improve treatments for common mental health problems. Although we have effective treatments including classic CBT, there is considerable scope for improvement, with better, more sustained treatments for depression and anxiety still a major challenge for the field. Identifying and targeting important mechanisms such as rumination is part of the process of addressing this contemporary need. Further, with growing evidence that rumination is a transdiagnostic vulnerability factor, developing better ways to tackle this mechanism across disorders is a pressing priority. This manual represents a step along the path to responding to these challenges. I hope the reader will find that it not only enhances his or her clinical practice and improves the outcomes for his or her patients, but also inspires further therapeutic and research developments along the way.

Acknowledgments

Just as science progresses through dwarves standing on the shoulders of giants, it is not possible to create anything completely new in the world of therapy. I am therefore deeply indebted to many people over the 20 years of clinical practice and research in which rumination-focused cognitive-behavioral therapy (RFCBT) has evolved.

From the beginning, three people—Susan Nolen-Hoeksema, John Teasdale, and Ruth Williams—have been critical to the birth of RFCBT, each of whom has inspired me in different ways, and whom I cannot thank enough.

There would have been no work focused on treating rumination without the seminal work of Susan Nolen-Hoeksema. Susan instigated the ground-breaking experimental and longitudinal studies that put rumination on the map as a major vulnerability factor for depression. For me individually, Susan was an inspiring and insightful collaborator, and we shared many fascinating conversations. Our whole field is diminished by her premature passing. I hope this work takes a step toward her dream of effectively tackling rumination. This book is dedicated to her memory and spirit.

Just as critically, the development of RFCBT would not have been possible without the mentorship of John Teasdale and Ruth Williams, my PhD supervisors, who instilled in me the values and skills on which this work has been built. John encouraged my enthusiasm for clinical research and my career-long focus on "unpacking" mechanisms, and he inculcated rigor, focus, and clarity in my research. Anything good in my own experimental research is due to John's exacting standards and wisdom. Ruth introduced me to cognitive-behavioral therapy with her unique combination of precision, compassion, and humanity. It is no coincidence that these are core aspirations within RFCBT: Ruth can take credit for the best bits of what has emerged in the therapy. No less important than their expertise, John and Ruth both embody warmth, humor, integrity, and modesty. I am privileged to have been guided not just by the best of clinical researchers but by the best of people. Thank you both so much.

Of course, treatment development is not a solo effort, and a team of people have been central to reaching this point. I was extremely fortunate at the start of this journey to have the best possible postdoctoral researchers in Nick Moberly and Michelle Moulds to take forward the rumination research. It is impossible to imagine that I could have found anyone smarter, more energetic, or more productive than either Nick or Michelle, each in their different ways. It is a real pleasure to see them move on to their own independent successes and to continue to collaborate with such excellent colleagues. Thank you, Nick and Michelle.

A special thank you goes to Jan Scott, who provided useful guidance at the critical stage of first testing RFCBT and has been a fantastic cheerleader for this work. Equally important was the dedication of the researchers and therapists within the RFCBT treatment trials, who helped complete this work on a shoestring budget: Thank you to Katharine Rimes, Herbert Steiner, Neil Bathurst, Rachel Eastman, Janet Wingrove, Sandra Kennell-Webb, and Yanni Malliaris.

RFCBT also benefits from excellent collaborators around the world, including Thomas Ehring, Maurice Topper, Morten Hvenegaard, Stine Moeller, Morten Kistrup, Steven Linton, Maria Tillfors, Winnie Mak, and Patrick Leung, who, I hope, will write the next step of its development.

This work would not have been possible without large-scale funding. I am grateful to the Wellcome Trust and the Medical Research Council UK for funding the experimental science that underpins RFCBT, and to the National Alliance for Research on Schizophrenia and Depression for funding the initial trial of RFCBT.

I have also benefited from many fruitful conversations with colleagues in the depression and cognitive-behavioral therapy fields. This is a wonderfully collaborative and supportive community, so I am not able to list all who have influenced my thinking and whose ideas have informed this book. However, notables include Paul Gilbert and Christopher Martell, with special thanks for their enthusiasm and insights into compassion and behavioral activation, respectively, and Mark Williams, Mark Freeston, Tom Borkovec, David M. Clark, Steve Hollon, Rob DeRubeis, Paula Hertel, Allison Harvey, Jutta Joormann, Colin MacLeod, Anke Ehlers, Colette Hirsch, Filip Raes, Emily Holmes, Dirk Hermans, Pierre Philippot, Ernst Koster, Rudi De Raedt, and Christopher Fairburn.

I also want to express my permanent gratitude to Eugene Mullan, a fantastic supportive colleague whose unfailing optimism has helped me through darker days. Your ability to continue to see the opportunities to make things better, even in the most challenging of times, is a lesson for us all.

Jim Nageotte, Senior Editor at The Guilford Press, was the force behind making this book happen. Thank you, Jim, for your vision to bring this project together, for all your support and encouragement, and for your constant good editorial judgment that has helped to shape a much better and clearer book. Thanks too for going the extra mile to get just the right image for the book's jacket. Senior Assistant Editor Jane Keislar, Senior Production Editor Anna Nelson, and copy editor Rosalie Wieder were superbly detailed, thorough, and precise—without being fussy—and persistent in their reminders, without nagging.

The most important people in this whole endeavor are the individuals who suffer from rumination and depression who have graciously and courageously given of their time to volunteer for our studies and engage in RFCBT. Their openness to share their experiences and life lessons has been invaluable to the development of this therapy. I have learned so much from hearing the perspectives of those in the throes of rumination, and from working together with them to find out what works. I am so grateful to all of the participants and patients who were involved. I hope their altruism has in some part been repaid by personal benefits and by contributing to the recovery of others who experience depression.

Finally, on a personal note, I could not have done any of this without the love and support of my family, and especially my wife, Jo. Thank you, Jo, for putting up with me with amazing patience, tolerance, and humor, and for wrangling the kids when I was absent at the writing desk. Every day I count my blessings to have such a wonderful partner, whose very company is the best cure for rumination I know.

Contents

PART II. RUMINATION-FOCUSED COGNITIVE-BEHAVIORAL THERAPY

Purchasers of this book can download and print
the handouts at *www.guilford.com/watkins-forms*
for personal use or use with individual clients.

PART I

RUMINATION PROCESSES IN PSYCHOPATHOLOGY AND TREATMENT

CHAPTER 1

Why a Treatment Targeting Rumination?

This manual details a novel form of cognitive-behavioral therapy (CBT) designed to treat depression and its common comorbid disorders by targeting ruminative thinking. In Part I, I introduce the rationale behind developing the therapy and the theoretical and clinical principles that underpin it. A guiding principle in my work has been that we need to do better at treating and preventing depression. Understanding and targeting key mechanisms causing depression is an effective means to do this.[1]

Addressing a Major Treatment Gap

Depression Is a Major Global Challenge

Depression is a highly prevalent disorder, affecting 20% of women and 10% of men in their lifetimes. Further, it is a chronic, debilitating, and recurrent disorder (Kessler et al., 1994). The medical, social, economic, and personal costs of depression are enormous, as it erodes quality of life, reduces productivity in the workplace, impairs fulfilment of social and familial roles, increases the risk of suicide and self-harm, and substantially increases global disease burden (World Health Organization, 2008).

---

[1] A key distinction at the outset is between unipolar depression and bipolar disorder. Unipolar depression, which is the principal focus of the rumination-focused treatment work, includes only depressive conditions occurring in the absence of current or past mania or hypomania. The treatment described in this manual has to date only been developed and evaluated in the context of unipolar depression. The use for patients with mania or hypomania would not be advised.

In this context, depression principally refers to the diagnosis of major depression within agreed guidelines, such as the *Diagnostic and Statistical Manual of Mental Disorders* (DSM), now in its fifth edition (DSM-5; American Psychiatric Association, 2013), and the *International Classification of Diseases*, now in its 10th edition (ICD-10; World Health Organization, 1992). The essential features of major depression include seriously compromised mood (at least 2 weeks of continuous depressed mood or loss of interest/pleasure/motivation, such as anhedonia) and at least four additional cognitive, behavioral, or physical symptoms. Individuals must show the symptoms all or most of the day, nearly every day for at least 2 weeks. In order to be diagnosed, the episode must be clinically significant, in terms of causing distress or impaired functioning in the person's typical social or occupational roles. Furthermore, alternative causes for the symptoms, such as bereavement (although this has been removed in DSM-5) or the direct physiological effects of medical illness (e.g., hypothyroidism), medications, and substance misuse need to be ruled out before a diagnosis of a major depressive episode can be reached.

Major depression produces the second-largest burden of disease in the world today and is by far the leading cause of disability (World Health Organization, 2001); it is estimated that by 2020 it will have the second-highest disease burden across all disorders (Murray & Lopez, 1996).

Other forms of depressive disorder include dysthymic disorder, which is diagnosed if symptoms persist for at least 2 years, although there might be brief periods of normal mood lasting no more than 2 months. Additionally, in order to be diagnosed, dysthymic disorder must be seen to cause significant distress or disruption in the person's significant areas of functioning. Minor depressive disorder is diagnosed for at least 2 weeks of symptoms but with fewer than the five symptoms required for major depressive disorder. Recurrent brief depression refers to episodes lasting 2 days to 2 weeks, occurring at least once a month for a year. Combined together, these different forms of depression are the most common presentation of mental health difficulties, accounting for 38% of all outpatient diagnoses in the United States. Each is associated with distress and disability.

A Major Treatment Gap

Critically, despite the high frequency and impact across all forms of depression, we still face a major treatment gap. Most people with depression do not receive treatment, about one-third of those who do receive treatment do not respond to current approaches, and over half of those who experience a first onset of a major depressive episode will experience one or more recurrences. Thus, although we have effective treatments such as antidepressant medication and CBT (Hollon et al., 2005; Nathan & Gorman, 2007) there is still considerable scope to improve treatments. Limitations of current effective therapies include substantial rates of partial or non-response (greater than 40%) and disappointing rates of remission (less than a third; Hollon et al., 2005; Nathan & Gorman, 2007). Moreover, even effective treatments have high rates of relapse and recurrence (50–80%), such that few patients actually enjoy sustained recovery (Bruce et al., 2005; Judd, 1997). Improved relapse prevention has been identified as a priority for treatment research in depression, because a significant proportion of people with depression experience a chronic or recurrent life course. We need to improve the efficacy and sustained effects of our treatments.

For example, after patients with major depression are treated with recommended doses of antidepressant medication, approximately 30% experience partial remission, that is, no longer meet criteria for major depression but still have elevated depressive symptoms, which cause significant distress and disability (Cornwall & Scott, 1997; Paykel et al., 1995). This subtype of depression is characterized as residual depression, and sometimes called treatment-refractory or medication-resistant depression. It is a chronic and persistent form of depression. Residual depression is important because of its frequency and because residual symptoms increase the likelihood of future relapse and recurrence of depression. In prospective longitudinal studies, elevated residual symptoms provide one of the best predictors of future depressive relapse (Fava, 1999; Judd, 1997; Judd, Paulus, & Zeller, 1999; Paykel et al., 1995). Furthermore, treatments that reduce residual symptoms reduce the risk of relapse (Fava, Zielezny, Savron, & Grandi, 1995). Chronicity of depression is also associated with substantial distress, high rates of comorbidity, marked functional impairments, and increased health care utilization. Randomized controlled trials (RCTs) of CBT suggest that it is effective at reducing subsequent depressive relapses when it is effective at reducing acute symptoms, but that it is less effective at achieving remission in chronic depression. Finding treatments for depression that are better at tackling residual depression and treatment-refractory chronic depression, and at achieving remission and preventing recurrence, is a pressing need.[2]

How Do We Make Our Treatments Effective and Lasting?

It is thus evident that improving the efficacy and sustained effect of psychological interventions requires better reduction of residual symptoms in

---

[2]Technically, the diagnosis of residual depression in a patient is operationalized as experiencing an episode of a major depressive disorder in the last 18 months while not meeting criteria for major depression in the last 2 months, but nonetheless having depressive symptoms (scores of at least 8 on the 17-item Hamilton Rating Scale for Depression [HRSD] and 9 on the Beck Depression Inventory [BDI]). Participants also need to have been taking antidepressant medication for at least the previous 8 weeks, with 4 or more weeks at a minimum clinically recommended daily dose (e.g., equivalent to at least 125 mg of amitriptyline).

depression. There are many common residual symptoms, including irritability, anxiety, loss of confidence, insomnia, and a tendency to worry and ruminate about difficulties. One potential approach to enhancing treatments is to identify and specifically target these residual symptoms.

In parallel to targeting key residual symptoms, recent recommendations to improve psychological treatments have emphasized the value of targeting an identified psychopathological mechanism to enhance treatment efficacy (Barlow, 2004). While CBT for depression is effective and influences depressogenic information processing (Hollon et al., 2005), it has changed little from the seminal treatment manual (Beck, Rush, Shaw, & Emery, 1979), despite considerable subsequent psychopathology research. In contrast, CBT for anxiety has evolved in response to psychopathology research, resulting in new and more effective interventions (e.g., the work of David Clark and Anke Ehlers in panic disorder, social anxiety, and posttraumatic stress disorder [PTSD]). There is thus scope to improve psychological interventions for depression by focusing on underlying mechanisms, as recommended in the recent Research Domain Criteria initiative from the U.S. National Institute of Mental Health (Sanislow et al., 2010, p. 631).

The treatment presented in this book does just that. In particular, it focuses on the mechanism of rumination. Happily, focusing on ruminative thought in depression has the potential to kill two birds with one stone, as it targets both a residual symptom of depression (Roberts, Gilboa, & Gotlib, 1998) and a key mechanism implicated in its onset and maintenance (Nolen-Hoeksema, 2000; Nolen-Hoeksema, Wisco, & Lyubomirsky, 2008; Watkins, 2008). To be precise about our terms, rumination is here defined as recurrent and repetitive thinking on symptoms (e.g., fatigue, low mood), feelings, problems, upsetting events, and negative aspects of the self, typically with a focus on their causes, meanings, and implications. More specifically, Susan Nolen-Hoeksema defined rumination as "passively and repetitively focusing on one's symptoms of distress and the circumstances surrounding these symptoms" (Nolen-Hoeksema, McBride, & Larson, 1997, p. 855).

Rumination as a Primary Therapeutic Target

There are good reasons to choose rumination as a primary therapeutic target. First, it is a common residual symptom, remaining elevated after both partial and full remission from depression (Riso et al., 2003; Roberts et al., 1998). Both currently depressed and formerly depressed patients report elevated levels of rumination compared to those who have never been depressed (Roberts et al., 1998). Moreover, elevated rumination is associated with less responsiveness to both antidepressant medication and cognitive therapy (Ciesla & Roberts, 2007; Schmaling, Dimidjian, Katon, & Sullivan, 2002), suggesting it may contribute to partial remission.

Second, there is extensive and robust evidence implicating rumination in the onset and maintenance of depression (Nolen-Hoeksema et al., 2008; Watkins, 2008). Prospective longitudinal studies have found that self-reported rumination, typically assessed on the Response Styles Questionnaire (RSQ; Nolen-Hoeksema, 1991; Treynor, Gonzalez, & Nolen-Hoeksema, 2003), predicts (1) the future onset of a major depressive episode across a range of follow-up periods in initially nondepressed individuals (Just & Alloy, 1997; Nolen-Hoeksema, 2000), with Spasojević and Alloy (2001) finding that rumination mediated the effect of other risk factors on onset of depression; (2) depressive symptoms across a range of follow-up periods in initially nondepressed individuals, after controlling for baseline symptoms (Abela, Brozina, & Haigh, 2002; Butler & Nolen-Hoeksema, 1994; Hong, 2007; Nolen-Hoeksema, 1991; Nolen-Hoeksema, 2000; Nolen-Hoeksema, Parker, & Larson, 1994; Nolen-Hoeksema, Stice, Wade, & Bohon, 2007; Sakamoto, Kambara, & Tanno, 2001; Smith, Alloy, & Abramson, 2006); and (3) depressive symptoms in patients with clinical depression, after controlling for baseline depression (Kuehner & Weber, 1999; Nolen-Hoeksema, 2000; Rohan, Sigmon, & Dorhofer, 2003).

In addition, experimental studies provide convergent evidence that rumination plays a causal role in a range of unconstructive outcomes associated with depression, including exacerbating negative mood and increasing negative thinking. These studies used a standardized rumination induction, in which participants are instructed to spend 8 minutes concentrating on a series of sentences that involve rumination about themselves, their current feelings and physical state, and the causes and consequences of their feelings (e.g., "Think about the way you feel inside") (Lyubomirsky & Nolen-Hoeksema, 1995; Nolen-Hoeksema & Morrow, 1993). As a control condition, a distraction induction is typically used, in which participants are instructed to spend 8 minutes concentrating on a series of sentences that involve imagining visual scenes unrelated to the self or to current feelings (e.g., "Think about a fire darting round a log in a fireplace").

Compared to the distraction induction, the rumination induction is reliably found to have negative consequences for mood and cognition. Critically the differential effects of these manipulations are found only when participants are already in a sad mood before the manipulations, indicating a moderating role of existing mood. Under these conditions, compared to distraction, rumination exacerbates negative mood (Lavender & Watkins, 2004; Lyubomirsky & Nolen-Hoeksema, 1995; Morrow & Nolen-Hoeksema, 1990; Nolen-Hoeksema & Morrow, 1993; Watkins & Teasdale, 2001); increases negative thinking (Lyubomirsky & Nolen-Hoeksema, 1995); increases negative autobiographical memory recall (Lyubomirsky, Caldwell, & Nolen-Hoeksema, 1998); reduces the specificity of autobiographical memory retrieval (Kao, Dritschel, & Astell, 2006; Park,

Goodyer, & Teasdale, 2004; Watkins & Teasdale, 2001; Williams et al., 2007); increases negative thinking about the future (Lavender & Watkins, 2004); impairs concentration and central executive functioning (Lyubomirsky, Kasri, & Zehm, 2003; Watkins & Brown, 2002); impairs controlled memory retrieval (Hertel, 1998); and impairs social problem solving (Donaldson & Lam, 2004; Lyubomirsky & Nolen-Hoeksema, 1995; Lyubomirsky, Tucker, Caldwell, & Berg, 1999).

Taken together, the prospective and experimental studies strongly implicate rumination in the onset and maintenance of depression. Third, depressive rumination partially accounts for the 2:1 rates of depression in women relative to men: once we statistically adjust for the greater tendency for women to ruminate, there is no longer a difference between men and women in rates of depression (Butler & Nolen-Hoeksema, 1994; Grant et al., 2004; Nolen-Hoeksema, Larson, & Grayson, 1999).

Fourth, clinical experience suggests that rumination is a key and often neglected component of patient's phenomenology in depression. For patients, depressive rumination often involves dwelling on past losses, analyzing past mistakes, and making social-evaluative judgments and comparisons. This thinking often includes "why" questions, such as "Why did this happen to me?"; "Why do I feel like this?"; "What went wrong?"; "Why can't I get things right?" Depressive rumination is often characterized by evaluative thinking, with patients making negative comparisons between themselves and others ("Why do I have problems other people don't have?"), between their current state and desired state ("Why can't I get better?"), and between the current self and past self ("Why can't I work as well as before?"). Patients report rumination as unintended, hard to stop, persistent, and repetitive. It is experienced as distressing and with a sense of being hard to control. There is the sense of being driven to ruminate, with a quality of "having to do it." The common reported consequences of rumination are increased sadness, distress, and anxiety, reduced motivation, insomnia, and increased tiredness, procrastination, self-criticism, pessimism, and hopelessness.

Thus, the logic of this approach is that successfully targeting rumination would both tackle a residual symptom of depression and reduce an important mechanism contributing to its onset and maintenance, thereby improving treatment outcomes.

Rumination as a Transdiagnostic Process

There is one further potential benefit of targeting rumination within psychological treatments. Rumination has been identified as a transdiagnostic or cross-cutting process, which means it is a mechanism that is (1) shared across multiple disorders and (2) causally contributes to the onset, maintenance, recurrence, or recovery from multiple disorders (Harvey, Watkins,

Mansell, & Shafran, 2004). There is evidence that rumination is common to multiple emotional disorders, in particular, depression, generalized anxiety disorder (GAD), social anxiety, PTSD, and eating disorders (for reviews see Aldao, Nolen-Hoeksema, & Schweizer [2010]; Ehring & Watkins [2008]; Nolen-Hoeksema & Watkins [2011]; Watkins [2008]), and causes both depression and anxiety disorders.

For example, Aldao et al. (2010) examined the relationships between emotion regulation strategies, including rumination, and symptoms of psychopathology across anxiety, depression, and eating- and substance-related disorders from 114 studies. There was a large effect size for rumination across all psychopathologies. Moreover, two large-scale longitudinal studies found that rumination explained the concurrent and prospective associations between symptoms of anxiety and depression (McLaughlin & Nolen-Hoeksema, 2011). In other studies, rumination prospectively predicted substance abuse (Nolen-Hoeksema et al., 2007; Skitch & Abela, 2008), alcohol abuse (Caselli et al., 2010), and eating disorders (Holm-Denoma & Hankin, 2010; Nolen-Hoeksema et al., 2007), after controlling for initial symptoms. Nolen-Hoeksema et al. (2007) examined the relationship between rumination and symptoms of depression, bulimia, and substance abuse in 496 female adolescents followed prospectively over time. Rumination predicted future increases in bulimic and substance abuse symptoms, as well as onset of major depression, binge eating, and substance abuse. This evidence suggests that rumination is a strong candidate to be considered a transdiagnostic process that contributes to psychopathology.

Consistent with the tenets of the transdiagnostic approach (Harvey et al., 2004), targeting rumination may thus have the further advantage of addressing comorbid presentations. After all, it is more common than not that a patient seeking help for depression will actually be suffering from multiple disorders—that is, presenting with two or more comorbid conditions. Most typically, such patients are dealing with both anxiety and depression. There are high rates of such comorbidity. Twelve-month rates of comorbid anxiety and/or depression are estimated as high as 40–80% (Kessler, Chiu, Demler, & Walters, 2005).

In practice, this means that a key decision for clinicians is how to treat comorbidity. As a therapist, you no doubt have frequently had patients present with a mixture of symptoms and difficulties. Further, one of your first and often hardest decisions is determining which difficulty or disorder to target first. If a patient has both social anxiety and depression, should you focus first on treating the social anxiety or on the depression? To date, we don't really have good empirical guidance for this all-too-common situation. The majority of our therapy models, for example, cognitive-behavioral treatments, have focused on individual distinct diagnoses, with evidence showing worse outcomes for patients with comorbidity.

Using a transdiagnostically focused treatment, which acts to reduce multiple emotional disorders simultaneously, may be one way to address comorbidity. One approach is to build a treatment package that has a range of therapeutic components integrated together, with a view to addressing multiple disorders. The best example of this approach is the Unified Protocol for Transdiagnostic Treatment of Emotional Disorders, developed by David Barlow and his colleagues (Barlow, Allen, & Choate, 2004; Wilamowska et al., 2010). This treatment essentially takes all the common elements across different CBT treatments for anxiety and depression and combines them into one package. For example, this treatment includes reducing avoidance, with exposure to external feared stimuli and to interoception; increasing behavioral activation (BA); and thought challenging. Preliminary evidence indicates this approach may have benefit (Wilamowska et al., 2010). Similarly, transdiagnostic treatment packages for eating disorders have been developed with some success by Christopher Fairburn and his colleagues (Fairburn, Cooper, & Shafran, 2003).

An alternative transdiagnostic treatment approach, as proposed by Harvey et al. (2004) and Mansell, Harvey, Watkins, and Shafran (2008), is to identify transdiagnostic mechanisms that cut across multiple disorders and then to target those mechanisms explicitly. It has been argued that a transdiagnostic approach to treatment may provide an efficient means to address comorbidity. Mansell et al. (2008) proposed several potential advantages of a treatment focused on identified transdiagnostic processes. First, it potentially enables us to match interventions to the specific vulnerabilities and processes that are relevant to the individual. For example, if an individual was assessed and found to be highly prone to rumination, it would be sensible to select treatment elements that reduce rumination. Second, it directly targets fundamental active mechanisms, rather than symptom clusters, and, as such, is hypothesized to improve treatment efficacy (Barlow, 2004; Sanislow et al., 2010). Third, it enables a flexible treatment approach that can be applied across a range of presentations, including comorbidity. Indeed, such a transdiagnostic treatment has the potential to produce more potent interventions that better address comorbidity than treatments based on diagnoses or disorders (Mansell et al., 2008).

Because rumination is found to causally contribute to both anxiety and depression, there is a strong case for selecting rumination as the focus of a transdiagnostic intervention (Topper, Emmelkamp, & Ehring, 2010). Successfully reducing rumination should reduce both anxiety and depression. The treatment described in this book is one of the first attempts to develop and evaluate such a transdiagnostic process intervention. It is important to note that to date this therapy has only been evaluated in RCTs for acute treatment or prevention of depression. However, the theoretical and transdiagnostic rationale behind an intervention for rumination suggests that it should provide a useful therapeutic module to include in psychological interventions for other disorders that include repetitive negative thought, including GAD, PTSD, and social anxiety.

Summary of Rumination-Focused Cognitive-Behavioral Therapy

Before going into more detail about the principles, rationales, and techniques of rumination-focused cognitive-behavior therapy (RFCBT), I briefly overview what it involves and how it compares to existing psychological therapies for depression. RFCBT is a manualized CBT treatment, typically consisting of up to 12 individual sessions scheduled weekly or biweekly.

The therapy is theoretically informed by experimental research indicating that there are distinct constructive and unconstructive forms of rumination (Watkins, 2008). This research suggests that there are distinct styles of rumination, with distinct functional properties and consequences: a helpful style characterized by concrete, process-focused, and specific thinking versus an unhelpful, maladaptive style characterized by abstract, evaluative thinking (Treynor et al., 2003; Watkins, 2004a; Watkins & Baracaia, 2002; Watkins & Moulds, 2005; Watkins & Teasdale, 2001, 2004). Building on these findings, the therapy is designed to coach individuals to shift from unconstructive rumination to constructive rumination, through the use of functional analysis (FA), experiential and imagery exercises, and behavioral experiments. FA is an approach aimed at determining the functions and contexts under which desired and undesired behaviors occur and thereby finding ways to systematically increase or reduce target behaviors. It is focused on studying the variability and context of behavior within an individual's personal experience and using this to guide interventions.

These adaptations distinguish RFCBT from standard CBT for depression (Beck et al., 1979), which focuses on modifying the content of individual thoughts, by placing a greater emphasis on directly modifying the process of thinking. Although still grounded within the core principles and techniques of CBT for depression (Beck et al., 1979; e.g., collaborative empiricism, Socratic questioning, behavioral experiments), RFCBT involves several additional, novel elements.

First, it incorporates the functional-analytic and contextual approach developed in the BA treatment that resulted from a component analysis of CBT (Addis & Martell, 2004; Jacobson et al., 1996; Jacobson, Martell, & Dimidjian, 2001; Martell, Addis, & Jacobson, 2001). This approach is based on the view that rumination is a learned habitual behavior that has developed through negative reinforcement. RFCBT incorporates the functional-analytic and contextual principles and techniques of BA (Martell, 2003), but explicitly and exclusively focused on rumination. Within BA and

RFCBT, rumination is conceptualized as a form of avoidance, and FA is used to facilitate more helpful approach behaviors.

Second, RFCBT makes much less use of thought challenging than standard CBT does. Socratic questioning in RFCBT tends not to focus on the evidence and accuracy of thinking or on generating alternative interpretations, but rather on the function, purpose, and usefulness of thoughts and behaviors. There is a focus on the pattern and sequence of thoughts rather than the meaning of individual thoughts. This shift in focus has the advantage of avoiding the risk of getting into disputes and arguments with patients over the meaning and interpretation of thoughts, events, and situations.

Third, a key innovative element within RFCBT is the focus on shifting a patient's processing style from unconstructive forms of thinking to more constructive forms of thinking, using FA, imagery, and experiential approaches. RFCBT uses FA to help individuals realize that their rumination about negative self-experience can be helpful or unhelpful and to coach them in how to shift to a more helpful style of thinking. In addition, patients use directed imagery to re-create previous mental states when a more helpful thinking style was active, such as memories of being completely absorbed in an activity (e.g., "flow" or "peak" experiences). Shifting to these states acts directly counter to rumination.

Empirical Evidence

RFCBT has been investigated in three clinical studies: a case series of individual RFCBT for patients with residual depression (Watkins et al., 2007), an RCT of individual RFCBT for patients with residual depression (Watkins et al., 2011, funded by the National Alliance for Research on Schizophrenia and Depression [NARSAD]), and an RCT of group RFCBT and Internet-based RFCBT to reduce and prevent depression in a high-risk group of young adults selected for having elevated levels of worry and rumination (Topper, Emmelkamp, Watkins, & Ehring, 2014). There have also been trials of concreteness training, which is a specific element within the RFCBT treatment package (Watkins et al., 2012; Watkins, Baeyens, & Read, 2009, funded by the UK Medical Research Council). All of these treatment evaluations have had positive findings, indicating that RFCBT and its components are efficacious at reducing rumination and depression. This section briefly summarizes each of the relevant studies.

Case Series of Individual Face-to-Face RFCBT for Residual Depression

A case series investigated 12 weekly 60-minute sessions of RFCBT for 14 consecutively recruited patients meeting criteria for medication-refractory residual depression (Watkins et al., 2007). Treatment produced significant improvements in depressive symptoms and comorbid disorders: mean reduction in Beck Depression Inventory of 20 points, pre- to posttreatment within-subject effect size (Cohen's *d*) of 2.5, 50% of patients achieving full remission from depression, and a 71% reduction in comorbid Axis I diagnoses. Importantly, RFCBT significantly reduced self-reported rumination, with rumination at pretreatment equivalent to that found in currently depressed patients but the range of scores at posttreatment equivalent to levels of rumination observed in never-depressed participants. This study provides initial evidence that RFCBT may be an efficacious treatment for depressive rumination and that it can tackle both depression and comorbid disorders.

Phase II RCT of Individual Face-to-Face RFCBT for Residual Depression

The study (Watkins et al., 2011) was approved by the U.K. National Health Service South London and Maudsley Research Ethics Committee and was conducted in community mental health teams and psychological treatment services in South East London and Devon, United Kingdom. Patients who were referred to outpatient services for depression and/or on the waiting list for psychological therapies were approached, and those who met inclusion criteria and gave written informed consent to participate were randomly allocated to treatment as usual (TAU) alone or to TAU plus RFCBT. TAU consisted of ongoing antidepressant medication and outpatient clinical management. Randomization was performed by an off-site researcher using computer-generated random numbers and stratified according to gender and the duration of the index episode of major depression. All participants were assessed by research staff masked to treatment allocation at intake baseline assessment and again 6 months later. Patients were included in the trial if they were over 18 years old and met criteria for medication-refractory residual depression, defined as meeting diagnostic criteria for major depression within the past 18 months but not in the past 2 months and with elevated residual symptoms of depression, and taking antidepressant medication at a recommended therapeutic dose. Patients were excluded from the trial if they had a history of bipolar disorder, psychosis, current drug or alcohol dependence, intellectual disability, or organic brain damage or were receiving concurrent psychotherapy at point of entry to the study. There were no exclusion criteria with respect to comorbid anxiety disorders or Axis II personality disorder diagnoses. Forty-two patients were randomized in the trial and followed up.

Adding RFCBT to TAU significantly reduced residual symptoms and improved remission rates relative to TAU alone, with a mean difference in change in symptoms from pre to post-treatment of 7.57 between the treatments on the Beck Depression Inventory scores (95% confidence interval = 1.86–19.08). The between-treatment effect size (standardized mean difference) was $d = 1.11$, which is good for a psychological treatment. Furthermore, there was a significant effect of treatment condition on rates of treatment response (TAU 26% vs. RFCBT 81%), rates of remission (TAU 21% vs RFCBT 62%), and rates of relapse between baseline and postintervention assessments (TAU 53% vs. RFCBT 9.5%). RFCBT therefore significantly outperformed continuing with maintenance antidepressants alone.

The outcomes found for 12 sessions of RFCBT (remission rates of 62%; between-treatment effect sizes of 0.94–1.1) for patients with residual depressive symptoms compare favorably with 20 sessions of standard CBT for depression (Paykel et al., 1999; remission rates of 25%; between-treatment effect size of 0.3) in an identically defined sample of participants with residual depression. Moreover, we found that the addition of a psychological intervention beneficially augmented pharmacotherapy, in contrast to other recent trials (e.g., Kocsis et al., 2009). Although we have to be cautious when comparing between differently powered studies, the outcomes for our TAU condition closely match the outcomes for the TAU arm in the Paykel et al. (1999) trial. In the absence of a definitive large-scale RCT of RFCBT with a larger sample and a longer follow-up, these results raise the possibility that the modifications made to CBT in RFCBT may engender better treatment outcomes in residual depression.

The number of comorbid Axis II diagnoses at study end, covarying for initial rates, was significantly less in the RFCBT group than the TAU group (TAU: $M = 0.67$, $SD = 0.97$; RFCBT: $M = 0.24$, $SD = 0.44$). There was also a similar, but nonsignificant trend for fewer comorbid Axis I disorders in the RFCBT group than the TAU group at follow-up (TAU: $M = 1.05$, $SD = 0.97$; RFCBT: $M = 0.62$, $SD = 0.86$, $p = .068$). Thus, consistent with the transdiagnostic hypothesis, there is some evidence that targeting rumination reduces both depression and other comorbid disorders.

Moreover, RFCBT significantly reduced self-reported rumination more than TAU, and the treatment effects on depression were mediated by change in rumination, although this was only measured concurrently. This provides evidence that the treatment reduced rumination as intended. It was also found to significantly reduce worry, as assessed using the Penn State Worry Questionnaire (PSWQ).

Concreteness Training

Consistent with a causal relationship between processing mode and individual differences in rumination, a proof-of-principle randomized controlled treatment intervention trial found that training depressed individuals to be more concrete when faced with difficulties reduced depression, anxiety, and rumination relative to a no-treatment control (Watkins et al., 2009).

The concreteness training involved repeated practice at asking "How?" and focusing on specific details when thinking about recent difficulties.

In a Phase II RCT, concreteness training was found to be superior to TAU in reducing rumination, worry, and depression in patients with major depression recruited in primary care (Watkins et al., 2012). Thus, shifting depressed patients into a more concrete processing mode reduced rumination and associated symptoms.

RCT of Group RFCBT and Internet-Delivered RFCBT to Target Rumination and Prevent Depression and Anxiety

This recently completed treatment trial (Topper, Emmelkamp, Watkins, & Ehring, 2016) examines two adaptations of RFCBT (a group format and an Internet-delivered format; see Chapter 13 for further details) as an intervention to prevent depression and anxiety. Because of the extensive evidence that rumination predicts the onset and maintenance of depression, individuals with elevated tendency to rumination are at greater risk to develop depression. This makes the targeting of high ruminators a plausible strategy for preventing the initial onset of depression, as rumination increases the likelihood of someone developing depression, is easily identifiable, and is a tractable psychological process (Topper et al., 2010). Topper et al. (2010) recently made a strong case for treatments that explicitly target rumination as a potential approach to preventing depression. Moreover, because of the evidence that rumination is a transdiagnostic process, targeting rumination may also help to prevent anxiety disorders, eating disorders, and substance and alcohol misuse.

A completed randomized trial comparing the group and Internet versions of RFCBT found that both RFCBT adaptations were effective relative to waiting-list control groups for reducing depression, anxiety, worry, and rumination in young adults selected for their vulnerability to worry and rumination, in a high-risk prevention intervention design conducted in Amsterdam ($n = 251$, project team: Prof. Thomas Ehring, Prof. Paul Emmelkamp, Dr. Maurice Topper, Prof. Ed Watkins, supported by ZonMw funding to Principal Investigator Prof. Thomas Ehring; see Topper et al., 2016). This study selected both males and females ages 15–21 with elevated worry and rumination scores but no current major depression or anxiety disorder, and randomized them to Internet RFCBT, group RFCBT, or waiting-list control and then followed up for 12 months. Intent-to-treat analyses showed that both versions of RFCBT intervention significantly reduced worry and rumination (controlled effect size Cohen's $d = 0.53$ to 0.89), as well as symptom levels of anxiety and depression (Cohen's $d = 0.36$ to 0.72) at postintervention, relative to the waiting-list control, with these effects maintained at 1-year follow-up. There were no differences between the group and Internet online versions of RFCBT on any of the outcome measures. The interventions also resulted in a significantly lower 1-year incidence rate of major depression (group intervention 15.3%, Internet intervention 14.7%) and GAD (group intervention 18%; Internet intervention 16%), compared to the waiting list (32.4% and 42.2%, respectively). However, these findings are based on caseness cutoffs on well-established self-report measures rather than structured diagnostic interviews, and further replication using diagnostic interviews is necessary to confirm the findings on preventing depression. Nonetheless, these results provide proof of principle that rumination increases the risk for the onset of major depression and GAD, given the elevated incidence rates in the untreated group of people with elevated levels of worry/rumination relative to the general population. The findings also provide further evidence that RFCBT can be an effective intervention to reduce worry and rumination, and that it can be effectively delivered in both group and Internet-based formats. Moreover, the findings are consistent with the transdiagnostic hypothesis of rumination, as targeting rumination reduced both depression and anxiety.

Case Series of Individual Face-to-Face RFCBT for PTSD

A version of RFCBT has also been used to tackle persistent PTSD in a population of young survivors of the 1994 genocide in Rwanda (Sezibera, Van Broeck, & Philippot, 2009). The rationale for using RFCBT in this population is that rumination has been identified as a major maintaining factor in PTSD (Michael, Halligan, Clark, & Ehlers, 2007), consistent with its hypothesized transdiagnostic role. In this study, all the participants were orphans of the Rwandan genocide in 1994 who met criteria for PTSD assessed on self-rating scales 11 years after the genocide and again 13 years after the genocide, indicating that the PTSD was persistent. Twenty-two individuals ages 15–18 years were treated (54.5% female). The treatment incorporated elements from RFCBT, including psychoeducation and FA of rumination, as well as narrative exposure to trauma reminders, and lasted for 10 weekly sessions of maximum duration 2 hours. The intervention was associated with a reduction in PTSD symptoms, with gains maintained at 2-month follow-up. Although this is an uncontrolled study and therefore needs to be interpreted with caution, it provides further evidence that targeting rumination may have transdiagnostic benefit.

Group RFCBT for Residual Depression

A further independent trial (Teismann et al., 2014) has confirmed that group-delivered RFCBT improved depressed mood and reduced rumination relative to a waiting-list condition in patients with residual depression, with treatment gains maintained over 1-year follow-up. This RCT assigned 60 patients with residual depression to a group-delivered RFCBT treatment incorporating elements of both RFCBT and metacognitive therapy versus a waiting-list control. Group RFCBT outperformed waiting list (remission rates 42% vs. 10.3%), with effects maintained for 1 year. This study provides an important confirmation of the potential benefits of RFCBT from an independent research group.

Comparisons between RFCBT and Other Treatments

CBT for Depression

Despite the growing evidence that rumination is an important mechanism in depression, the original CBT for depression (Beck et al., 1979) did not explicitly focus on treating rumination in detail. There is a brief mention of rumination in the seminal 1979 book *Cognitive Therapy of Depression*, but no specific elaborations on how to address it, presumably under the assumption that repeated challenging of negative thoughts would suffice.

The clinical experience my colleagues and I have accumulated in our clinic through treating highly ruminative chronically depressed patients over the last 20 years has shown us that the classic CBT approach for depression (Beck et al., 1979) can sometimes be effective, but that it has a number of limitations and difficulties. First, focusing on challenging individual thoughts is not effective when dealing with a strong and habitual stream of negative thoughts, as is characteristic of depressive rumination. Trying to stop one thought does not prevent the full flow of rumination, because the first negative thought is simply followed by another thought in the chain, often in the form of a "Yes, but" thought.

The clinical experience of using a classic CBT approach with patients who ruminate can be like trying to stop a waterfall by catching one drop of water at a time. The difficulty of changing rumination is entirely consistent with conceptualizations of rumination as a habitual response (Nolen-Hoeksema, 1991) because habits are argued to be difficult to change by challenging beliefs. Our experience was that thought challenging can be helpful for rumination but only under two specific circumstances. It can prevent rumination when it catches the start of the chain of ruminative thoughts and nips it in the bud. Alternatively, when patients conscientiously practised thought challenging so that it became a habit in its own right, it could displace the habit of ruminative thinking.

Second, thought challenging can itself act as a further trigger to rumination. For example, once you have successfully challenged the evidence for a negative automatic thought with a depressed patient, the patient may then dwell on the thought "Why couldn't I do that before?" or "Why am I so stupid?," and the cycle of recurrent thinking is off and running again.

To effectively treat rumination, we hypothesized that it may be better for patients to step back from the thought process itself, rather than from any individual thought.

Third, with patients highly prone to rumination, any form of discussion and disputation can become focused on *talking about* what has happened and what it might mean to the patient. When that happens it is easy to become trapped in ruminating aloud with the patient, where sequences of negative thinking are repeatedly discussed in detail without any therapeutic change. For patients who ruminate, there is also a strong press toward thinking about and talking about the causes, meanings, and implications of their symptoms and difficulties. This can easily become the focus of the treatment session, with the patient bringing up difficulties to reflect on each week. One indicator of such "corumination" is the realization that large amounts of a treatment session have passed without any sense of progress. This was my experience with the first few patients I treated where rumination was a prominent difficulty. We would have often interesting and engaging discussions about the big issues in the patient's life and what they might mean, but little therapeutic progress was made, and symptoms did not improve.

Outcome evidence finds that standard CBT interventions are less effective at treating depression in high ruminators compared to low ruminators (Ciesla & Roberts, 2002; Schmaling et al., 2002). Furthermore, to date, there is no reported evidence from RCTs that standard CBT can reduce rumination.[3]

RFCBT uses standard CBT approaches, organization, and components such as a structured format, here-and-now focus, collaborative empiricism, agenda setting, use of feedback and summaries, homework, guided discovery, and behavioral experiments. However, as mentioned earlier, there are adjustments and alterations from the standard CBT protocol.

Behavioral Activation

There are emerging interventions that more directly target rumination than classic CBT, although direct evidence for their efficacy at reducing rumination is still lacking. BA was originally one component of the full CBT intervention, consisting of activity monitoring and activity scheduling. A trial comparing the different components of CBT found that BA alone was as effective at reducing symptoms as BA plus thought challenging and as the full CBT protocol (Gortner, Gollan, Dobson, & Jacobson, 1998; Jacobson et al., 1996). As a consequence, BA was elaborated into a stand-alone treatment, focusing on understanding the function and context in which depression occurs and targeting avoidance behaviors in depression (Martell et al.,

---

[3]Of course, we need to be careful about interpreting the current trials because until recently rumination was not an outcome measure in the majority of treatment trials.

2001). In a large-scale RCT, BA has been found to be an effective intervention for depression, producing outcomes as good as pharmacotherapy and better than CBT for severe depression (Dimidjian et al., 2006). However, to date, its effect on rumination has not been formally assessed.

As noted earlier, the RFCBT described in this book shares a number of similarities with BA, as well as several key differences. Both approaches incorporate a functional-analytic and contextual approach to behaviors. The development of RFCBT has been informed by the work within BA and by dialogue with leading proponents of BA, such as Christopher Martell. Within both BA and RFCBT, rumination is conceptualized as a form of avoidance, and FA is used to facilitate the reduction of this avoidance and to replace it with more helpful approach behaviors. Like BA, RFCBT treats rumination as behavior, even if covert, which can be contextually and functionally understood. However, RFCBT has greater elaboration in its approaches to rumination than BA. Moreover, an additional novel element not shared with either BA or standard CBT is the explicit focus on shifting thinking style during rumination, derived from my experimental research. The experiential exercises in RFCBT designed to shift thinking style (e.g., concreteness training, absorption work, compassion work) are not found in BA, although they are consistent with its functional-contextual principles.

Mindfulness-Based Cognitive Therapy

Another recent treatment that is explicitly designed to reduce rumination is mindfulness-based cognitive therapy (MBCT). MBCT incorporates elements of a mindfulness-based stress reduction program (Kabat-Zinn, 1990) into CBT to create a relapse prevention treatment for recurrent depression (Teasdale, Segal, & Williams, 1995). MBCT is delivered in weekly group training sessions, in which participants practice and develop a moment-by-moment awareness of sensations, thoughts, and feelings through the use of formal and informal meditation exercises, such as watching the breath and the body scan. The theoretical rationale behind MBCT is that training patients to step back and observe their thoughts and feelings as mental events and to become connected with direct experience in the present moment would reduce evaluative ruminative thinking.

In two RCTs, for patients with a history of three or more episodes of major depression but who were currently symptom-free, MBCT significantly reduced risk of relapse and recurrence over 1 year compared to TAU (Ma & Teasdale, 2004; Teasdale et al., 2000). Kuyken et al. (2008) demonstrated that MBCT has similar rates of relapse over 1 year follow-up to continuation antidepressant medication for patients with recurrent depression.

Consistent with the proposed theoretical underpinnings, mindfulness approaches have been found to reduce rumination, although not all studies randomized to treatment condition or used clinical populations. In an experimental analogue study, Feldman, Greeson, and Senville (2010) compared mindful breathing, progressive muscle relaxation, and loving-kindness meditation on negative reactions to repetitive thoughts in undergraduates and found that the association between frequency of repetitive thoughts and degree of negative reaction to thoughts was significantly less in the mindful breathing condition relative to the other two, suggesting that mindfulness reduced the impact of rumination. Two studies comparing pre-to-post change in rumination in mindfulness versus a matched waiting-list control (mindfulness meditation, Chambers, Lo, & Allen, 2008; mindfulness-based stress reduction [MBSR], Ramel, Goldin, Carmona, & McQuaid, 2004) demonstrated a reduction in rumination in the treatment group, although neither study randomized to condition. A randomized trial of mindfulness meditation versus relaxation in a nonclinical sample demonstrated a reduction in rumination (Jain et al., 2007). In an RCT, Geschwind, Peeters, Drukker, van Os, and Wichers (2011) found that MBCT reduced self-reported rumination pre- to postintervention relative to waiting-list control in patients with a history of major depression and current residual symptoms. However, Kuyken et al. (2008, 2010) failed to find that MBCT reduced rumination more than continuation antidepressant medication in patients with a history of recurrent depression.

RFCBT differs from MBCT in its suggested target population and treatment content and style. To date, MBCT has been shown to be effective in preventing relapse in people who are not currently depressed but have a history of recurrent depression (three or more episodes). It is not known whether MBCT is of value for patients in an acute episode of depression when rumination is at its most fierce. It may be that it is difficult or counterproductive to try to meditate when experiencing acute depressed mood and strong rumination. Future research will need to determine whether MBCT is effective for patients with acute symptoms of depression.

In contrast, RFCBT is designed to be used with patients experiencing acute symptoms of depression and rumination, whether in a major depressive episode or with residual symptoms. Indeed, one further advantage of targeting rumination is that it is observed to be elevated as a risk factor prior to the onset of depression, during episodes of major depression, in partial remission, and in full remission from depression. Elevated rumination is thus found at all points in the course of depression. Targeting rumination thus has potential for primary prevention, acute treatment, and prevention of relapse and recurrence, gaining further efficiency from the treatment (see Chapter 13).

RFCBT is a much more direct intervention than MBCT. It is explicit about what it is trying to achieve and how it is trying to coach patients into more helpful ways of coping through active practice of exercises. In contrast, MBCT is more indirect and involves patients learning more gradually through their own experience during meditation.

CHAPTER 2

Understanding Rumination

This chapter describes the theoretical and experimental background that underpinned the development of RFCBT. Understanding the theoretical background to the treatment methods will improve mastery of the therapy and improve its implementation. This chapter will be of particular interest to researchers and scientist-practitioners who want to understand more about the reasoning behind the development of the therapy. The chapter is split into sections that address key theoretical concepts concerning the mechanisms underpinning depressive rumination.

Rumination Is a Normal Process Driven by Unresolved Goals

It is important to recognize that rumination is a common, normal, and sometimes helpful response not limited to people with psychological disorders. We have all had the experience of ruminating about personal losses such as bereavements or breakups, trying to understand why they happened to us. However, for most people, such rumination is relatively brief.

As a brief thought experiment, reflect on your own experience in the following situations. Spend a few moments considering each situation in turn.

After making an easily avoidable but public mistake
After the unexpected end of a relationship
After the death of a loved one
Before going to the dentist
Before a meeting with someone who is confrontational and aggressive

Did you recognize that in at least one of these situations you would dwell (or did dwell) on what had happened or on what might happen next?

In my experience, these kinds of situations trigger worry and rumination in nearly all people. This highlights how rumination is a common and normal response. Moreover, in some of these situations, rumination may be helpful. Dwelling on what might happen before meeting an aggressive person may help you to develop better plans and prepare for the meeting. Dwelling on the loss of a loved one is a natural part of the bereavement process, which may help you to come to terms with the loss.

Current theoretical models hypothesize that unresolved concerns or unattained goals initiate recurrent thinking in order to facilitate effective self-regulation toward the goal (Martin & Tesser, 1996a, 1996b). Thus, rumination is conceptualized as an attempt to make sense of an upsetting event or to solve a problem. For example, Martin and Tesser (1996a, p. 7) defined rumination as "a class of conscious thoughts that revolve around a common instrumental theme and that recur in the absence of immediate environmental demands requiring the thoughts." Within this conceptualization, rumination is repetitive thought on a theme related to unresolved personal goals and concerns, which can have either constructive or unconstructive consequences, depending on whether the rumination helps or hinders the progress toward the unattained goal that triggered the rumination.

Thus, rumination has been characterized as a self-focused attempt at problem solving, triggered by a perceived discrepancy between a desired goal and the current state of affairs. The rumination is maintained until the goal is either achieved or abandoned (Carver & Scheier, 1998; Martin & Tesser, 1996a; Pyszczynski & Greenberg, 1987; Watkins, 2008). Clinically, I often see patients start trying to solve a problem but then shift their attention to evaluating the meaning of the problem and ending up stuck in rumination.

This theoretical analysis suggests that people are likely to get stuck in rumination for two main reasons. First, excessive rumination is more likely when individuals set goals that are difficult to attain and hard to abandon. For example, individuals can set goals that are simply unattainable or beyond their control or capability. This is particularly likely in individuals with extremely high standards or who are perfectionists, because their goals are likely to be hard to achieve while at the same time being highly important to them and hard to abandon. It could also result from setting goals that are poorly defined or whose pursuit requires a longer time period, making it harder for progress on the goal to be realized. I often see patients asking unanswerable questions, such as why a particular negative event happened. In such circumstances, rumination is likely to persist.

Second, people may get trapped in rumination if they do not know how best to attain their goals, for example, because of poor problem-solving skills. Recent experimental research suggests that there are distinct styles of rumination, with distinct functional properties and consequences: a helpful style characterized by concrete, process-focused, and specific thinking versus an unhelpful, maladaptive style characterized by abstract, evaluative thinking (Treynor et al., 2003; Watkins, 2004b; Watkins & Baracaia, 2002; Watkins & Moulds, 2005; Watkins & Teasdale, 2001, 2004). This research suggests that when a depressed patient dwells on symptoms and difficulties, analyzing and evaluating the meanings and implications of his or her experiences (e.g., "What does this failure mean about me?") increases overgeneralization (e.g., "I can never get it right"), impairs problem solving, and exacerbates depressed mood. However, dwelling on symptoms and difficulties in a more concrete and specific way, reflecting on how to do something about the difficulties, improves problem solving and reduces depression. This difference between thinking styles appears to be one factor determining the duration and usefulness of rumination, because individuals prone to pathological rumination tend to be more abstract and evaluative. I will describe research into processing mode and rumination in a later section.

Lessons for Psychological Treatment

This research suggests a number of lessons for our psychological treatment of rumination. First, rumination should not be treated as always pathological, because it can be a normal and helpful response to difficulties. Second, it may be useful to normalize the experience of rumination to patients by emphasizing that it is something that we all do and not something weird or odd, or something that reflects weakness. Third, both patients and therapists would benefit from discriminating between when rumination is helpful versus unhelpful. It is advantageous to distinguish between problem solving versus dwelling on a problem that goes nowhere.

Clinically, I have found some useful heuristics to help patients and therapists decide whether a particular episode of rumination is constructive. Key rules of thumb are asking, "Is it an unanswerable question?" and "Is this leading to a useful decision or plan?" If the rumination seems to be focused on an unanswerable issue, such as explaining other people's behavior or one's own emotions, or addressing existential or philosophical questions, then it is unlikely to lead to resolution. Likewise, if the thinking is just leading to more thinking, rather than to a decision or plan, then it is also unlikely to be helpful.

Pathological Rumination as a Habit

Another important theoretical underpinning for RFCBT is the hypothesis that rumination is a mental habit. The principal theory concerning depressive rumination is the response styles theory (RST; Nolen-Hoeksema, 1991), which hypothesizes that depressive rumination is a stable, enduring, and habitual trait-like tendency to engage in repetitive self-focus in response to depressed mood (Nolen-Hoeksema et al., 2008; Watkins & Nolen-Hoeksema, 2014). Depressive rumination is hypothesized to be learned in childhood, either because it was modeled by parents who themselves had a passive coping style (Nolen-Hoeksema, 1991; Nolen-Hoeksema et al., 2008), because the child failed to learn more active coping strategies for negative affect as a consequence of overcritical, intrusive, and overcontrolling parents (Nolen-Hoeksema, Wolfson, Mumme, & Guskin, 1995), or because of early physical/sexual abuse. Consistent with this hypothesis, elevated rumination is associated with self-report of overcontrolling parents (Spasojević & Alloy, 2002). In addition, rumination is associated with reported physical, emotional, and sexual abuse (Conway, Mendelson, Giannopoulos, Csank, & Holm, 2004).

Habits are behaviors that are performed frequently in stable contexts (Ji & Wood, 2007). Wood and Neal (2007, p. 843) proposed that "habits are learned dispositions to repeat past responses. They are triggered by features of the context that have covaried frequently with past performance, including performance locations, preceding actions in a sequence, and particular people." Habitual behavior typically involves some automaticity (Verplanken, 2006; Verplanken & Orbell, 2003; Wood, Tam, & Witt, 2005). A behavior can be conceptualized as automatic on several distinct dimensions: lack of conscious awareness, not requiring extensive resources to be performed (e.g., performed equally well under cognitive load versus not under load), lack of control, and lack of conscious intent (Bargh, 1994). Verplanken, Friborg, Wang, Trafimow, and Woolf (2007, p. 526) proposed that a habit is "a behavior that has a history of repetition, is characterized by a lack of awareness and conscious intent, is mentally efficient, and is sometimes difficult to control."

As a response that occurs frequently, unintentionally, and repetitively in the same emotional context (depressed mood), depressive rumination fulfills all of these conceptualizations of habit (see arguments in Hertel, 2004; Watkins & Nolen-Hoeksema, 2014). Its gold standard measure, the RSQ (Nolen-Hoeksema & Morrow, 1991), assesses the frequency of repeated ruminative behaviors in response to the stable internal context of feeling sad, down, or depressed. Hertel (2004) noted that rumination is a habit of thought and that the initiation of an episode of rumination can often occur automatically, without conscious awareness or effort. Consistent with this conceptualization, individual differences in rumination are found to be stable across situations and repeated testing (Nolen-Hoeksema, Morrow, & Fredrickson, 1993; Nolen-Hoeksema et al., 2008), even when there are changes in the levels of depression. Depressive ruminators report that rumination occurs without conscious intent, and that they are unable to control it (Watkins & Baracaia, 2001). A self-reported index of habitual negative thinking assessing the relevant dimensions of habits (e.g., lack of conscious awareness, lack of conscious intent, mental efficiency, hard to control) is positively correlated with both trait and state rumination (Verplanken et al., 2007).

Considering rumination as a habit is also consistent with BA conceptualizations of rumination, which propose that rumination may become more frequent and extensive if it is a learned behavior with perceived positive consequences. This contextual-functional approach argues that rumination may be a response to particular environments learned in the course of one's life (Martell et al., 2001).

Wood and Neal (2007) propose that habits develop through a process of automatic association between a behavioral response (e.g., rumination) and any context that occurs repeatedly with performance of the behavior (e.g., sad mood). Such context cues become automatic triggers for the behavioral response, such that the behavior is controlled by the presence or absence of the cue, rather than via the mediation of an implicit or explicit goal. Thus, any response repeated frequently that is contingent on a particular context could result in the development of a habitual response to that context, consistent with classic stimulus–response theories of learning (for further details, see Watkins & Nolen-Hoeksema, 2014). The habit being directly cued by context means that depressive rumination can occur without direct intention and without effort, which is consistent with what I hear from my patients.

Wood and Neal (2007, p. 844) further argue that "habits arise from context-response learning that is acquired slowly with experience. As a result, habit dispositions do not alter in response to people's current goals or occasional counter-habitual responses." Habits are resistant to changes in goals, outcomes, and intentions, and difficult to restrain (Hertel, 2004). Because control of a habitual behavior is outsourced directly to those contextual cues that have been reliably paired with past enactment of the behavior, habits are enacted and performed without reference to goals or outcomes. The habit model suggests that once rumination becomes a habit, it will be hard to stop even if new behavioral goals are adopted, even if it has negative consequences, or even if the rumination is at odds with an individual's attitudes and intentions.

Lessons for Psychological Treatment

This habit analysis suggests a number of lessons for our psychological treatment of rumination. Interventions focused on changing individual's beliefs, attitudes, and intentions and providing new information are not effective at changing habitual behaviors (Verplanken & Wood, 2006; Webb & Sheeran,

2006) because they do not directly address the patterns of context-response learning. This in turn suggests that depressive rumination would resist interventions (Verplanken & Wood, 2006), such as changing goals, persuasion, cognitive restructuring, or psychoeducation. Hence, focus on thought content alone (e.g., thought challenging) is insufficient to stop rumination as a habit. Rather, successful habit change involves either (1) disrupting the environmental factors (time, place, mood, prior behavior) that automatically cue the habit, or (2) counterconditioning an alternative incompatible response to the triggering cues for the habit, which is, in effect, training a new helpful habit.

Wood and Neal (2007, p. 860) propose that "interventions to maximize habit change provide people with concrete tools for controlling habit cueing." The habit model suggests that habits can be broken by altering or avoiding exposure to the cues that trigger habit performance (Verplanken & Wood, 2006). For example, where the cueing context for rumination involves a particular location (e.g., bedroom), person, preceding behavior (e.g., sitting down for a coffee after work), or environmental feature (e.g., sad music), environmental modification to remove or avoid the triggering context ought to interrupt depressive rumination.

Another key implication is that directly targeting the automatic context-response association will improve the efficacy and durability of interventions for rumination and depression (see Marteau, Hollands, & Fletcher, 2012). For a treatment to be effective in reducing rumination, the unhelpful ruminative response to the cueing context needs to be replaced with a more helpful response, with the patient learning a new, more adaptive habit. This requires "counterconditioning or training to associate the triggering cue with a response that is incompatible and thereby conflicts with the unwanted habit" (Wood & Neal, 2007, p. 859). Such an intervention involves repeated practice at utilizing the alternative incompatible coping strategy (e.g., concrete thinking, relaxation) in response to the triggering cue (e.g., sad mood) to develop the new context-response association.

This theory has contributed to the development of RFCBT (see Watkins & Nolen-Hoeksema, 2014), and is consistent with BA approaches to depression. There is a strong emphasis within the therapy on spotting the warning signs and triggers that may act to cue the habitual rumination (the "antecedents"). FA is used to experiment with altering the environment to prevent the activation of rumination. The use of contingency plans and If–Then plans focuses on repeated practice of an alternative response to these warning signs, with the goal of training an incompatible functional response instead of rumination. I believe current treatments do not emphasize the learning of new habits sufficiently (see Marteau et al., 2012), and that making this explicit in RFCBT is one way to enhance treatment effects.

Functional Accounts of Rumination:
Rumination as a Form of Avoidance

Individuals may develop a tendency toward more frequent and extensive rumination because rumination has an instrumental benefit for them, either via instrumental learning and the effects of positive and negative reinforcement (e.g., Martell et al., 2001) and/or through formation of explicit metacognitive beliefs about the perceived pros and cons of rumination (e.g., Wells, 1995). These "functional" accounts hypothesize that reinforcing functions maintain and exacarbate elevated rumination but differ in the degree to which individuals are consciously aware of these functions.

Using such a functional account, theorists have conceptualized rumination as an avoidance behavior that is negatively reinforced by the removal of aversive experience (Borkovec & Roemer, 1995; Martell et al., 2001; Nolen-Hoeksema et al., 2008; Watkins et al., 2007). This model views rumination as unhelpful escape and avoidance behavior that has been reinforced in the past by removal of aversive experience (Ferster, 1973; Martell et al., 2001). Martell et al. (2001, p. 121) proposed that "although rumination may be experienced as aversive to the individual, it is possible that it is maintained by the avoidance of even more aversive conditions." Rumination may put off overt action and avoid the risk of actual failure and humiliation, or serve to avoid unwanted personal characteristics (e.g., becoming selfish) through constant vigilance and criticism of one's performance. Nolen-Hoeksema et al. (2008) hypothesized that rumination is reinforced by the reductions in distress that come from withdrawing from aversive situations and from being relieved of responsibility for outcomes.

Rumination is also a potential cause and consequence of avoidance. Thus, rumination typically leads to procrastination, which becomes avoidance. Conversely, not completing plans that have been made (i.e., avoidance of trying the plan out) can be a source of further rumination in patients.

Avoidance can be particularly problematic for the development and maintenance of depression. First, avoidance prevents an individual from coming into direct contact with an ongoing problem, resulting in no chance to fix it. Second, avoidance closes life down. Avoidance tends to generalize and spread to all aspects of life, leading to a closed, not very fulfilled life. Third, avoidance usually prevents exposure to new information that may disconfirm concerns or provide the opportunity for learning, resulting in little chance for change.

All of these properties are also common to rumination. Rumination reduces an individual's direct contact with experience because it leads him to focus on his thoughts and internal state, rather than what is going on in the world. This blocks learning from experience and the ability to fully engage in positive activities. Rumination involves being "stuck" in the head rather than being in the world.

Rumination is positively correlated with self-reported measures of avoidance (Cribb, Moulds, & Carter, 2006; Giorgio et al., 2010; Moulds, Kandris, Starr, & Wong, 2007), as well as with greater frequency of escape and avoidance behavior, such as cutting, bingeing, and drug and alcohol abuse (Nolen-Hoeksema et al., 2007). However, this correlation could reflect avoidance causing increased rumination, or both avoidance and rumination being related to a third factor, such as depression. To date, there is no direct experimental evidence of whether rumination acts as a form of avoidance. However, my clinical experience to date has indicated the value of examining rumination as a form of avoidance. Patients do report that rumination serves as avoidance for them (Watkins & Baracaia, 2001).

Rumination may also have perceived positive reward value as a means to increase understanding and insight into self, feelings, and problems (Lyubomirsky & Nolen-Hoeksema, 1993; Watkins & Baracaia, 2001). Lyubomirsky and Nolen-Hoeksema (1993) found that following a period of rumination, dysphoric individuals reported gaining insight into their problems relative to a period of distraction, even though rumination in depressed individuals is associated with poorer problem solving. Watkins and Baracaia (2001) and Freeston, Rhéaume, Letarte, Dugas, and Ladouceur (1994) found that high ruminators and high worriers reported perceived advantages of rumination that included increasing understanding and insight of self and depression, solving problems, learning from past mistakes, preventing future mistakes, increasing empathy, and not losing control.

There is also evidence that people prone to depressive rumination have elevated beliefs that rumination is useful for solving problems and resolving difficult emotions (Papageorgiou & Wells, 2001; Watkins & Baracaia, 2001; Watkins & Moulds, 2005). These positive metacognitive beliefs about rumination may lead these individuals to engage in excessive rumination. Recent studies have indicated that such appraisals and beliefs can causally drive rumination. A prospective longitudinal study found that beliefs that rumination is helpful for gaining understanding predicted increases in trait rumination over the next 2 months (Kingston, Watkins, & Nolen-Hoeksema, 2015; Kingston, Watkins, & O'Mahen, 2013). An experimental study found that manipulating appraisals of the usefulness of rumination influenced the amount of state rumination following an unexpected failure, with appraisals of rumination as helpful leading to more rumination relative to appraisals of rumination as unhelpful (Kingston & Watkins, 2015).

Hypothesized and clinically observed functions of worry and rumination include (1) avoiding the risk of failure/humiliation by thinking about rather than implementing behavior; (2) attempting to problem-solve or to understand current problems but without a concrete plan of action; (3) avoiding and minimizing criticism by anticipating potential negative responses from others; (4) controlling unwanted feelings; (5) avoiding unwanted attributes by motivating oneself (e.g., "keeping me on my toes"); (6) increasing instrumental understanding by trying to understand the reasons why something happened so as to better know what to do and to prevent future problems; and (7) reducing a sense of responsibility and increasing a sense of certainty about one's conclusions.

Within this functional-contextual account, early experiences may explain why some individuals get stuck in excessive and pathological rumination. Rumination can be learned as a coping strategy to deal with difficult and abusive childhood experiences. When faced with criticism or abuse, a child may spend a lot of time analyzing and evaluating other people's motives and signals in order to predict their behavior and to avoid criticism and punishment. In this context, rumination may be an adaptive strategy that reduces harm, such that it becomes reinforced, overlearned, and indiscriminately applied to other situations.

Rumination may also develop if a child is discouraged from expressing her thoughts and feelings or is powerless to influence the situation through her own actions, encouraging further turning inward. Similarly, if a child fails to learn active behavioral coping strategies for dealing with difficulties and emotions because his parents are overcontrolling, there may be increased risk of rumination (Spasojević & Alloy, 2002). Consistent with these hypotheses, reports of childhood sexual abuse, which involves hard-to-understand experiences, powerlessness, and prohibitions from talking about what happened, are associated with rumination (Conway et al., 2004). Finally, rumination may be modeled by a parent or significant carer. Many patients report that one or both of their parents were worriers and ruminators.

Lessons for Psychological Treatment

The avoidant account of rumination underpins the BA approach to rumination (Martell et al., 2001). It suggests the value of looking in detail at the potential functions of ruminative behavior, as exemplified by FA. These functions are likely to be idiosyncratic for each patient. Replacing rumination with an alternative behavior is likely to be more successful when the replacement behavior is reinforcing to the patient and serves the same function as the rumination. For example, if rumination is used as a means to avoid undesired feelings such as anger, alternatives to rumination are unlikely to stick in the person's repertoire unless they also reduce anger. The functional-analytic approach within RFCBT is designed to address this theoretical element.

Processing Mode in Rumination

An important variable identified as influencing the consequences of rumination is the processing mode or thinking style adopted during rumination (Borkovec, Ray, & Stober, 1998; Watkins, 2008). There is evidence that negative rumination characterized by an abstract processing mode has more unconstructive consequences than rumination characterized by a concrete processing mode. An abstract processing mode is conceptualized as focusing on general, superordinate, and decontextualized mental representations that convey the essential meaning, causes, and implications of goals and events, including the *why* aspects of an action and the ends consequential to it. In contrast, a concrete processing mode involves a focus on the direct, specific, and contextualized experience of an event, and on the details of goals, events, and actions that denote the feasibility, mechanics, and means of *how* to do the action.

The processing mode account of rumination (Watkins, 2008) proposes that the consequences of abstract versus concrete processing are determined by their relative sensitivity to contextual and situational detail. Relative to a concrete mode, an abstract mode insulates an individual from the specific context, making her less distractible and less impulsive, and enabling more consistency and stability of goal pursuit across time. It also allows both gainful and unhelpful generalizations and inferences across different situations. However, the abstract mode also makes the individual less responsive to the environment and to any situational change and provides fewer specific guides to action and problem solving because of its distance from the mechanics of action (Watkins, 2011). Thus, with respect to difficulties and negative events, a concrete processing mode will be adaptive relative to an abstract processing mode because it will result in (1) improved self-regulation focused on the immediate demands of the situation rather than its evaluative implications (Leary, Adams, & Tate, 2006); (2) reduced negative overgeneralizations to emotional events, wherein a single failure is explained in terms of a global personal inadequacy, which is implicated in increased emotional reactivity (Carver & Scheier, 1982, 1990) and vulnerability to depression (Carver, 1998); and (3) more effective problem solving by providing more elaborated and contextual detail about the specific means and actions by which to best proceed when faced with difficult, novel, or complex situations.

Elaborations of problems about which participants worry or ruminate are rated by independent and blind researchers as more abstract and less concrete than problems about which participants do not worry or ruminate (Borkovec et al., 1998; Stöber, 1998; Stöber & Borkovec, 2002; Watkins & Moulds, 2007). Further, using an experience sampling method in 31 undergraduates sampled eight times a day for 1 week, Takano and Tanno

(2009) found that individuals with increasing levels of depressive symptoms engaged in more abstract thinking in daily life. Moreover, consistent with the hypothesis that processing mode influences the consequences of rumination, self-focused rumination was only significantly positively associated with negative mood in the context of elevated abstract thinking.

Experimental studies have further demonstrated that manipulating processing mode influences the consequences of rumination consistent with the processing mode theory. Studies adapted the standardized rumination induction to retain the key original element of repetitive focus on self, symptoms, and mood, but with instructions to adopt different processing modes. In depressed patients, a rumination induction encouraging more concrete processing, in which participants were instructed to "focus attention on the experience of" feelings, mood, and symptoms, was compared to a rumination induction encouraging more abstract processing, in which participants were instructed to "think about the causes, meanings, and consequences" of feelings, mood, and symptoms. Compared to abstract rumination, concrete rumination reduced negative global self-judgments such as "I am worthless" (Rimes & Watkins, 2005), improved social problem solving (Watkins & Moulds, 2005), and increased specificity of autobiographical memory recall (Watkins & Teasdale, 2001). These findings suggest that rumination focused on the direct concrete experience of moods and feelings reduces patterns of cognitive processing implicated in increased vulnerability for depression, relative to rumination focused on the causes, meanings, and consequences of moods and feelings.

Experimental studies have also investigated whether manipulating participants to think repetitively in either an abstract or concrete mode influences the emotional response to analogue loss and trauma events. Relative to manipulations to engage in abstract rumination, manipulations that instructed participants to engage in concrete rumination produced faster recovery from negative affect and reduced intrusions after a previous negative induction (watching a distressing film: Ehring, Szeimies, & Schaffrick, 2009; failure on IQ test: Watkins, 2004a). Watkins (2004a) randomly allocated participants to expressive writing about a previously induced failure in either an abstract way (e.g., "*Why* did you feel this way?") or a concrete way (e.g., "*How* did you feel moment by moment?"). Processing mode influenced emotional recovery from the failure: At higher levels of trait rumination, levels of negative mood 12 hours after the negative induction (failure on the test) were greater, but only in individuals who wrote abstractly and not in individuals who wrote concretely. Further studies trained participants to think in an abstract or a concrete way through repeated practice at either abstractly evaluating the causes, meanings, and implications of emotional scenarios or imagining the concrete details of what is happening in each scenario prior to an unanticipated failure. Individuals trained to think about emotional events in a concrete way had reduced emotional reactivity (less sad mood) to a subsequent experimental stressor relative to those trained to be abstract (Watkins, Moberly, & Moulds, 2008).

Thus, processing mode may influence the outcomes of rumination in response to an upsetting or distressing event. In sum, these findings suggest that there are more constructive forms of rumination, characterized by a concrete thinking style, in contrast to unconstructive forms of rumination, characterized by an abstract style.

Lessons for Psychological Treatment

This research suggests a number of lessons for our psychological treatment of rumination. First, it suggests that targeting processing style may help individuals to shift from maladaptive repetitive thought to adaptive repetitive thought, from rumination to problem solving. Second, and more specifically, it suggests that being more concrete (asking "How?") is more adaptive when responding to negative situations than being abstract (asking "Why?"). Shifting processing style is thus a key component of RFCBT, directly translated from this basic science work.

The Relationship between Worry and Rumination

People often ask whether worry and rumination are the same. Within the scientific literature, there is a debate as to whether worry and rumination reflect distinct but related processes (e.g., Papageorgiou & Wells, 1999), versus the same underlying process applied to different disorder-specific contents (Segerstrom, Tsao, Alden, & Craske, 2000; Watkins, 2008).

Worry and rumination are highly related: there is typically a high correlation (.6–.7) between the standardized questionnaire measures of worry and rumination (PSWQ vs. RSQ, respectively). Moreover, structural equation modeling finds that these measures load on a common factor, and that both forms of repetitive thought are similarly related to symptoms of anxiety and depression (Fresco, Frankel, Mennin, Turk, & Heimberg, 2002; Segerstrom et al., 2000). In addition, when individuals rated personal examples of worry and rumination on a range of cognitive dimensions, few differences were found (Papageorgiou & Wells, 1999; Watkins, 2004b; Watkins, Moulds, & Mackintosh, 2005), other than that worry predominantly focused on the future, whereas rumination predominantly focused on the past. Experimental studies experimentally manipulating worry versus rumination have found similar effects on mood, with both increasing ratings of anxiety and depression relative to control conditions (e.g., Blagden & Craske, 1996; McLaughlin, Borkovec, & Sibrava, 2007). Thus, the convergent evidence indicates considerable similarities between the processes and consequences of worry and rumination. While we need to be cautious about reaching a definitive conclusion, the most parsimonious account consistent with this evidence is that worry and rumination share a common underlying process that differs in specific content. This account is consistent with goal-based models of repetitive thought (e.g., Martin & Tesser, 1989; Martin & Tesser, 1996a) which propose that worry and rumination occur in response to an unattained or unresolved goal and persist until the goal is attained or abandoned, with the thought content depending on the unresolved goal. Thus, worry may be triggered by unresolved goals related to threat and focused on the future, whereas depressive rumination may be triggered by unresolved goals related to self-identity and focused on the past.

In clinical practice, it is hard to precisely distinguish worry and rumination. Patients often use the terms interchangeably and may use "worry" as a label for depressive rumination as much as anxious worry. Moreover, people tend to dwell both on past events and future uncertainties, with one triggering the other. Thus, thinking about a past event that went badly is likely to lead into thoughts about what could go wrong in the future, and vice versa. Even if worry and rumination are assumed to be different, they thus merge and flow together dynamically in the moment-to-moment thoughts of patients.

Lessons for Psychological Treatment

The implication of the close parallels between worry and rumination is that interventions designed to reduce depressive rumination, such as those developed in RFCBT, should also be successful in reducing anxious worry. The evidence from the clinical trials discussed in Chapter 1 indicates that RFCBT reduces worry as well as rumination.

Potential Functions of Rumination

As noted earlier, rumination is conceptualized as escape and avoidance behavior that has been reinforced in the past by the removal of aversive experience or because it has perceived or actual functions. During 15 years of developing and evaluating RFCBT, I have observed a number of common and recurring functions for rumination in patients with depression and anxiety. The next section describes these commonly hypothesized functions. While sometimes patients may have a conscious sense of these functions, often they are unaware of the potential functions that may be operating to reinforce their rumination. Even if the patient initiated the rumination for another reason, if it has a reinforcing function, this results in the rumination becoming more frequent. As a therapist, I work collaboratively with the patient to hypothesize potential functions (see Chapter 6 on FA). Functions are not necessarily independent: they can be overlapping, and for any single patient, rumination may have several potential functions.

Seeking Understanding and Insight

Often rumination is focused on trying to understand the causes and meanings of difficult events, feelings, and behaviors, as exemplified by asking "why" questions about events. Some individuals who ruminate are preoccupied with analyzing situations until they can work out the reasons for what happened. Such analytical thinking may have an instrumental design in terms of finding ways to prevent bad things from happening again and to provide a sense of control or of certainty. It may feel safer for some people to try and work out things in their head, rather than in the real world.

Self-Motivation

Patients often report that they need to dwell on their difficulties, shortcomings, and negative characteristics as a means to motivate themselves and put pressure on themselves to improve performance. Patients talk about reminding themselves of their limitations in order to spur themselves on and avoid lapsing into unwanted behaviors (e.g., saying "I am lazy, I am not trying hard enough, I should be able to do this"). This is similar to the motivational approach of exhorting, criticizing, and shouting at oneself to push oneself forward. One patient gave the example of having a critical internal voice like a sergeant major shouting over his shoulder, to spur himself on. This approach may work in the short term to produce a brief burst of increased activity but is unlikely to be productive in the longer run, as it will lead to more negative self-evaluations. A more constructive alternative may be adopting a more encouraging and compassionate stance toward oneself.

Planning and Preparation

Repetitive thought, particularly about unresolved problems or anticipated future events, can be an attempt to plan and prepare for these events, for example, by imagining what will happen and running through possible responses. Such preparation and planning is a common feature of worry. It can be adaptive and useful, leading to better performance and improved problem solving. However, attempts at preparation and planning may not be helpful and may not generate useful solutions. Moreover, even if it has useful elements, in some patients, the rumination can become overextended and repetitive, as the scenarios are played over and over again, and the plans repeatedly tinkered with, but never actually put into action. In this instance, the attempt at planning and preparation becomes a way of avoiding engaging with the actual situation, as the ruminator strives for total confidence in his plan before putting it into action. Encouraging problem solving and concrete thinking are good alternatives to rumination that address the function of planning and preparation. Asking if the rumination leads to a decision or a plan, and whether thought leads to action, is a useful heuristic to determine if the patient is getting stuck in overextended rumination.

Avoiding an "Unwanted Self"

Related to the function of self-motivation, some rumination appears to serve the function of avoiding becoming the particular kind of person the patient fears being. For example, an individual who worries about being an arrogant person ruminates about instances when he has been pushy or self-centered and berates himself for such behavior. In this case, the individual fears that without the rumination putting a brake on his behavior, this unwanted self will materialize. Constantly pointing out unwanted aspects of himself acts as a reminder to act differently. Reports of a difficult parent that the patient does not want to emulate are one clue that this function is present (e.g., a woman who describes her mother as difficult and selfish and is greatly concerned with not being selfish herself).

Avoiding the Challenges of a Job or the Tedium of the Daily Grind

Rumination involves going inward mentally and focusing on the internal world of memory, images, and thoughts. At times, this can be a way of distracting attention away from boring, difficult, or unpleasant events in the external world. A good example of this is daydreaming about good things that might happen. Even if focused on positive outcomes, this could be detrimental if it becomes frequent and prolonged. This may be particularly prevalent when a patient is faced with job challenges or a repetitive and boring daily routine.

Avoiding the Risk of Failure or Humiliation

Rumination often involves repeated thoughts about situations that are perceived as challenging, difficult, or risky, such as meeting new people, asking someone out for a date, asserting oneself, talking to one's manager, taking a test, attending an interview, or trying something new. The rumination and worry involves prolonged dwelling on these situations—on what might happen, what they might mean, and what the consequences might be. The act of thinking at length about such situations often means that the individual is not actually taking action but rather procrastinating and putting off engaging with the situations. While such extensive thinking might be initiated as an attempt to make plans or resolve goals, it can be maintained because it avoids the risk of actual failure or humiliation. Thinking about what could go wrong may be preferable and feel safer for some patients than trying things out in the real world and facing the risk of things actually going wrong, especially if the feared outcome is seen as catastrophic. Some patients report that they use rumination instead of confronting problems in actuality.

Preempting Another's Criticism and Anticipating Potential Negative Responses

Rumination is often focused on social and interpersonal themes, and may have the function of influencing other people's responses and limiting the impact of how other people act. Hence, a lot of rumination and worry focuses on trying to anticipate and preempt other people's negative responses or criticism. This can take the form of trying to mind read and of second-guessing what might happen next. For example, a child whose parents are highly critical and sometimes physically aggressive becomes very sensitive to signs of criticism and ruminates about what she is doing that might provoke a response from her parents. Such rumination may help her to anticipate when her parents are more likely to be critical and aggressive and, thus, to reduce these negative responses and to avoid actual criticism. In this developmental context, rumination about how others are responding may become habitual. Rumination would be functional in this original context but then may be maintained and applied indiscriminately to other situations as an adult. Rumination may also serve the function of trying to minimize the negative impact of criticism and rejection by internalizing and anticipating such responses, such that the patient feels prepared and is not impacted so much by subsequent criticism.

Control of Feelings

Rumination has been conceptualized as a form of (ineffective) emotion regulation. Nonetheless, it is clear that ruminating on emotional topics can both exacerbate emotions consistent with the focus of rumination, and diminish emotions that are inconsistent with it. One function of rumination is therefore to control feelings and emotions. A person who is feeling down and negative about himself may ruminate on how his difficulties are all due to other people and reflect on others' inadequacies and conspiracies, which would cause him to shift from feeling down to feeling angry, with an accompanying increase in energy and self-justification. Such effects on emotion would reinforce the rumination. Often, we see complex and dynamic patterns of emotions associated with rumination that develop into reciprocal loops (e.g., a patient feels down and ruminates in a way that makes her angry, but then she ruminates about her anger and how insensitive she is, and then begins to feel guilty and down, and so on).

Making Excuses and Generating Rationalizations

Dwelling on all the difficulties and problems that a patient faces can provide excuses and rationalizations for not changing things or not getting started on things. One patient reported to us that "I am doing something about it by thinking about it." Of course, thinking about problems can be helpful and productive, which is why RFCBT seeks to shift patients into productive thinking rather than keeping them from thinking about problems. However, if the thinking only leads to more thinking, rather than to decisions or actions, it is likely to not be helpful.

Gathering Evidence and Generating Justifications

In a similar vein, mental rehearsal of arguments about why things should be a certain way, evidence in support of a certain viewpoint, and generating justifications for behavior can be a potential function for rumination. This function may be particularly associated with rumination involving extreme standards and anger toward people who do not match those standards. Here the individual would keep dwelling on instances in which her standards have not been met, and why things should be the way she wants them to be. The patient may feel that to not keep thinking about her standards would be to relax them.

CHAPTER 3

Key Components
and Principles of RFCBT

Key Components of RFCBT

RFCBT has a number of principal components, which are outlined below. There is no step-by-step delineated protocol that calls for particular components to be used in a certain order or in certain sessions—there is no recipe book for doing RFCBT. The particular treatment components used depend strongly on the assessment, FA, and formulation for each individual patient. Nonetheless, RFCBT does follow a loose structure. The first sessions concentrate on assessment and socialization, as well as introducing one or two simple active interventions, such as adjusting environmental contingencies, practicing relaxation, listening to a recording of the session, or reading educational handouts. The later sessions then focus on replacing avoidance with approach and problem solving, and coaching in identifying and shifting thinking style. The final sessions then consolidate these changes, deal with termination, and make plans for the future, including relapse prevention.

Throughout the therapy, RFCBT uses standard CBT elements and organization, including a structured format, here-and-now focus, collaborative empiricism, agenda setting, feedback and summaries, homework, guided discovery, and behavioral experiments (e.g., as described in Beck et al., 1979). The key changes from standard CBT for depression are an increased emphasis on the function and usefulness of thoughts and behaviors (rather than examining their accuracy and evidence), the explicit focus on changing habits, and work on shifting thinking style.

The key components of RFCBT in the typical order they are used over the course of treatment are:

1. An idiosyncratic assessment tied to a clear rationale for the focus on rumination and avoidance, building on the idea that rumination is a learned behavior. It is important here to incorporate the patient's developmental history into the rationale.

2. Practice at spotting rumination, avoidance, and early warning signs of each, using formal homework.

3. FA to examine the context and functions of rumination and avoidance. FA is an approach to determine the functions and contexts under which desired and undesired behaviors occur and thereby find ways to systematically increase or reduce target behaviors. It is focused on studying the variability and context of behavior within an individual's personal experience and using this to guide interventions.

4. Contingency If–Then plans involving the practice of more adaptive and helpful responses to early warning signs, instead of rumination. These alternative responses can include overt behavior or the use of imagery and visualization exercises.

5. Experiments to examine whether rumination is adaptive and to try out alternative strategies, for example, the Why–How experiment, in which patients compare thinking about an upsetting situation in an abstract way (asking "Why did it happen?") versus thinking about it in a concrete way (asking "How did it happen?") to learn that thinking styles influence the effects of rumination (see Chapters 2 and 9).

6. Increased activity and reduced avoidance, including the development of routines. This activity needs to be made as explicit as possible, targeting behavioral changes.

7. The use of experiential exercises and visualizations to provide functional experience of the adaptive use of attention as a counter to rumination. These exercises can include positive "absorption–concentration" memories and compassion exercises. The goal of these exercises and experiments is to establish an alternative constructive thinking style to replace the pathological abstract style found in rumination (see Chapters 9, 10, and 11).

8. A focus on the patient's values to minimize rumination about non-valued areas and to encourage activity in line with values.

9. Relapse prevention.

Therapy typically follows this sequence of treatment elements. However, because therapy is determined by the outcomes from the FA, assessment, and formulation, there is no set order in which the therapist administers the treatment elements. I encourage RFCBT therapists to be familiar with the principles of therapy and to be flexible in implementing interventions, such that clinical opportunities are seized when they come up. The selection of treatment components is based on the formulation arising out of the assessment and FA of each individual patient (see Chapters 4, 6, 7, and 8).

For face-to-face individual RFCBT, the treatment has typically comprised 12 sessions of approximately 1 hour's duration, with the therapy predominantly targeting rumination. In our treatment trials, we exclusively focused on treating rumination within the 12 sessions of the protocol because we were testing the hypothesis that targeting rumination alone is sufficient to reduce depression and anxiety. Moreover, because worry, rumination, and avoidance are associated with many difficulties and symptoms of anxiety and depression, this selective targeting felt like an efficient way to deliver therapy, which patients endorsed and found engaging.

However, it is not essential for rumination to be the only focus of therapy. The approaches and techniques discussed in this manual could be used as a stand-alone treatment for depression, or incorporated as a module focused on rumination or worry within a course of CBT that has other targets as well. Incorporating RFCBT into a broader treatment may be particularly helpful for patients who are not improving, and where worry and rumination are identified as a major difficulty.

Structure of Treatment Sessions

The general structure of each treatment session is as follows:

1. Brief review of time since last session.
2. Set agenda for session.
3. Feedback on previous session; discussion of the audio recording of the previous session. (To maximize the impact of therapy, I suggest you and your patient each listen to these recordings between sessions.)
4. Review of homework.
5. Main focus for discussion and further practice in the session. This central section of each session focuses on FA, behavioral experiments, experiential exercises, and homework planning. It is underpinned by the general principles of RFCBT (outlined later in this chapter), with a view to giving the patient the experience of alternative ways of responding to difficulties. In an ideal session, a difficulty is identified and mapped out in concrete detail, perhaps through FA, which suggests a potential helpful change. That change is then experientially tested through an exercise or behavioral experiment

in the session. If this change in behavior or thinking style proves to be beneficial in the session, plans are made to practice it further and apply it in daily life, perhaps as an If–Then plan.

6. Summary of issues explored and what was learned.
7. Setting new homework tasks.
8. Feedback on session and arranging the next session.

Principal Techniques Used in RFCBT

RFCBT uses a range of treatment interventions and techniques, including standard ones from existing cognitive-behavioral treatments, as well as some novel ones derived from the basic research described in Chapter 2. There is no standard order or formula for the selection of a particular technique. Rather, the selection of techniques follows from the assessment of the patient, the FA, and the formulation. Chapter 7 discusses in more detail how treatment components are selected.

The therapist and patient develop an intervention plan using any of the strategies listed below. Strategies should be selected on the basis of how they fit the FA and formulation and how consistent they are with the patient's presenting problems and goals. Thus, the interventions that should be prioritized are those that are most likely to alter rumination and avoidance in a manner consistent with the formulation, and that are consistent with the patient's goals. As a general principle, any intervention will be more effective if:

- A plan is drawn up, with both patient and therapist taking notes.
- The patient practices the intervention repeatedly in session and during homework.
- The intervention is made as precise and as concrete as possible.

The principal techniques used within RFCBT include the following.

Antecedent–Behavior–Consequence Analysis

The antecedent–behavior–consequence (ABC) analysis is a central technique within FA, with rumination as the target behavior. The ABC approach involves asking patients what comes before an episode of rumination (antecedents: potential triggers and cues), what happens during the rumination (the content and sequence of thoughts), and what follows after the rumination (consequences), such as changes in behavior and feelings (e.g., was it helpful or not?). We want to know how the rumination develops and evolves over time, and to get a sense of how one thought flows into another thought. Rumination is not static but a dynamic process, with thoughts, feelings, and actions interacting, so it is important to examine these components and how they feed into each other. Understanding the antecedents or triggers to the rumination provides clues as to what purpose it may serve and helps to plan where and when to make changes to reduce the habit. Knowing its consequences provides clues to its use and functions and helps the therapist and the patient to consider what alternative actions might usefully replace rumination. In other words, what is the use or purpose of the behavior? When a person is ruminating, what effects does that rumination have? The answers to these questions form a central part of the formulation and conceptualization of rumination within RFCBT; the hypothesis as to the function or purpose of rumination strongly informs how the therapist will try to change it.

CUDOS Analysis

CUDOS is a mnemonic for Context, Usefulness, Development, OptionS. It is a parallel and complementary way to conduct functional analyses. It looks for information that relates to both the function of rumination (as examined by the ABC analysis) and also the variability and situationality of the target behavior. More specifically, the analysis looks for the following:

- Context that influences the rumination and associated behaviors (what, when, where, how, with whom it happens or does not happen).
- Usefulness of the rumination (function and effects; when it was helpful or unhelpful).
- Development of the behavior (when it started).
- OptionS to try instead of rumination (what happened when it stopped; see Chapter 6 for further details).

The Context and Usefulness components of CUDOS overlap with the ABC analysis in looking at antecedents and consequences of target behaviors such as rumination. However, CUDOS has a greater focus on looking at changes in circumstances between when rumination does or does not occur and between when it has differential outcomes. In essence, the CUDOS approach to FA asks under what conditions the target behavior (e.g., rumination) occurs and under what conditions it does not occur. The contextual factors that influence rumination are split into external environmental factors, such as aspects of the world (time, place, setting, other people), and internal patient factors, such as the patient's mood, tiredness, alertness, or mental state, as well as how she is responding to the world (How is she behaving? What is she paying attention to?). In other words, the therapist is looking for what influences or moderates the frequency, effects, or duration of rumination.

Self-Monitoring Forms

Patients monitor their rumination and its antecedents and consequences to inform the FA and to identify positive activities to increase.

Activity Scheduling

The patient and therapist collaboratively schedule activities, typically approach activities that are hypothesized to be rewarding. The focus is on increasing approach behaviors and reducing avoidance. The rationale given to patients is of "opening up to life" and "recharging batteries" by increasing positive activities.

Mastery–Pleasure Activities

Patients identify activities that increase their sense of mastery and pleasure and schedule these activities as further homework. Diary records are often used to identify suitable activities to increase.

Graded Task Assignments

Activities are broken down into smaller steps to make them more manageable and planned as homework tasks.

Verbal Rehearsal of Assigned Tasks

The therapist and patient talk through tasks and practice them in the therapy session to increase the likelihood of their being implemented in daily life.

Managing Situational Contingencies

Plans are made to increase the likelihood of desired activities occurring, for example, by setting them in a schedule, telling other people about them, and setting up physical surroundings that are conducive to their occurring.

Role Playing and Therapist Modeling

The therapist and patient practice alternative behaviors in the session to increase the likelihood of their being enacted in daily life.

Environmental Control

Potential cues and triggers for habitual rumination are identified and modified by changing the external environment or patterns of patient behavior. For example, if rumination is triggered by listening to sad music in the car, then the patient would replace the sad music with other music. If rumination is associated with a particular routine (e.g., coming home after work and sitting down for a smoke), then the patient changes her routine.

Contingency Plans (If–Then Plans)

These plans are strategies to break up the patient's rumination and associated avoidance by interrupting his thinking habit, as well as to replace the rumination with a constructive alternative. This alternative will be determined with reference to the patient's repertoire and values, what is empirically and experientially found to be helpful, and to the clinical formulation. Each of the other techniques and strategies listed in this section can be applied as part of these If–Then plans.

Applied and Progressive Relaxation

The patient practices tensing and relaxing muscle groups and making breathing slower and deeper to reduce anxiety and physiological arousal (see Bernstein & Borkovec, 1973, Borkovec & Costello, 1993, and other standard texts on relaxation techniques).

Problem Solving

The patient practices steps to define the problem, generate a range of possible solutions, select the solution most likely to succeed, implement the potential solution, and evaluate the outcome.

Concreteness Training

The patient practices verbal and imagery approaches to shift away from an unhelpful abstract style of thinking to a more helpful concrete style of thinking (see Chapters 2 and 9).

Absorption Training

The patient uses imagery and visualization exercises to recapture the experience of being immersed and absorbed in activities as a means to provide a counter-experience to rumination and shift processing style. Absorption work also includes identifying and building in activities that the patient finds absorbing and immersing (see Chapter 10).

Compassion Training

The patient uses imagery and visualization exercises, building on past experience to develop feelings of compassion toward the self and others, as a means to provide a counter-experience to rumination and a functional alternative to motivate and encourage herself. Compassion work also includes identifying activities that need to be increased and activities that need to be decreased to take care of oneself (see Chapter 11).

Visualization Exercises

In addition to the visualization exercises used for concreteness training, idiosyncratic imagery and visualization exercises may be used within RFCBT.

Communication and Assertiveness Training

The patient learns and practices ways to improve communication and assertiveness with others, typically focused on finding more effective ways of expressing his or her opinion, making requests of others, and saying no to others. Many ruminators find it hard to say no to other people and as a consequence become put upon by others and feel taken for granted, which can be draining and a source of further rumination.

Behavioral Experiments

The therapist and patient collaboratively plan for the patient to try different ways of doing things in the therapy session and in the real world to learn more effective approaches. Many patients who ruminate tend to try to work difficulties out in their heads and rely on logical rational analysis as an approach to fixing problems. This overreliance on thinking about difficulties feeds into rumination and tends not to be effective for the major emotional problems that people experience, such as resolving their own feelings and getting on well with other people. In these situations, learning through direct experimentation, through experience, and through trial and error may be more effective than rational analysis.

Emotional Exposure

The patient is exposed to an upsetting or fearful event (either in imagination or in reality) until he or she habituates to the event and discomfort is reduced. One of the triggers for rumination can be intrusive memories or thoughts about past upsetting events, which are often unresolved and have not been fully worked through and come to terms with by the patient. Having a tendency toward an abstract thinking style in rumination often leaves a patient dwelling on the meanings and implications of past upsetting events, but not on the details of what actually happened and how the patient actually felt. This abstract style can distance the patient from the direct experience of the past upsetting event and slow any habituation to it. Exposure to past upsetting events can therefore be helpful in reducing these triggers. Exposure is often combined with reexperiencing the specific and concrete details of what happened, facilitating effective exposure and habituation to the past event.

Homework

In order to facilitate self-help and the consolidation of learning, it is important to emphasize the importance of homework. Patients need to make notes and record plans during sessions. As patients enter treatment, therapists need to spell out explicitly that they expect them to complete between-session plans and actively take notes in therapy, and they need to encourage patients to listen to audio recordings of treatment sessions between sessions. Some therapists find it useful to provide a patient with pen and paper to facilitate note taking and a folder in which to store notes and records. I found it helpful to audio-record each session and ask patients to listen to it before the next one, originally with audiotapes and more recently with digital files. I also recommend that the therapist listen to the recordings between sessions in order to review how interventions could be made more effective. Standard consent forms for recording can be used.

It is simpler and more efficient to plan homework tasks as the session progresses rather than allocating them all at the end. It is important to ask patients to summarize the purpose and details of the homework to make sure they know what they are doing and how it will be useful. When agreeing on homework plans, it is essential to make the plans simple, explicit, and concrete. Specifying how, when, where, and with whom the plan will be implemented not only increases the likelihood that it will happen but also models a more concrete, specific style of thinking. Ideally, homework plans also incorporate predictions of what the patient expects to happen, so that the plan can be set up as a behavioral experiment. Encouraging an experimental approach to difficulties and problems, which involves active testing in the real world, will reduce the tendency to work everything out in one's head and hence reduce rumination. Furthermore, carrying out these experiments builds up an evidence base of times when the patients' predictions are not accurate. This evidence will be useful for encouraging approach behavior on later occasions when patients predict that bad things will happen if they try new things.

RFCBT and Negative Thinking

To keep the therapy simple for the patient and make the most of 12 sessions, RFCBT usually avoids the explicit discussion of negative automatic thoughts, dysfunctional assumptions, and core beliefs that is typical in standard CBT. Therapists hypothesize these cognitive structures and integrate them into their formulation and conceptualization of the patient. But they are not an explicit part of the treatment protocol; sessions are not set aside to work on dysfunctional assumptions. That's not to say that challenging beliefs is prohibited within RFCBT. I recommend doing whatever will facilitate the change in rumination and avoidance. If talking about beliefs and reviewing their advantages seems helpful in initiating behavioral change, please use that approach. At times, it may be useful to briefly talk about the rules that people have learned with respect to their rumination and avoidance. Likewise, it may be useful to explicitly link changes in behavior with challenging and testing these rules. In summary, at clinical discretion, these concepts may be discussed, but in the service of reducing rumination and avoidance. Nonetheless, my experience has been that this is not often necessary (and at times can be counterproductive), and that adopting a functional-analytic approach to repeated negative cognitions can be effective without requiring explicit thought challenging.

In the same way, specific periods of time are not set aside for challenging negative thoughts and testing out the evidence for or against them. Rather, in RFCBT, the work on negative automatic thoughts focuses on training patients to spot them and to replace them with a different thinking style. However, within each therapist's clinical judgment, there may be times when direct challenging of thoughts facilitates therapy. Thus, in general, the therapy encourages a guided discovery approach to the process of thinking, rather than a "changing thoughts" approach. It is my experience that with more severe, chronic patients, particularly when there are high levels of rumination, there is a risk that discussion of thought content can easily develop into within-session rumination, which is usually counterproductive. Therefore, as a general rule of thumb, I recommend avoiding discussion of thought content where it does not also inform thought process.

Key Principles in RFCBT

RFCBT focuses on increasing effective behavior. The goal of therapy is not necessarily to stop rumination, but rather to shift repetitive thinking about real problems so that it becomes adaptive and functional, and thereby to reduce depression. We want patients to learn better ways to tackle their difficulties, instead of unconstructive rumination.

RFCBT is grounded within the core principles and techniques of CBT for depression (Beck et al., 1979) with three key adaptations. First, the therapy adopts a contextual–functional-analytic perspective similar to that of BA (Addis & Martell, 2004; Martell et al., 2001), but more explicitly focused on internal behaviors, including ruminative thinking.

Second, building on the research described in Chapter 2, there is an explicit focus on shifting from unhelpful styles of processing to more adaptive styles of processing (Watkins, 2008). Third, there is a much greater emphasis on treating depressogenic cognition as a habit, and utilizing techniques designed to change habits within the treatment (see Chapter 2 for background).

There are a number of key principles that form the core of RFCBT. These principles derive from the basic science underpinning the treatment development (see Chapter 2) and from the lessons learned by myself and my colleagues over 15 years of using the therapy. This section briefly summarizes these principles and their application within the components described earlier. They are reapplied in greater detail throughout specific sections of the treatment.

Principle 1: Normalize the Patient's Experience of Rumination

It is critical to help patients to see the experience of rumination as normal rather than as a sign of weakness, inadequacy, or oddness. The therapist explicitly discusses how rumination is a frequent, common, and sometimes useful way of responding to difficulties. It is helpful to recognize that everyone ruminates and that it is a natural way of responding to unresolved goals or problems. Indeed, rumination is reframed as indicating to the patient the importance of his ruminative concern and his desire to make headway with it. The idea that rumination is driven by unresolved goals (see Chapter 2) is a useful starting point for discussion with patients.

Furthermore, despite recognizing the negative effects of rumination, many patients find it difficult to contemplate stopping it. For example, for a woman ruminating about her painful divorce, there is a strong investment in trying to understand why it happened and to make sense of why her ex-partner treated her this way. Asking her not to think about this event is not realistic and likely to be counterproductive. It is useful to validate her experience and to acknowledge that it is normal to dwell on such an event and that therapy will seek to find a more helpful way to do this.

Likewise, an individual whose rumination involves a hectoring and critical voice that highlights the imperfections and mistakes in her work, and who describes the rumination as "spurring me on and stopping me from becoming a good-for-nothing" will be resistant to direct attempts to reduce it. By acknowledging the normality and potential usefulness of rumination, we improve engagement with patients and avoid getting into arguments about changing valued behaviors.

Normalizing rumination can also reduce the secondary negative response to rumination itself, or "rumination about rumination" (e.g., "Why do I keep dwelling on my problems?"). Once a patient and therapist have reached a shared collaborative view of the advantages and disadvantages of rumination, they have a greater scope to review more useful alternatives. Chapter 5, which describes the therapy rationale, provides a detailed example of how rumination may be normalized.

Principle 2: Make Rumination an Explicit Target of Therapy

I find it helpful to be explicit about rumination as a target of therapy. When discussing the goals and problems of a patient (see Chapter 4 on assessment), I look out for examples of worry and rumination and link this behavior to the difficulties the patient is experiencing. I highlight that one of the goals of the therapy is to reduce unhelpful rumination. Talking in detail about rumination can be helpful for engaging patients, many of whom recognize their tendency to dwell on problems but have not talked about it with others or had it as a focus of therapy before. Further, many patients feel previous treatments have not tackled this problem, so highlighting it as a focus of treatment can help patients to feel confident about the approach and enhance their hope about recovery.

It is important at the start of therapy to directly address the likelihood of rumination interfering with the therapy itself. Patients who are prone to rumination are almost certain to ruminate about the therapy before, during, and after treatment sessions, for example, on how they are coming across to the therapist ("Does he think I'm boring and stupid?") or on the progress of therapy. Before the session, anticipatory rumination may increase anxiety and reduce attendance. During the session, rumination may obstruct engagement and new learning, as the patient is able to attend to only a fraction of what is being discussed. After the session, postmortem rumination may result in unhelpful misinterpretations and interfere with homework plans. In the first session, you should therefore discuss the fact that rumination is likely to occur during therapy and ask the patient to report it whenever he notices it, while noting that if you as the therapist think the patient is ruminating during a session, you will also point it out. Identifying and naming rumination as it happens in session provides a golden opportunity to increase direct engagement, identify what triggers rumination, and to directly experiment with alternative responses.

Because my colleagues and I expect rumination to occur in the treatment session and to interfere with concentration and memory, we recommend audio-recording the treatment sessions and giving the patient a copy of the recording to listen to each week. This technique has a number of advantages. First, it helps the patient to identify moments in the session when she may have been caught up in her head and missing what was being discussed. This recognition can inform future discussions about the triggers and nature of rumination and improve awareness of the ruminative habit.

Second, the recording provides an opportunity for the patient to rehearse and refresh her memory of what was discussed and practiced, consolidating gains from a session and improving recall of the therapy. Listening to sessions helps patients to reflect actively on what they have learned and highlight potential points of disagreement, misinterpretations, and omissions to review in future sessions.

Third, listening to recordings of sessions gives patients useful direct feedback on how they are coming across. Many patients report that it is useful to hear how they go over and over the same thing. Fourth, if an experiential exercise was practiced in the session and was successful, then having the recording enables the patient to repeatedly practice the exercise from the recording. For patients who are avoidant of their emotions, listening to the tapes can provide a form of useful exposure. Fifth, when assembled across the course of the treatment, the recordings provide a resource that patients can use to remind themselves of the therapy once it has been completed.

Principle 3: Encourage Active, Concrete, Experiential, and Specific Behavior—The ACES Rule

A central tenet of RFCBT is that we encourage thoughts and behaviors that are action focused, concrete, specific, and directly engaged in experience (summarized in the mnemonic ACES: Active, Concrete, Experiential, Specific). Individuals who ruminate tend to be passive, abstract, and evaluative, focused on analyzing and intellectualizing events in their life, and characterized by overgeneralizations and global thinking, in which failure on one task leads to assumptions of fixed trait-like deficiencies across multiple situations. Patients can also be focused on a series of problems without looking at solutions. When talking about a problem or difficulty, there is a tendency for those who ruminate to move into abstract thinking focused on meanings and implications, even when prompted for specific details. For example, when you ask a patient to describe a recent difficult event, the patient may start talking about the meaning of an event, rather than what happened.

It is easy to get into long discussions about the patient's history and problems, trying to understand why these are the way they are, but such discussions tend to be unproductive and can become a form of ruminating aloud together. When this happens, a whole session can pass without any useful progress being made.

When treating patients with elevated rumination, such as those with chronic or residual depression, try to keep the therapy as focused, solution orientated, specific, and concrete as possible. The therapist needs to both explicitly and implicitly work on encouraging a specific, concrete, and solution-focused mode. This can be done explicitly by providing psychoeducation on rumination, working through the specific concreteness exercises (see Chapter 9), asking patients to redescribe situations in more detail, starting sessions by rehearsing being concrete (see Chapter 9), and by assigning relevant homework. Implicitly, the therapist models a specific and concrete approach, and discourages long unfocused discussions.

Therapy needs to shift patients away from the abstract–evaluative pattern by directly coaching them to be more concrete, specific, and grounded in experience. The therapist models this behavior by making plans and asking questions that are action focused, concrete, specific, and that pertain to direct here-and-now experience rather than meaning.

The ACES principle is also used to direct therapist questions and strategies. Given the choice between talking about something versus trying something out in an experiential or imagery exercise or behavioral experiment, choose the latter, as it shifts the patient away from the thinking style associated with unhelpful rumination. I recommend experimenting with exercises and engaging in new experiences rather than further discussion of problems. The emphasis here is on the patient *doing* things differently (e.g., making plans, doing experiential exercises, trying out behavioral experiments in session, exploring what happened) rather than *talking about* things. When a hurdle or problem comes up in therapy, it is usually more helpful to take a step back and try an action, or experiment with a new way of doing things, or focus on the details of the concrete experience, instead of trying to understand and analyze the problem. Analysis and attempts at abstract understanding are what the patient is doing all the time, without much success, so the therapist needs to deliberately try something else.

Similarly, when exploring a recent event, the focus needs to be on the specific and precise details of how it happened moment by moment (i.e., a micro-level analysis), rather than on a general summary or consideration of its meaning. The therapist wants to know exactly what happened, when it happened, where it happened, how it happened, and with whom it happened, down to the level of the actual behaviors conducted. The goal is to get sufficient detail to understand what is happening, to move the patient away from an abstract way of describing events, and to get events into perspective and improve problem solving. This shift in attention and focus can be difficult to achieve at first, as it goes against the grain for the ruminating patient, who has learned to be abstract and evaluative. It requires persistent efforts from the therapist. The therapist gradually shapes and socializes the patient into being more concrete and specific by repeatedly asking for more detail, by using more concrete and experiential language, and by modeling being concrete and specific.

The phrasing and questions used by the therapist make a big difference in how specific and concrete a patient will be in describing situations. Vague and general questions are unhelpful ("What kind of thoughts do you have?"), as are questions about meanings and implications (asking "Why?"; "Why do you think he did that?"; "What do you think that means?"). It is more productive to ask questions about exact behaviors and about the sequence of events ("How did it happen?"). More concrete questions refer to a specified behavior within a particular context and at a narrowly defined time, for example, "What did he say then?"; "How did he say it?"; "What did you do just after you noticed you were getting angry?" Such questions focus the patient on the details of the situation and steer him to more specific responses.

It is often necessary to ask follow-up questions, seeking more detail and information, until your patient gives you a detailed, specific, and concrete answer. Questions like "What exactly did he do?"; "What were the exact words?"; and "What physical sensations do you notice when you are angry?" lead a patient to greater specificity and concreteness.

The language used also prompts a more concrete and specific way of thinking and responding. Asking "How?" is more useful than asking "Why?" Language that describes the actual behavior conducted is more useful than language that uses vague, generic, interpretative, and implicational terms. For example, when you say, "John kicked the ball," you provide a clear description of the actual physical behavior and the mechanics of the actions involved. This description also produces a clear image of what happened. However the statement "John moved the ball" is much less precise; it is not clear how he moved the ball. He could have moved it with his hands or feet. You could imagine multiple images of what happened. Asking, "What did he do?" is more helpful than asking, "What do you think he was doing?"

There are some useful rules of thumb to determine if the patient has been concrete or specific enough, and whether you need to work harder at encouraging an ACES response. First, when a patient describes a situation, do you know exactly what was done and how it was done, or is there still some level of interpretation involved? For example, a patient might report that a difficult event occurred during the week when a friend insulted her or when a family member ignored her. Both of these descriptions involve interpretative verbs that leave ambiguous exactly what happened. In this situation, the therapist does not know what the friend did that the patient found insulting. Did the friend say something rude, act in a demeaning way, or make an insulting gesture? This is where it is helpful to ask, "What exactly did your friend do?" The therapist seeks to know the actual behavior that occurred rather than relying on the patient's interpretation of what happened. The therapist seeks to drill down to a description that makes clear who did what. The detailed description of what happened may enable the therapist to suggest a different interpretation and help the patient to gain perspective on the situation. Similarly, the therapist wants to move away from descriptions of events and situations that use adjectives and replace them with descriptions using verbs focused on behavior. For example, if the patient describes himself as having been "stupid" during a difficult situation, then it is helpful to ask about the particular behavior that the patient thought was stupid. Focusing on behaviors rather than character traits affords more opportunity for learning and flexibility to change.

Second, it is helpful to check on what mental image the patient's description conjures in your own mind as a therapist. If you are getting a vivid picture of what happened and how it happened, then the description is reasonably concrete, specific, and experiential.

Principle 4: Take a Functional-Analytic Approach

Within RFCBT, rumination is conceptualized as escape and avoidance behavior that has been reinforced in the past by the removal of aversive experience, or because it has perceived or actual functions (see Chapter 2). Understanding the idiosyncratic functions and contexts in which rumination occurs for each patient is therefore an important part of the treatment. In RFCBT, we view rumination as a set of actions in context and as understandable and predictable given a person's life history and current context. A key element in a formulation is that rumination is typically maintained because it avoids short-term pain, although it leads to longer-term negative consequences.

The functional-contextual approach focuses on function rather than form, and on process rather than content. The same behavior may have different uses or purposes and lead to different consequences in different situations or at different times. For example, complaining to another person could serve the function of trying to solve a problem at one time but reflect an attempt to avoid taking responsibility at another time. Likewise, two different behaviors may have the same use or function. Lying in bed doing nothing versus being busy fulfilling a hectic schedule are different in form, but both could be ways of avoiding facing up to a difficult situation. The focus of therapy is therefore not on what the behavior looks like (its form) but rather on its uses and consequences (its function).

The ABC analysis and CUDOS mnemonic are used to guide questions to determine the functions of rumination, the conditions in which it occurs, and what may influence its variability in duration and usefulness.

This analysis of function involves asking about the content of the rumination—the moment-by-moment thoughts that go through the patient's mind during an episode of rumination—in order to trace the sequence of it. We can't find out about thought process without discussing thought content. To do this, the therapist uses Socratic questions exactly as in standard CBT. Moreover, the content of the rumination gives the therapist information about the concerns and issues facing the patient, as well as her style of thinking about things (e.g., Is it abstract? Is it self-critical?). However, unlike in standard CBT, we are less interested in examining the accuracy and evidence for each individual thought in the sequence, but rather focused on mapping out the whole sequence and helping the patient to shift it. Rather than trying to challenge a single thought, we want the patient to spot the whole sequence of thinking and find ways to shift away from this pattern of thinking. This approach reflects my clinical experience that challenging individual negative thoughts is not always effective, as often patients just move on to another negative automatic thought in the sequence. In RFCBT, the priority is to disrupt or shift the *whole cycle of thinking*, rather than change a single thought.

This information then guides the introduction of specific treatment strategies (see Chapters 6 and 7). Thus, FA and self-monitoring help patients to recognize the warning signs and triggers for rumination. The FA is used to identify and alter any environmental and behavioral contingencies maintaining rumination. Using this information to alter routines and environments can reduce rumination. For example, if rumination is triggered first thing in the morning just after waking up, it may be useful to look at ways of changing the early morning routine, such as getting up and being active rather than lying in bed brooding. In general, increasing structure and activity and, especially, shifting the balance of activities from routine chores and obligations toward more self-fulfilling and absorbing activities reduces rumination. Encouraging patients to slow things down, focus on only one thing at a time, and pace their activities without taking on too much may help, as this reduces the sense of rushing around and being under pressure, which feeds into rumination.

Experiments derived from an understanding of the possible function of the behavior allow the therapist and the patient to manipulate identified variables to find better ways for the patient to handle situations. FA in RFCBT examines if these planned changes reduce rumination, reduce symptoms of anxiety and depression, and increase successful pursuit of the patient's goals. If they do, this confirms the hypothesized formulation of rumination, suggesting the therapist should extend and consolidate these changes. If they don't, then the therapist should review the changes, refine the ABC and functional formulations, and try out other changes.

FA is also used to develop alternative strategies and contingency plans (ones that are more functional) to replace rumination. Where appropriate, the alternative strategy also serves the original function of the rumination. For one patient, the function of ruminating on her failings was to avoid becoming lazy, complacent, and arrogant. This was consistent with her warning signs and triggers for rumination: tiredness, inactivity, and irritability. Rumination was effective at preventing her from becoming complacent and arrogant but at the cost of making her depressed, reducing her motivation, and eroding her self-confidence. Treatment focused on helping her to recognize the warning signs for rumination and on developing an alternative response to rumination that more constructively served the same function, in this case, the use of imagery and visualization exercises designed to increase feelings of compassion, first to others and then to herself. The training in compassion provided an effective and beneficial alternative to rumination, since it is antithetical to laziness and arrogance, yet at the same time positive and calming, and provided an experience counter to her beliefs about being "a bad person."

For another patient, the function of rumination was to reduce angry and aggressive feelings. Whenever he became angry, even when justified, he would ruminate on why he overreacted and blame himself for being oversensitive, which would replace his anger with depressed mood. This patient was particularly afraid of losing control of his anger and becoming like his father, who was violent, aggressive, and abusive. For him, the use of relaxation and assertiveness was an effective replacement for rumination. Rumination is often tied up with avoidance of an unwanted or feared self, and treatment interventions need to address this powerful motivation.

It is important to remember that FA is a method that can be applied to any problem or difficulty that comes up in therapy. For any hurdle or obstacle, such as a patient not completing homework, or not finding a particular exercise helpful, FA can be useful. Examining the variability in the desired outcome (when a behavior is effective versus ineffective) and associated contexts often suggests potential points of leverage to influence behavior and outcome, which can then be experimented with. In effect, everything is grist to the mill for FA.

Principle 5: Link Behaviors to Triggers and Warning Signs

As noted above, an important element of FA is identifying the context in which rumination occurs, with a particular emphasis on spotting triggers and warning signs for the onset of rumination. This is particularly critical when trying to reduce habitual rumination, because it will be automatically triggered by these cues. As discussed in Chapter 2, identifying and then removing the cues to habits is an effective way to reduce unwanted habitual behaviors.

Principle 6: Emphasize the Importance of Repetition and Practice

Reflecting the hypothesis that pathological rumination is often habitual (see Chapter 2), a key element of the treatment is the counterconditioning of alternative responses to rumination-triggering cues. This counterconditioning involves the learning of new helpful habits. It requires repeated practice over multiple occasions of alternative responses to the cues that normally trigger rumination. The literature on habit formation suggests that it may take as many as 60–100 repetitions for a new behavior to become habitual. This indicates that the level of repetition and practice required to replace rumination may be much greater than that typically employed in cognitive-behavioral therapies.

My experience with therapy is that "less is more": it is better to introduce fewer elements into therapy but to repeat them more frequently in order to consolidate changes. For the same reasons, persistence by the therapist is an important aspect of therapy. Change is possible, but it can take time, effort, and repetition. The therapist needs to be positive and supportive about helping patients to keep practicing until benefit is achieved.

Principle 7: Shift to an Adaptive Style of Thinking

Within RFCBT, there is a focus on shifting the style or mode of thinking in order to counter rumination. RFCBT uses experiential and imagery exercises and behavioral experiments designed to facilitate a shift into a more helpful thinking style. Patients use directed imagery to vividly re-create previous states when a more helpful thinking style was active, such as memories of being completely absorbed in an activity (e.g., "flow" or "peak" experiences of being creative, immersed in sensory experience, or involved in highly focused physical activities like rock climbing or skiing). Alternatively, patients may focus on experiences of being compassionate, tolerant, and supportive to themselves or others. These mental states are characterized by a concrete, process-focused thinking style and by reductions in evaluative, abstract, and judgmental thinking. Therefore, such exercises generate mental states at odds with rumination and so can be used as a functional alternative strategy in response to warning signs for rumination (see Chapters 6 and 7). The effective generation of these alternative styles of processing involves vividly imagining all the elements contributing to the original experience and desired mode: thoughts, feelings, posture, sensory experience, bodily sensations, attitudes, motivations, facial expressions, and urges. The patient recalls a vivid memory or generates an image that captures the desired experience and is then guided into a deeper, more elaborated experience via therapist questions focusing the patient's attention and imagination on each detail of the experience. The patient is encouraged to imagine the event in the present tense and from a field perspective, as if he or she were looking into the scene right now (see Chapters 10 and 11).

In parallel work, Paul Gilbert has been developing a compassionate mind training intervention in which patients use imagery and visualization to develop self-soothing and self-nurturing skills (Gilbert, 2009, 2010; Gilbert & Irons, 2004; Gilbert & Proctor, 2006). Given the high incidence of shaming, self-critical, and intolerant thoughts in rumination, and considering the positive outcomes for RFCBT, Gilbert's approach is also likely to be an effective intervention for rumination.

Principle 8: Focus on Nonspecific Factors— Warmth, Empathy, Optimism, Validation, Persistence

As for all therapies, in RFCBT, therapists need to pay attention to nonspecific factors such as genuineness, warmth, empathy, and developing a good therapeutic alliance with patients. These factors are particularly important when treating patients with persistent and severe depression. For therapy to be successful, it is important that therapists develop a kindly attitude to the difficulties and frustrations of this patient group. Severe depression can make therapy difficult by impairing energy and concentration, and progress can be slow. Furthermore, patients can be detached and distant from therapists, or may be oversensitive, scanning for any signs of therapist hopelessness or annoyance. Often in the past, such patients have been considered to be lacking in motivation or to have personality disorders, or even to be deliberately thwarting the therapist's best efforts at help. It is important to remember that these patients are suffering a great deal of distress and have often had very unhappy lives, faced with difficult experiences and situations.

Furthermore, in the RFCBT model, patterns of thinking and behavior that patients learned in the past obstruct their recovery. It is the therapist's job to work creatively and empathically to help patients find ways of shifting out of these patterns of thinking and behavior. The unhelpful ways of responding that patients use are generally habits that have developed through their earlier circumstances, and not aspects of their personalities.

Empathy involves conveying an understanding of how the world looks through the patient's eyes. Validating the patient's experience is an important step in helping him to feel better and preparing him to move toward active change. The therapist also needs to be persistent, to keep working and pressing for change in the patient. The therapist needs to provide a model of appropriate optimism, hope, and engaged action. Successful treatment of depression requires that therapists don't get caught up in the pessimism of their patients and give up in the face of difficulties and lack of improvement, but rather persevere and stick to the task, constantly looking for ways to navigate the problems that patients experience. A sense of engaged commitment and realistic confidence from the therapist can provide a major boost to a depressed patient.

Similarly, in patients suffering from residual depression, we need to pay deliberate attention to the regulation of affect. Patients with chronic depression often show particularly extreme patterns of affect regulation, either experiencing emotion as regularly overwhelming or presenting as somewhat numb and cut off, having blocked off emotion. To make therapy as effective as possible, we seek to activate emotion sufficiently that patients can learn to handle it at meaningful levels. We want emotional arousal to be clinically relevant but manageable for the patient. Thus, the therapist will need to either heighten the patient's emotional experience or take steps to stem its flow when emotion is overwhelming. The teaching of relaxation and imagery strategies early in therapy may help direct emotional experience in either direction: relaxation and imagery of coping or of distracting situations may help to stem the flow of emotion, whereas imaginal rehearsal of potentially emotional events may provoke emotional experience.

PART II

RUMINATION-FOCUSED COGNITIVE-BEHAVIORAL THERAPY

CHAPTER 4

Initial Assessment

Assessment is central to the conduct of RFCBT. The choice of interventions and the form they take depends a great deal on the initial and later assessments, with particular emphasis on FA. Since RFCBT is a relatively brief treatment intervention, the formal assessment period should be relatively concise, with continuous assessment and information-gathering occurring throughout the therapy.

In the first two sessions, the critical information is gathered for assessment as follows:

1. *Brief orientation to the patient's background, situation, and problems.* We want to know the patient's major concerns, goals, and issues. This includes current status, main symptoms, overview of his or her childhood, and major events. This is by necessity brief, while ensuring that no important information has been missed. More detailed work will occur during subsequent assessment of rumination and avoidance.

2. *Outline of the current episode of depression.* This includes onset, maintaining factors, and main symptoms and problems. This part of the assessment provides an opportunity to look for where rumination and avoidance may fit into the patient's difficulties so that a more complete personal rationale can be developed later in the session. This assessment includes drawing up a problem list with the patient.

3. *Initial evaluation of rumination and associated avoidance,* focusing on a general understanding of its more general properties and consequences, and review of its triggers, moderators, and functions. This is the first iteration of FA, which continues throughout the course of therapy.

Goals for the initial assessment include establishing that rumination is a major problem (i.e., the patient reports extensive unproductive dwelling on negative thoughts) and establishing that it has negative consequences. This provides the platform for collaboratively agreeing on rumination as the target of therapy and as a treatment goal. A key objective of the initial assessment is to derive suitable information to explain what rumination is to the patient, using examples from her own experience.

Further goals of the first sessions are engaging and socializing the patient into the treatment model, and giving the therapist a route map for therapy. In Chapters 6, 7 and 8, I discuss the more detailed use of FA and how it informs treatment formulation and the selection of interventions.

The assessment needs to help the therapist understand the patient's problems and background and provide an initial analysis of rumination and avoidance. To help with that initial analysis, the therapist asks the patient to complete self-report monitoring forms in the period between the screening assessment and the start of therapy.

Brief Orientation to the Patient's Background, Situation, and Problems

The assessment briefly explores the development of problems and the patient's personal history, including social and environmental factors potentially contributing to depression. The overview briefly asks about the patient's current situation and environment. Furthermore, the therapist assesses the onset and development of the current depression and the patient's view of depression as an illness and its treatment. This is important to understand the context relevant to the patient's presenting problems and to begin to build a therapeutic relationship with her.

Questions to ascertain current relationships, family, work, finance, housing, health, and legal issues include:

> "It would be helpful for you to briefly tell me something about your current situation. Who do you live with? Who do you regularly spend time with each week? How do you get along with them?"
> "Are you working/employed? What does your work involve? How do you find your work?"
> "Where do you live? Are there any problems there?"
> "Are there any financial concerns?"
> "Do you suffer from any physical health problems or concerns?"
> "How, if at all, do any of these areas contribute to your difficulties or help you overcome your difficulties?"

It can be useful to obtain a quick overview of the patient's background and childhood. This can be a difficult area to ask about and a difficult one for patients to talk about. It is useful to warn the patient that you may ask some probing questions and to give her permission to stop at any time or to decline to answer questions should she wish to do so. It is also helpful to get patients to reflect on their experience of talking about their childhood. This discussion of background can be helpful for clarifying how patients may have learned to adopt certain dysfunctional coping styles, such as rumination and avoidance. Framing rumination and avoidance as learned behavior can be very helpful in socializing patients into the treatment approach. Knowing about background and childhood experiences helps the therapist to formulate potential causes underpinning the development of the patient's rumination.

Typical questions include:

"Where were you born and brought up as a child?"
"How many siblings do you have?"
"How would you describe your childhood?"
"What did/do your parents do for a living?"
"What sort of person is/was your mother/father? How did you get on with him/her?"
"What values did your parents emphasize in your childhood?"
"Did you suffer any serious illness as a child?"
"What was your experience of going to school?"
"Did you ever have any unwanted sexual experiences as a child or adolescent?"
"When did you start to worry or ruminate about things? What was happening at that time?"
"Could you have learned to worry from anyone else in your family?"

The therapist then seeks a quick overview of the patient's view of him- or herself. Some useful things to ask include:

"How would you describe yourself as a person?"
"How would you compare yourself to other people?"
"What aspects of yourself do you like/dislike?"
"What do you see as your strengths/shortcomings?"

An Overview of the Patient's History of Depression and of the Current or Most Recent Episode

It is important to get a sense of the patient's depression, reviewing the current episode and the history of depression. The therapist then determines a problem list collaboratively with the patient. It is important to ensure that problems related to rumination and avoidance are explicitly on the problem list. Such problems should naturally emerge through discussion of the patient's symptoms, particularly as many are linked to rumination (e.g., procrastination, insomnia, negative mood, tiredness, anxiety, irritability). Problems on the list should be operationalized and defined as clearly as possible. Describing the problems as concretely and specifically as possible (1) makes it easier to assess progress in dealing with the problems, (2) makes the problems seem more manageable, and (3) models being specific and concrete to the patient.

Important questions when reviewing the history of depression include:

"How old were you when you first experienced depressive symptoms?"
"What was going on in your life around that time?"
"How did the illness affect you then?"
"How long do your episodes of depression tend to last?"
"When did the most recent episode start? What was happening then?"
"How did the depression develop over time?"
"What were the main difficulties that came with the depression?"
"What has changed about your life since the depression started?"
"What has made the depression better/worse?"
"What have you found helpful/unhelpful in trying to get better from depression?"
"What is your understanding of why you get depressed?"
"What are the problems that you have at the moment that you would most like to deal with?"
"Can you describe the situations where those problems occur in more detail?"

Throughout this manual, I will return to a number of case vignettes to illustrate the therapy, to give detailed examples of patient–therapist dialogue, and to illustrate the reasoning behind therapist decisions.

Here we introduce several of these cases, providing a summary of patients' responses to these initial questions about background, problems, goals, and depression. These examples are based on amalgams and generic composites across a number of real-life patients seen in treatment trials, with any potential identifying details altered and verbatim material paraphrased. Hopefully, they give a flavor of the common elements as well as the heterogeneity of presentations for patients struggling with rumination.

Case Example: Ruth

Ruth is a 40-year-old woman presenting with major depression and some anxiety including symptoms of agoraphobia and social phobia with concerns about being judged negatively by others. She described herself as a perfectionist and described her mother as being critical and unsupportive. She has two children, both girls, and is separated from their father. Her goals for therapy were to increase her confidence, to not respond in such an extreme way to events, to be less self-critical, and to plan where to go with things in her life. She works for a local charity and has done so for several years.

Case Example: Jenny

Jenny is a 21-year-old woman presenting with depression and anxiety. She reported a history of recurring major depression, with the first episode when she was 13 years old. She also met criteria for GAD, characterized by the tendency to worry more days than not in the last 6 months.

Her parents' long-standing marriage broke up some years ago. Since then, she has had little contact with her mother, and she remains angry about her mother's treatment of her father. Jenny felt sad about the lack of belief in her shown by her parents. She worked in an administrative role in an office. There is a repeated family history of depression, including her parents and grandparents.

In her initial assessment, she described wanting to move on, feeling stuck in the past since she was a teenager, constantly thinking about things that happened when she was 12 years old. She said that she finds it easy to dwell on the past over things that she cannot change. She also wanted to manage her thoughts better. She reported being bullied at school when she was 12 or 13 both physically and verbally: a gang of girls picked on her, and she was often scared, causing her to avoid school and hide in the bathrooms. She felt she had no real support at home and that was difficult. She did not get along with her older sister.

Case Example: Paula

Paula is a woman in her 60s who presents with ongoing feelings of grief and loss after the death of her husband 2 years earlier. She described feeling lonely and a dread of being left a lonely old lady. She reported that she had a very close relationship with her husband and that most of her friends were his friends. She also reported low self-esteem going back many years. Since being on her own, she worried about not doing the right things. Her main fear was that she could not cope with life. As to her goals, she wanted to feel good about herself and to stop blaming herself for her loss.

Paula met the criteria for a history of major depression and social anxiety (particularly fears of eating in front of others and of not doing the right thing at work). She also met criteria for GAD, characterized by uncontrollable worry more days than not.

Both her parents were dead. He father had died when she was a child. She described her mother as very strict, bossy, bad tempered, and very critical and nasty to her as both a child and as an adult. Paula did not enjoy school, where she felt that teachers and peers picked on her—she felt that there was something wrong with her that annoyed other people.

She had lived with her husband for nearly 40 years. Her main concerns were loss, feeling guilty about the passing of her husband, feeling isolated, low self-esteem, trying to have a social life, and selling her property to move to a new house. She often had feelings of worthlessness and failure; she would like to have more of a social circle.

Case Example: John

John is a 53-year-old man who reported several presenting issues. He described himself as a quiet, introspective person with a lack of confidence and self-worth. He said that he found it difficult to enjoy life. He believed that he does not have much to say to others; he reported being quiet in social situations.

He had a strained relationship with his teenage son, often finding his son's behavior frustrating, which led to arguments. He has always been self-critical and always disappointed himself with his lack of achievements. He reported that he managed his depression quite well in the past, but since an attempted suicide last year, he recognized that he needs help to sort himself out.

He presented with a history of reoccurring major depression. He has a past history of alcohol dependency, which lasted for 5 years, about 10 years ago. He also described social anxiety characterized by fear of being scrutinized in social situations. He described himself as always being shy and quiet, particularly when meeting new people.

He described his father as an opinionated, difficult, and domineering man. Although they had been very close when he was young, their relationship became strained as John sought more independence during his teenage and young adult years. His biggest fear was that he would end up like his father. He reported that he always thought his father was the problem but now recognizes that his mother also played a part in his behavior. He described her as timid, shy, and always worrying.

During his childhood, the family moved many times as his father relocated for his work, which he found unsettling and which made it difficult to make friends. He has been married for 25 years and has a good and loving relationship with his wife. He described her as considerate and quiet. He felt that she didn't confront problems, which he found difficult, and wanted to know what she thought so they could sort things out. He has worked as a postman for the last 25 years.

Initial Evaluation of Rumination and Associated Avoidance

The goals of this initial evaluation of rumination are to:

1. Begin to understand the experience of rumination for the patient and, thereby, orient the therapist to what may be relevant for the patient.
2. Identify the antecedents and consequences of rumination and begin to consider a possible case formulation. Case formulation in RFCBT is based on understanding the antecedents and consequences of rumination, identifying possible moderators of rumination, and hypothesizing possible functions for the rumination. This formulation then begins to inform potential interventions for the patient and the next steps in the therapy (see Chapter 7).
3. Inform the therapist's socialization and engagement of the patient.

Questions start by being focused more generically on the experience of rumination (e.g., "When do you tend to ruminate?"; "When is it better?"; "When is it worse?"). The therapist then explores in more detail one or two specific episodes of rumination that have occurred in the last week or two, to get a sense of the sequence and contents of rumination for that individual. This information guides the starting formulation of the patient's rumination, which in turn guides the selection and implementation of treatment approaches.

Useful opening questions to get an overall sense of rumination from the patient include:

"How often do you find yourself ruminating or dwelling on your problems and difficulties?"

"What do you tend to ruminate about?"

"How long does this rumination tend to last?"

"When do you tend to find that you are worrying and ruminating more?"

"When do you tend to feel worse?"

"What are the consequences of your rumination?"

"What effect does it have on you?"

"When does it tend to be better?"

"When does it tend to be worse?"

"What do you notice about your feelings that might be warning signs for your worry?"

"Are there situations, times, or places where it tends to happen more often?"

"How long have you been ruminating?"

"Can you remember when it started? When did it start?"
"What tends to stop your ruminating? When does it come to an end?"
"Is there someone you could have learned it from in childhood?"

It is important to work within the patient's phenomenology and vocabulary. Throughout the text, I use the word *rumination* as the simplest common label for repetitive negative thinking. However, each patient will have his or her own term or label to describe this negative thinking, whether it be dwelling, brooding, ruminating, worry, "chewing things over," or pondering. I recommend using the term that is acceptable and makes sense to each individual when discussing rumination.

It is useful to get a sense of what the patient is ruminating about. Often this will involve particular problems and difficulties in his or her life. Situational and environmental factors that can influence depression include relationships, problems at work, problems at home, life events (redundancy, unemployment, bereavement, divorce, jail sentence, other losses, trauma), and illness.

In these initial sessions, the therapist also checks on more general life events that are often common themes within rumination:

"Are there any particular events that have happened in your life that are relevant to how you feel?"
"Are there any memories that repeatedly come back to you now even if they happened a long time ago?"
"Are there any events that make you feel strongly sad, anxious, guilty, regretful, ashamed?"

An Example of General Orientation to Rumination: Jenny

THERAPIST: How often do you find yourself ruminating or dwelling on your problems and difficulties?

JENNY: I can always find something to worry about. I seem to do it nearly all the time. It overwhelms me.

THERAPIST: It sounds like worry is a major difficulty for you and one well worth addressing. What do you tend to worry about?

JENNY: I always expect the worst from situations; if something happens I always worry it will go wrong.

THERAPIST: That must be very tough for you. What effect does the worry have on you?

JENNY: It makes me feel more stressed. I have extreme mood swings from feeling very happy to feeling very sad or feeling very irritable. My mood changes quickly in response to what happens around me—I constantly feel I am overreacting to what is going on and never get the chance to feel more relaxed. I then often become verbally aggressive toward people that I love, which then makes me feel guilty.

THERAPIST: OK, from what you say, it seems as if worry tends to exacerbate your sadness and anger and makes it hard for you to stay on an even keel. Is that right?

JENNY: Yes.

THERAPIST: How long have you been worrying like this?

JENNY: I have always been a worrier.

THERAPIST: Can you remember when this first started?

JENNY: I was probably around 12 or 13—when I was being bullied at school.

THERAPIST: Did the worry start around the same time as the bullying?

JENNY: Yes, I worried about what would happen when I went in to school, and I started to avoid going in. What made it worse was that I had no real support at home. My parents didn't believe me when I told them I was worried about going back to school on a Monday.

THERAPIST: Is there anything else that might have contributed to your worry, for example, learning to worry from someone else?

JENNY: My mother was always worrying a lot. It didn't help that my dad always compared me negatively to my older sister. This knocked my confidence and made me worry about how I looked. No one said positive things about me, so I started to believe it.

THERAPIST: When do you tend to find that you are worrying and ruminating more? When do you tend to feel worse?

JENNY: I feel worse when I am making comparisons, when I compare myself to others and wonder how other people see me. Am I funny? Am I boring? Am I strange? I often think that I come off worse, and I make comparisons, which sets things off.

THERAPIST: What do you notice about your emotional feelings or physical sensations that might be warning signs for your worry?

JENNY: I feel tense and have a knot in my stomach. I get stomach pains and headaches.

Inside the Therapist's Mind

In this initial assessment, the therapist looks for clues as to the triggers and functions of the rumination to inform his case formulation and what he may do next. The therapist looks for points of contact to feed into the idiosyncratic treatment rationale. The basic treatment principle is that the therapist looks for points where there is leverage for change—points where the assessment indicates that rumination can shift under different circumstances—to then exploit these as fully as possible in within-session experiments, contingency plans, and homework. The therapist then selects one of the interventions (outlined in Chapter 4 and discussed in more detail in the subsequent chapters) based on what is learned.

Let's see how these ideas apply to Jenny. The formulation for her is based on understanding the antecedents and consequences of the target behavior of rumination. What aspects of the environment or of her actions increase or reduce it? What are possible functions for the rumination? This formulation then suggests potential interventions for her and next steps in therapy.

The formulation and the associated working plan are an ongoing iterative process best considered as a hypothesis to test. Predictions and interventions arise from the hypotheses, which are then tested and refined as therapy progresses. Treatment plans provide an experimental design to evaluate and refine the hypotheses.

For Jenny, this initial brief interview establishes that rumination is an important problem for her that she recognizes. The therapist can feed this into the rationale he gives her for the therapy. It also suggests potential causes for the development of unhelpful rumination through the combination of bullying at school and lack of support and criticism at home. The therapist could next explain that it makes sense that she has gotten into the habit of ruminating because of those early experiences where there was a good reason to anticipate what might happen to avoid getting bullied or to avoid criticism. Further, the therapist could explain that through repetition, this became a habit that still carries on.

The tense knot in the stomach may be a good early warning sign to link to alternative behaviors. The therapist encourages Jenny to pay attention to this sign and notice what happens when she starts to get tense.

The content of the rumination (negative self-comparisons, thinking the worst) and the context in which it occurs (social evaluation) suggest the hypothesis that the rumination may serve the functions of preempting and preparing to prevent unwanted outcomes and, in particular, to avoid negative judgments and responses from other people by checking on herself in advance. Further assessments focused on specific examples will need to look for evidence consistent and inconsistent with this formulation to further refine it.

This hypothesis also suggests potential techniques and approaches that may benefit Jenny, such as enhanced problem solving, self-compassion, and approach behaviors.

An Example of General Orientation to Rumination: Paula

THERAPIST: You mentioned dwelling on the past and on your problems as something you found yourself doing. How much of a problem is this for you?

PAULA: Recently, it has been a big problem. I have always got stuck on things, but it has been much worse over the last week.

THERAPIST: When did it start?

PAULA: I have always been a worrier, and I often hide and withdraw from others.

THERAPIST: What kind of thoughts go around and around in your mind?

PAULA: I find it difficult to be open with people. I often dwell on whether I am going to be criticized or rejected by other people. I spend a lot of time worrying about how other people react. When I am home on my own, I am worrying about what is going to happen when I go to see people. When I am out I want to get back to safety. There is a fear of being rejected and not being accepted. After I have got back from seeing people, I will replay what has happened over and over again in my mind. I feel I am being punished for doing things wrong, for getting irritable, for losing my temper. If things go wrong, then I think, "What have I done to deserve this?"; "Why am I so useless?"; "Why doesn't this work?" I feel a lot like I have caused it in some way.

THERAPIST: What is the effect of the dwelling on these thoughts, asking yourself questions like "Why am I so useless?" or "Why doesn't this work?" over and over again?

PAULA: I become totally overwhelmed. I feel down and useless. If I do one thing wrong, I start to feel that I am useless. Things get completely blown out of proportion, which makes things worse. I know I should do something, and it is better to do something than to think something, but I find it really hard. This reduces my confidence and energy.

THERAPIST: Have you noticed anything that often comes up just before you start to ruminate?

PAULA: I have negative thoughts—being unsure about other people, not sure about them. I do not always believe what people say. I ask "Are you sure?"; "I'm sorry to be a nuisance"; and I am checking "This is not going to be an inconvenience," and that often makes me feel unsure about what is going to happen and whether people really want to help. Why do I always think the worst?

THERAPIST: When does this tend to happen more or less?

PAULA: It is easy to get into it when I am feeling low. It happens more at home than at work.

THERAPIST: When do you feel better?

PAULA: I feel better when I am busy concentrating on things.

THERAPIST: What tends to stop your ruminating? When does it come to an end?

PAULA: Sometimes it ends on its own, or something interesting might take my mind off it. I might be distracted by a TV documentary.

THERAPIST: Can you remember when this started as a child?

PAULA: My mother always told me I was useless, that I could not do anything right. She blamed me. She always felt I was not capable and not as good as anyone else. And after my father died, I wanted to be the same as everyone else. I remember that when I was younger, I was worried about not fitting in, so I was spending a lot of time worrying that I was so useless at everything. It would go round and round in my mind.

Inside the Therapist's Mind

For Paula, this initial interview establishes that rumination is an important problem for her that she acknowledges, so the therapist can discuss this as a key and potentially helpful target of the treatment. It also suggests potential causes for the development of unhelpful rumination through the long-standing criticism in her childhood. The therapist can explain that it is not surprising that Paula learned to ruminate in this context.

Paula's answers suggest the hypothesis that the rumination may have the function of trying to help her fit in by trying to work out and understand what is going on, particularly with other people before, during, and after social interactions. More specifically, there is a sense that she might be ruminating as a means to reduce uncertainty and to gain control through understanding. Further assessments focused on specific examples will need to look for evidence consistent and inconsistent with this formulation to further refine it.

It appears that a key trigger for her rumination may be doubtful thoughts about other people, followed by attempts at reassurance seeking. This suggests that a potentially useful behavioral experiment may be for Paula to try an alternative, more assertive response in these situations.

It is also useful for the therapist to mentally note and record the large number of "why" questions that Paula is asking herself. These provide an indication of the abstract, analytical thinking that is characteristic of her rumination. It suggests that a potential intervention is to shift her to more concrete thinking, for example building on a Why–How experiment (see

Chapter 9). It may be useful to highlight to Paula how many "why" questions she is asking herself by enumerating this list, and to consider alternatives she could try. This suggests the value of trying an experiential experiment in session to see if becoming more concrete works for Paula. If it does, then that would suggest the value of practicing this technique in response to doubtful thoughts as an ongoing plan.

It is also worth noting that her responses suggest that rumination can end when she becomes absorbed in other activities. This suggests a potential point of leverage for change that can be encouraged, for example, through planning absorbing activities and through absorption exercises using mental imagery. This response prompts the therapist to look out for other examples of this shift as therapy progresses. Examples of absorbing activities that Paula reports already doing and that are practically convenient would be considered as a possible intervention.

From this example, you can see that a brief set of questions can begin to set off a range of possibilities for further investigation and consideration as the therapy proceeds. These possibilities are worth keeping in mind as you move to discussing specific examples of rumination, as this might guide your questions and, if confirmed in further questioning, feed into the first steps for treatment planning.

An Example of General Orientation to Rumination: John

THERAPIST: Is there anything in particular that you are dwelling on that is more recent?

JOHN: I remember an episode at work, about a month ago, where I got into an argument with this guy at work who often belittles me. There was just a bad atmosphere, and he said something. I didn't respond for a while, although I was stewing over it and could feel myself getting wound up. Even though I was telling myself to just let it go, it all came up again, and I had a go back at him. After that, I kept thinking over what happened, wishing I hadn't said what I did. I have been dwelling on it most days since it happened.

THERAPIST: What thoughts have been going through your mind since then?

JOHN: I think "I am not popular, no one likes me, I don't want to be at work"; "Why am I doing this?"; "Why am I making myself feel so bad?"

THERAPIST: What effect do these kinds of thoughts have on you?

JOHN: I feel more isolated. It winds me up and gets worse and worse. I ended up taking a week off work sick. It gets me down. I get quieter, withdrawn, nobody else would be worrying about it—I wish I could be a more popular person. I don't see myself as likable. I should be likable.

I don't feel as though I have a lot of friends. I wish I had something more interesting to say. I have nothing to say. I am quiet. I wonder why this is so difficult. These thoughts go round and round in my head. It makes me feel worse. It brings me down, it doesn't help, I get into a situation where I do not think I can win.

THERAPIST: It sounds like this tendency to get caught up in thoughts that go round and round is pretty insistent and powerful for you—and what's more, that it has a strong negative effect, getting you down and making you take time away from work. Is that right?

JOHN: Yes, it has taken over my life.

THERAPIST: OK, I am hearing that this is having a big impact on you and is definitely worth us tackling together. When did this tendency for thoughts to go around and around in your head start?

JOHN: I have done it since I was a teenager at least.

THERAPIST: When do these kinds of thoughts tend to be worse?

JOHN: Whenever there is a fear of what to do, of not making the right decision, of being isolated. It tends to happen during any quiet moment. I try to work out what is going to happen when I am with other people, how I will get along with them. I have never felt like I've been particularly popular or well liked. When I go places, I feel like a spare part—my thoughts justify that I am going to get rejected. There is a feeling that it might go totally wrong, that I am a quiet person and I do not put out my opinions. I have a distinct feeling that other people will not want to talk to me, that they would want me to go off separately and keep to myself.

THERAPIST: Does this happen a lot in situations where you are meeting up with other people or going to new places?

JOHN: Yes, all the time. It starts before I can help it.

THERAPIST: It sounds like worry and rumination have become a habit, needing to get it right, second-guessing other people, thinking it is easier not to say things, trying to work out in your head how it might turn out.

JOHN: Yes, that's right.

THERAPIST: Could you have learned this habit from someone?

JOHN: My father was not very likable, he was so opinionated and down on life; nothing was ever right in his eyes. He was such a pessimist. Everything was black to him—nothing was worth doing. I don't want to be like my father. I often ruminate about my past. Why do I do this? Why do I think like this? Why do I blame others? Why can't I find things to make myself a happy person? Why is it so hard for me? Why do I make such a big deal out of all this stuff?

THERAPIST: Are there times where you think you can work through things?

JOHN: It is easy with practical things. I can work through those. It is much harder with problems with people, working through problems with people. If I do something practical, that makes my mind off the problem.

Inside the Therapist's Mind

For John, this initial interview establishes that rumination is an important problem, so the therapist can discuss this as a priority of the treatment. It also suggests a potential cause for the development of unhelpful rumination through his experience of his father and his attempts to not be like him. The attempt to avoid an unwanted self is a common motivation behind rumination; here it reflects a concern about not becoming a negative, opinionated person. All the questions John asks himself about his past and about how he comes across to others could serve the function of avoiding becoming such an opinionated person, while also reflecting some of the negativity that may have rubbed off from his father. Further assessments focused on specific examples will need to look for evidence consistent and inconsistent with this formulation to further refine it.

His answers are very consistent with his rumination being a habit, and it is thus a good idea for the therapist to directly check this with him. It appears that key triggers for his rumination may be when he is alone or has to express an opinion. This suggests elements of his environment that could influence his rumination.

It is also useful to note and record the large number of "why" questions John is asking himself. This suggests that concrete thinking may be a potential intervention for him. It is also worth noting that his rumination tends to stop when he is engaged in practical problems. In this situation, he is good at generating solutions. This suggests a possible useful counterpoint for the times when he gets stuck, which might be used to introduce variability in a future FA. The therapist may examine what John does when he solves a practical problem and how this differs from his thinking and response for a problem involving other people. This comparison may help John learn better ways of responding that build on his own established repertoire. In other words, the therapist is actively looking for times when a patient copes well because these provide points of leverage to introduce positive experiences into the treatment.

Examining a Specific Episode of Rumination

Having gotten a sense of how rumination occurs generally for a patient, it is useful to talk through at least one specific example of a recent episode of

Self-Test: Thinking through the Formulation for Ruth

Here is a summary of the information provided by Ruth in answer to the orienting questions.

Ruth recognized rumination as an involuntary habit that occurred frequently and described often having thoughts like "Why didn't I finish this?" and "Why haven't I done more with my life?," leading to a sense of failure. She described how she has a pattern of getting very upset very quickly. She can feel very flat and that can be a trigger to ruminate. Sometimes when she hears news, her thoughts can start running on and build up, taking things to more extreme levels.

She reported that the rumination varied in how frequently it happens. She does not do it at all if she is feeling OK; for example, when she is at her arts course and she is enjoying and absorbed in it then she tends not to ruminate.

She identified the following as common warning signs: reminders of her childhood; when she is reminded that she hasn't completed things (e.g., when she thinks about the fact that she did not complete her studies and is not sure what she wants to do next, and she thinks, "Why didn't I carry on?"; "If only I had carried on"). When things are quieter at work and there is less going on it tends to get worse. When she is on her own and the children are in bed, she starts to think, "What I am going to do with my day?"; "What have I done?"; "What have I achieved?" Rumination follows the sequence of "Why didn't I do that?"; "Why am I too scared?"; "What is stopping me from doing things?" There are also worries about her depression influencing her children and the effect that it might have on them, as well as thoughts like "What will other people think of me?"

When asked about the consequences of the rumination, she recognized that it tends to take up her energy and time. It makes her feel like a failure, irritable, depressed, and useless, reducing her motivation.

She describes ruminating on and off since she was a teenager and describes moving when she was younger and not fitting in and starting to ask questions like "Why do I find this difficult?"; "Why am I not happy?"

Use this information to create an initial formulation for Ruth, taking into account that your goals are to identify antecedents and consequences of rumination, identify potential moderators, and hypothesize possible functions for the rumination.

Useful questions to reflect on include:

- What comes before the rumination?
- Does this suggest possible changes in environment or patient behavior to reduce cueing of rumination?
- What follows the rumination? What are its effects?
- How might the rumination have developed?
- How might this knowledge contribute to the rationale given to the patient?

- What does this suggest about possible functions of the rumination?
- How can I further test this hypothesis?
- What other information do I need? What do I need to check in more detail when discussing specific examples?
- What next steps might be possibilities for interventions?

See the box on pages 86–87 at the end of this chapter for some potential answers.

rumination. This will help to give a sense of potential triggers to the rumination (antecedents), of the nature and process of the thoughts that occur (behavior), and of the consequences of the rumination (consequences). This feeds into the therapist's conceptualization of what is happening with the rumination and informs the rationale given to the patient. This initial assessment then leads into socialization into the therapy and the provision of the treatment rationale.

This exploration starts by asking the patient to recall a recent time—in the last few weeks—when she has noticed that she is caught up in dwelling on her feelings or problems. Having identified an example, the therapist prompts the patient to recall it as vividly and in as much detail as possible, starting from what happened just before the rumination started. The ACES principle is particularly important when reviewing these examples of recent episodes of rumination. A good strategy is to ask the patient to recall the event in detail but to slow it down, as if running a film in slow motion or one frame at a time, so that together you can map out what happens moment by moment during the sequence of rumination. The therapist further promotes this by asking questions that are focused and tightly defined in terms of place, time period, sequential order, and element of observed experience. If patients begin to lump together steps in the sequence or compress minutes of the rumination into a single description (e.g., "I just kept dwelling on what happened"), then the therapist asks further questions to split these up into smaller steps.

It can be useful to draw out the sequence of the rumination on a board or piece of paper to illustrate the thinking process. Here are some sample questions:

"What happened just before you started to ruminate?"
"What was the very first thought you noticed?"
"What sensation did you notice in your body in the seconds immediately after that?"
"After you noticed that, what did you do next?"
"When you had that thought, how did you feel right afterward?"

"When you started to feel anxious, what did you think next?"
"After you had that thought, what went through your mind in the next
    second?"
"Where exactly were you focusing your attention just then?"

By using questions like this, the therapist draws out a detailed, second-by-second outline of the sequence of rumination, starting with the initial trigger and moving through the sequence of thoughts, feelings, sensations, and actions, and begins to map out the process of rumination for the patient. This informs the therapist about the kinds of questions the patient asks him- or herself and the key themes of the rumination. It is useful to keep a close eye out for more abstract and evaluative questions such as "Why me?" This can indicate entry and exit points into and from the bout of rumination, which gives clues to possible points of intervention. It also provides a concrete example of the effects of rumination on particular symptoms and difficulties for the patient, which can be fed directly into the therapy rationale.

Drawing Out a Specific Example of Rumination: Paula

THERAPIST: Let's go through an example in a bit of detail and see if we can understand what is happening. Can you think of a recent time when you were starting to worry?

PAULA: A few days ago I was concerned about asking to take time off work.

THERAPIST: As you remember that time, let's slowly go through it moment by moment as if things are in slow motion so we can learn as much as possible about what happened. What did you first notice?

PAULA: I started to feel a bit agitated and tense.

THERAPIST: Where did you notice that you were tense?

PAULA: I was tense across the shoulders.

THERAPIST: What was going through your mind as you started to feel tense?

PAULA: I was thinking about what would happen. I was imagining what would happen if I asked, thinking they would probably say no.

THERAPIST: What did you imagine exactly?

PAULA: I saw my boss looking at me as if I was stupid and telling me no, and imagined myself feeling shamed.

THERAPIST: What happened when you started to think that?

PAULA: I started to feel tenser.

THERAPIST: And then what happened immediately after that?

PAULA: It stopped when I actually asked the question and got the answer.

THERAPIST: What happened then?

PAULA: My boss actually agreed to my request.

THERAPIST: It seems important to note that things did not turn out quite the way you expected. Let's take a step back—what happened between imagining the worst and asking the question? I am guessing that there was more going on there.

PAULA: I was saying to myself I have got to ask the question; there is no point putting it off. It is now or never. I was getting very self-critical. "It is pathetic, I am a failure."; "Can I be grown up enough and go and ask?" I just felt worse and worse and it got harder and harder to get started.

THERAPIST: OK, it sounds like there is a lot going on there. Let's try and slow that down to capture the sequence of what happened more precisely. As best you can, run what happened through your mind in slow motion, like watching a film frame by frame. You have just imagined your boss saying no and started to feel the tension grow in your shoulders. What was the very next thought that you had?

PAULA: I need to make this appointment—it is urgent.

THERAPIST: OK, and the next second after thinking that, what are you saying to yourself?

PAULA: I tell myself that I can't put it off—I have to ask now.

THERAPIST: And how do you feel right then?

PAULA: I am getting tense, feeling under pressure and stressed.

THERAPIST: And what goes through your mind just then?

PAULA: I ask myself, "Why can't I do this?"; "Why is this so difficult?"

THERAPIST: And what follows the instant after asking those questions?

PAULA: That's when I criticize myself and think how pathetic I am.

THERAPIST: What follows that thought? What effect does it have on you?

PAULA: I begin to feel down and lacking in motivation.

THERAPIST: And what follows immediately after that?

PAULA: I keep dwelling on why do I find it so hard to do these easy things and why am I such a failure? Why do I keep doing this? Why is everything so difficult?

THERAPIST: How does this make you feel?

PAULA: More and more depressed.

THERAPIST: What happened next?

PAULA: I kept criticizing myself, but then I would return to the thought that I need to make this appointment.

THERAPIST: What happened then?

PAULA: The same thoughts would run through my mind again.

THERAPIST: OK, let me check I understand this correctly. You had thoughts about asking to have time off to make this appointment but then imagined your request going wrong, which makes you feel anxious, and then you remembered how important it was and wondered why you weren't doing it and why it was so hard, and then these thoughts would lead into thoughts of being a failure, making you feel down, before returning back to the thought that I need to ask about taking time off. And then the whole sequence would repeat itself. Is that right?

PAULA: Yes.

THERAPIST: How long did this repeating sequence of thoughts carry on when you were at work?

PAULA: It went round and round in my head for about an hour.

THERAPIST: That sounds like it was a difficult hour for you, making you feel much worse, but on a positive note, you did manage to break out of it and go and ask the question. What happened just before you did this?

PAULA: I thought to myself that this is just getting worse and I am making no progress and I need to do something different about it. I decided I needed to ask the question, and focused on what I would say.

THERAPIST: And that led to you asking your boss, who agreed—after which the rumination stopped. Is that right?

PAULA: Yes, I felt a huge relief and a lifting of the tension.

THERAPIST: So to summarize, it seems that taking an action rather than thinking about it, that actually asking the question rather than checking it out in your mind seemed to be helpful?

PAULA: Yes—that's right.

Inside the Therapist's Mind

This dialogue illustrates several common issues. It indicates how the therapist needs to push and prompt to track the full sequence of thoughts in concrete and specific detail from moment to moment. This includes breaking down global descriptions into smaller specific segments and slowing down the description of what happened. This is critical because it helps to reveal the dynamic process of rumination—how it can become self-perpetuating, but also where it may break down.

This dialogue shows how it is important for the therapist to summarize and provide feedback on the thought cycle as it emerges in order to check that it is correct. This helps to highlight the flow of thoughts to the patient.

This step-by-step unpacking of a specific example provides further information to refine the initial formulation of Paula's rumination. It confirms the interpersonal focus of her rumination and how the rumination is focused on understanding and trying to improve her sense of certainty about actions.

Finally, this example suggests possible moderators of the rumination and alternative responses such as making a decision to do something or asking rather than thinking. The therapist will want to highlight these because they indicate points of leverage that could be further elaborated in later sessions.

Drawing Out a Specific Example of Rumination: Jenny

THERAPIST: Have there been any particular examples when you started to worry last week? Anytime where we could go in to a bit more detail? When were you worrying the most this week?

JENNY: I was starting to worry about going out on a date.

THERAPIST: When was the date going to be?

JENNY: That was on Friday night.

THERAPIST: And when did the worry start?

JENNY: On the Tuesday, I was getting ready to go off to work and I started to feel anxious. On the way to work, my head starts to fill up with all of these thoughts about what could happen.

THERAPIST: What did you start to worry about?

JENNY: Thoughts were running through my head about what could happen, what could go wrong. I wondered if we had anything in common. Will he think I am interesting, funny, and pretty? Will I embarrass myself?

THERAPIST: What was the effect of that thinking and those worries about embarrassing yourself?

JENNY: I felt much tenser and wound up. I found it hard to concentrate.

THERAPIST: What was the effect of that like?

JENNY: It was really tiring and exhausting.

THERAPIST: What went through your mind next after asking those questions about how he will react to you?

JENNY: He might think I am boring. This goes on a loop, and I get more and more wound up because for an hour I am imagining and thinking about all of the things that could go wrong.

THERAPIST: How long did the worry last in total?

JENNY: It went on most of the day.

THERAPIST: And how did it come to an end?

JENNY: I went out with a friend in the evening. Then it started again the next day, and I just went with it. I had taken all the fun out of it, and I had spent all of my time worrying.

THERAPIST: And how did the date turn out?

JENNY: The date was really good. However, by the time I got around to it, I was feeling really drained and afterward I was replaying some of it over and over again.

THERAPIST: Is there anything that you can do to reduce the worry?

JENNY: I could think about what we could talk about, and I could plan what I could wear.

THERAPIST: What happens then?

JENNY: I feel like I've got a little more control, but then another worry takes over.

THERAPIST: What could you talk about on the date?

JENNY: We could talk about music. But then maybe we would have nothing left to say.

THERAPIST: What else could you talk about?

JENNY: Books and films.

THERAPIST: When we think about what you could say, how does that make you feel?

JENNY: I feel a bit better. In my head I want to be in control of the whole conversation, and to be able to think of something to say. I am always concerned about running out of things to say. What I could do wrong, what I could do to embarrass myself? I am really worried about being clumsy or spilling things. I am imagining doing something embarrassing and having thoughts like "What if I spill a drink?"; "What if I trip?" I have images of doing these things.

THERAPIST: So it sounds like part of the process of thinking all these things through is to try and preempt it, prepare for it, think about what could go wrong and then find ways to do something else. Does that sound right?

JENNY: Yes.

Inside the Therapist's Mind

This dialogue illustrates several common issues. First, it gives a good sense of the flow of thinking for Jenny and how the thoughts build on each other. It also gives a good feel for the content of her rumination and the kinds of concerns that keep coming up. It provides further evidence of how the rumination may be unhelpful.

Second, it illustrates how it can be useful to directly ask about what may change or influence the rumination. Jenny is aware that she can reduce the worry and rumination if she is focused on what she can concretely do. This suggests a number of possible interventions that may be helpful for her (e.g., concrete thinking, problem solving, role playing).

Third, this step-by-step unpacking of a specific example provides further information to refine the initial formulation of the function of her rumination. It suggests that the worry has a preparatory function in order to try and prevent future difficulties, particularly around not knowing what to do with other people. The possible functions of the rumination can be collaboratively discussed with patients and this dialogue illustrates how the discussion can be started, building directly from the patient's responses.

Drawing Out a Specific Example of Rumination: Ruth

THERAPIST: Let's go through an example in a bit of detail and see if we can understand what is happening. Can you think of a recent time when you were starting to ruminate? As we think of that time, let's slowly go through it moment by moment as if things are in slow motion so we can learn as much as we can about what happens.

RUTH: I was getting stressed and wound up after coming home with the children on Tuesday, and found myself dwelling on things.

THERAPIST: It is helpful to identify exactly what happened just before the rumination started—to see if we can spot the triggers. What happened just before you started getting stressed?

RUTH: I had been to my class and then I took the children to the park.

THERAPIST: How were you feeling then?

RUTH: I felt good and positive.

THERAPIST: OK, when did you notice the dwelling on things begin to start?

RUTH: It was after we had all gotten home. About an hour after we got home, I noticed my mood starting to go down and I was feeling fed up.

THERAPIST: OK, that sounds like an important time to focus on in detail. Let's try and look at that second by second. What were you doing during that first hour home?

RUTH: I got going on some chores around the house, tidying up, and ironing.

THERAPIST: And what else was happening around you? For example, what were the children doing?

RUTH: My oldest daughter was watching TV, and my youngest daughter was sitting at the kitchen table and supposed to be doing her homework.

THERAPIST: OK, so you are working around the house and the children are sitting watching TV or doing their homework, and to start with you are feeling OK, is that right?

RUTH: Yes.

THERAPIST: When do you notice your mood drop?

RUTH: As I was doing the housework, I was thinking how I hated being a housewife and was getting fed up with all of those things.

THERAPIST: Can you remember exactly what thoughts went through your mind just then? What was the first thought you noticed?

RUTH: I thought I am going back to the daily grind.

THERAPIST: And how did that thought make you feel?

RUTH: I felt tired, bored, irritated.

THERAPIST: And what thoughts came immediately after the thought about going back to the daily grind?

RUTH: I thought, "I can't be bothered. This is dull, repetitive, and irritating."

THERAPIST: What effect did these thoughts have?

RUTH: My mood got worse, more down and irritable.

THERAPIST: What happened next?

RUTH: I was in the kitchen and my daughter was not concentrating on her homework, and this made me even more irritated.

THERAPIST: What went through your mind just then?

RUTH: She is not even trying properly.

THERAPIST: What did you do just then?

RUTH: I told her to concentrate on her homework, but she didn't concentrate any more.

THERAPIST: What did you think then?

RUTH: I thought, "What is the point? I am not getting respect from anyone. No one listens to me."

THERAPIST: And when you had these thoughts, what effect did it have on how you felt?

RUTH: I got more and more irritated.

THERAPIST: What did you do or say just then?

RUTH: I started to nag my daughter and just left the room feeling really irritated.

THERAPIST: What went through your mind just then?

RUTH: I can't even be a good parent. Why can't I even do that well?

THERAPIST: How did you feel then?

RUTH: Irritated and down and flat.

THERAPIST: And what followed that?

RUTH: My thoughts continued to spiral into the same negative thoughts over and over again. Thoughts like "Why do I let it get to me?"; "Is my past going to come back and haunt me?"; "Is it my fault?"; "Why am I so pathetic?"

THERAPIST: How long did this last?

RUTH: It went on until I went to bed.

Inside the Therapist's Mind

This example again indicates how the therapist needs to push and prompt to track the full sequence of thoughts in concrete and specific detail, from moment to moment. This includes breaking down global descriptions into smaller specific segments and slowing down the description of what happened. Doing this is critical because it helps us to see the dynamic process of rumination, how it can become self-perpetuating, but also where it may break down.

This dialogue helps the therapist to identify possible warning signs and cues for Ruth's rumination. It looks as if having thoughts like "I'm going back to the daily grind" and feeling bored are a risk point for triggering a period of rumination. Knowing this could help in planning when it would be best for Ruth to practice alternative responses and what triggering cues to link these with. It suggests that the therapist and Ruth should look out for this warning sign and similar signs in future examples.

This interaction also gives clues as to possible functions for Ruth's rumination. One possibility is that the rumination is focused on helping to understand past problems and prevent them from recurring. Another possibility is that the rumination may serve the function of trying to avoid an unwanted outcome—in this case Ruth's sense of herself as someone who has not achieved anything and is just a housewife. There may be a motivating aspect to the rumination that involves dwelling on what she has not achieved to put pressure on herself to do more.

It is also useful for the therapist to note and record the large number of "why" questions that Ruth is asking herself. These provide an indication of the abstract, analytical thinking that is characteristic of her rumination. It suggests that a potential intervention is to shift her to more concrete thinking, for example, building on a Why–How experiment. It may be useful to

RUMINATION-FOCUSED COGNITIVE-BEHAVIORAL THERAPY

point out to her how many "why?"-type questions she is asking herself by going over this list, and to consider alternatives she could try.

Self-Test Answers: Reflection on the Formulation for Ruth

- **What comes before the rumination?** Potential antecedents and triggers for Ruth's rumination include reminders of her childhood, reminders of not completing things, when she is less busy or occupied, when she is on her own, when her children are in bed, when she is concerned about life passing her by without achieving anything.

- **Does this suggest possible changes in environment or patient behavior to reduce cueing of rumination?** It suggests that some changes in her routines might be helpful (e.g., rumination often starts when her children have been put to bed, so it may be useful to plan an activity to do then). There seem to be strong triggers such as thoughts and memories about not achieving things, so it may be effective to use these as warning signs in a contingency If–Then plan, with a positive alternative behavior to be practiced in response to those signs.

- **What follows the rumination? What are its effects?** It produces a sense of failure, increases irritability, and reduces motivation.

- **How might the rumination have developed?** It may have developed because of a sense of not fitting in and trying to work this out as a teenager.

- **How might this knowledge contribute to the rationale given to the patient?** There is good evidence to feed into the rationale that rumination is unhelpful and that it is a habit. This can provide some background as to how it is an understandable reaction that may have started as a response to her difficulties as a teenager.

- **What does this suggest about possible functions of the rumination?** The focus of the rumination is on thinking "Why haven't I done more with my life?" Potential reinforcing functions of the rumination include (1) an attempt to understand why things happened this way to prevent it continuing; (2) making sure that incomplete tasks in the past are not forgotten and are focused on to stop her from slipping up in the future (reminders to keep the pressure on).

- **How can I further test this hypothesis?** Collaborative discussion with Ruth; looking at specific examples of rumination to see if patterns of thinking are consistent; behavioral experiments to see if providing alternatives reduces rumination.

- **What other information do I need? What do I need to check in more detail when discussing specific examples?** There is information on potential reinforcing consequences from the examples of rumination. You could ask Ruth about what might rumination avoid or prevent from happening, what would happen if she stopped ruminating? Such questions might give insight into particular functions.

- **What next steps might be possibilities for interventions?** (1) As noted above, the contingency If–Then plans can be developed with alternative responses to the identified triggers; (2) because of the preponderance of abstract, analytical "Why?" questions, practice at thinking in a more concrete way may be helpful; (3) because of the focus on completing tasks, explicit focus on activity scheduling and goal setting may be helpful as an alternative to rumination; (4) if the hypothesis about rumination as a form of spur to the self to avoid future failures (albeit an unsuccessful one) is correct, then providing an alternative, more constructive way for Ruth to motivate and encourage herself might be helpful (e.g., self-compassion work); (5) the examples Ruth provided indicated that her rumination was lessened when she was doing creative work such as her arts course. This raises the possibility that absorption work may be helpful.

CHAPTER 5

Therapy Rationale
and Goal Setting

In addition to assessment, the first few sessions need to socialize the patient into the RFCBT model, provide a rationale to explain depression, rumination, and how therapy will work, and incorporate some brief interventions to give patients some positive experiences early in therapy. Developing a detailed and convincing rationale is important for two reasons. First, a good rationale for therapy can help the patient feel there is a chance that therapy will be helpful, reducing hopelessness. Second, patients who ruminate are often spending a lot of mental energy trying to understand why things are the way they are. A convincing rationale and account for their depression may temporarily help to reduce this particular aspect of rumination.

The Therapy Rationale

Socialization needs to start within the first session. Discussing a recent example of a problem or episode of rumination is helpful in developing the therapy model for patients, using their own experience and their own words. Thus, socialization into the therapy naturally follows from the initial assessment. Socialization should focus on showing the link between antecedents, behaviors, and consequences. It is particularly useful to draw simple diagrams based on the patient's own experience. It can also be helpful to summarize the process of rumination, drawing out the sequence of an episode of rumination and discussing this as a common pattern. It is important to have rumination (however labeled in the patient's own words) and avoidance on the diagram, and shown to contribute to the maintenance of the depression. Putting specific examples of these behaviors on the diagram can also be helpful. The handout on rumination (see Handout 1, Key Facts about Rumination, in the Appendix) is used to support this psychoeducation.

The more the patient's symptoms and experiences can be normalized, the better, since many people who suffer from extreme rumination tend to believe that they are odd, different, and deficient, and are focused on making negative comparisons between themselves and others. It is helpful to stress the internal logic of the patient's responses (e.g., "If I believed this, I would also act in this way"; "If this happened to me, I would find it hard to get it out of my mind"; "Given these consequences, it makes sense that rumination continues").

The key points to get across in the rationale are:

1. Recurrent negative thinking (worry, rumination) and avoidance maintain depression.
2. Both rumination and avoidance are quite normal and helpful in limited amounts under the right circumstances (i.e., "It is not surprising that you use them—everyone else uses them too").
3. However, when used excessively or when they are out of balance, they become problematic.
4. Excessive use occurs because of past learning, either from copying others or from previous occasions when you learned that rumination was a useful strategy, that is, where it had perceived benefit.
5. Rumination has become a habit learned from repeated use during past experience, which makes it automatic and often triggered without awareness.
6. Because it was learned, it can be replaced with a new more adaptive strategy, which is learned in its place.
7. Therapy will coach you in learning a new, more adaptive approach based on your own experience and benefiting from the therapist having a wider perspective.
8. Because rumination is a learned habit, changing the habit requires increasing awareness of what triggers the rumination and repeated practice to shift the habit. This can take time and effort but is doable.

These points are made in detail in the initial handouts on rumination and avoidance (see Handout 1, Key Facts about Rumination, and Handout 2, Avoidance). As in the standard CBT approach, regular feedback will be sought to check that this information makes sense and seems relevant to patients (e.g., "How does this fit your experience?").

The suggested scripts below provide a general guide to what is useful to say when providing a rationale, although each needs to be changed to incorporate particular examples from each patient's own words and experiences.

Rumination and Avoidance Maintain Depression

"We have seen that you spend a lot of time dwelling on negative thoughts, rehashing things in your mind. Furthermore, we have seen that the more you do this, the worse you feel and the less motivated you feel. We have also talked about how you avoid several situations. For example, as you became depressed, you stopped doing [give example from the patient's own experience].

"I am interested in these two aspects of your behavior because I believe they are involved in maintaining your depressed symptoms. There is evidence that dwelling on things and avoiding things can keep depression going. Does this make sense to you based on your experience?

"Can you see examples of this from your own experience? For example, as you stopped going out, you continued to feel sadder and sadder [perhaps refer to a diagram showing the relationship between thinking, behavior, and symptoms]. Further, despite spending long periods of time thinking about things to try and work them out, it seems that you rarely reach a useful conclusion and just feel worse and worse [use examples from the patient's assessment (i.e., of mood getting worse and worse as the patient ruminates—see examples in dialogues from Chapter 4 and this chapter)].

"Repeated dwelling on, worrying about, analyzing, and thinking about unpleasant events, feelings, and problems is called rumination. When prolonged, frequent, and extreme, rumination is problematic, contributes to anxiety and depression, reduces motivation, leads to procrastination, and reduces direct contact with the world. You have given me some recent examples of this [where possible, illustrate with examples from the patient's own experience]. In these ways, rumination, dwelling on negative things, can become a 'central engine' that keeps on fueling the depression.

"Likewise, avoiding risky and painful situations seems a sensible response, but over time it means that you do less and less, and you have fewer and fewer chances to have positive experiences or discover new ways to handle things. This too can further maintain the depression."

Rumination and Avoidance Are Normal

"Rumination is a normal response to difficulties, although it is usually relatively brief and limited to a particular concern. When there is a problem, it is natural to try and solve it, work it through, and make sense of it by thinking about it. Indeed, thinking about things can be helpful, for example, look at how it can solve practical problems. Indeed, most of the technological advances mankind has made are a consequence of dwelling on and analyzing things."

Rumination Can Become a Problem

"However, we find that 'thinking about' things can be unhelpful when:

- It is applied to inappropriate concerns or applied too widely.
- The balance between thinking and action is lost or thinking becomes an end in itself. Thinking is useful if it acts as a guide to action, and action then informs further thinking, such that one feeds back into the other. However, if thinking becomes much more frequent than action or replaces action, then we end up with procrastination and avoidance, and problems are not solved. For example, imagine that your car does not start. It is helpful to dwell on why it might not be starting and generate possible reasons for it not starting (e.g., problems with spark plugs, engine too cold, battery too low), and this thinking will help to solve the problem. But for this thinking to be helpful, you need to actively investigate (look under the hood, try out different things, etc.). Just thinking won't solve the problem. Likewise, just trying an action without dwelling on the problem probably won't solve the problem, for example, repeatedly turning the key in the ignition. So a balance is important.
- The style of thinking might be important too. Let's imagine the differences between asking 'Why isn't the car starting?' and asking yourself 'Why is this happening to me?' What is the effect of asking these two different questions? Which question is more helpful?"

We might then say something along the lines of the following:

Excessive Rumination Is Learned

"Excessive rumination should not be accepted as a normal response, nor as part of your personality. In fact, rumination is a particular learned response—a new, different response can be learned instead to replace it. Rumination was learned because it was taught to us, or because at some point there was some kind of payoff or benefit to doing it."

At this point, the therapist reviews the idiosyncratic development of rumination within the assessment to illustrate how the rumination may have been learned. This includes talking about how rumination may have been adaptive in some limited circumstances (e.g., to avoid getting into trouble;

to try and make sense of difficulties; to prepare for the worst). It is important here to normalize the patient's responses as the tendency to worry or ruminate is likely to be an understandable and normal response to a genuinely difficult situation or to chronic strains. The therapist acknowledges that these may be situations that would cause anyone to dwell on the problem or difficulty in an attempt to resolve it. One advantage of this approach is that it allows the therapist to empathize directly with patients and to explicitly recognize the genuine difficulties they face. In my experience, many patients with depression are faced with difficult life circumstances. There is value in acknowledging these genuine difficulties and validating the patient's experience rather minimizing or challenging her difficulties and moving straight into problem solving. Time spent acknowledging these real problems and why it is natural and understandable that the patient is spending time thinking about them over and over is a key step in developing a good therapeutic rapport. Failing to do this can make it hard for patients to trust the therapy or therapist.

Excessive Rumination and Avoidance Are a Habit

The therapist aims to communicate the following ideas. First, like any habit, rumination will be hard to change at first and will tend to recur when the patient is stressed. Second, like any habit, it is typically automatic and is triggered by internal and external cues, often outside of awareness. There will be periods when rumination comes back, and this is natural and not something the patient should criticize himself for when it happens. Instead, patients should be encouraged to just gently return to the new strategies they have learned and to see this as a further opportunity to practice breaking out of the habit.

> "We view worry as a habit. A habit is an automatic way of responding that has been learned across repeated occurrences and occasions so that it is triggered without awareness or intention. When a response such as worrying repeatedly occurs paired with the same kinds of situation, these situations can become automatic triggers that set off the habit. For example, a person who smokes a lot when socializing with friends in a bar can develop a habit, so that the next time she is in the bar, she finds herself lighting up without thinking. Similarly, worry can be automatically set off in situations where you have worried before, such as times of increasing stress. It sounds like feeling tense and making comparisons with others might be such a cue for worry for you. Is that correct?"

I have found that the language of "habits" is helpful to patients because it is simple, approachable, makes sense, and reduces stigma. Everyone can think of examples of having good habits and bad habits and can understand what it might take to change a habit, such as awareness of when it is happening and repeated practice. It also helps patients to consider rumination as something that is distinct from their personality and amenable to change. Many patients come into therapy saying "This is something I have always done. It is part of my personality." Framing rumination as a habitual behavior opens up the possibility of change.

The rationale then continues with the following point:

Rumination Can Be Replaced by Learning New Strategies

"The good news is that because worry is a learned habit, we can replace it with other more helpful strategies and responses, which are learned in its place. This therapy will concentrate on learning new responses, rebalancing action and thinking, and finding better strategies to reduce rumination and avoidance, and help you to achieve your goals and reduce your depression. We will focus on building from your own experience. There are times when you handle problems well and times when you don't handle problems so well, and we want to learn from the times that you handle problems well so that we can make that happen more often and more consistently."

This emphasis on learning from the patient's own experience is important because it affirms that the patient does have some resources and abilities. This empowers the patient by focusing on how the therapy will build on what he or she can already do. This approach is designed to validate the patient. This contrasts with therapy where the therapist acts only as an expert who gives the patient new solutions, which can make the patient feel stupid or weak for not having come up with the solution themselves. This approach helps with patient engagement and with building up optimism and confidence. It naturally leads to the therapist acting as a coach to support and guide the patient, with the patient having to put in the hard work of daily practice. It is consistent with and lays the groundwork for detailed FA work.

It is useful to ask patients about other habits they may have tried to change and their past experience with this, for example, "What did you learn from trying to change this habit?" Good examples of changing habits include learning a new routine, taking a new route to work, starting to exercise, or stopping smoking. Other helpful questions include:

"What helped you to learn these new skills? Did you learn them right away without mistakes? Were there periods where it seemed to go well and other periods when it did not go so well? Were there times when the old habit came back? What can you learn from those times? Did it take time for it to become more automatic, so that you did not need to think about it?"

These questions help to generate realistic expectations and improve planning for learning the habit. For example, for Jenny, the therapist might say:

"We can see from your own experiences that worry and rumination are major problems for you, which contribute to your anxiety and depression. You mentioned how you always find something to worry about and that this worry makes you more anxious, down, and more tired. This is a pretty common experience for people with depression and anxiety. Because of this, we see rumination and worry as a central engine that drives the onset and maintenance of depression and anxiety. This is supported by the most recent scientific evidence. If we can knock out this worry, this usually leads to a big improvement in symptoms but also helps to improve quality of life. Does this make sense to you?

"Is worry and rumination something that you have talked about before or tried to change before in therapy? Our experience is that often people haven't directly focused on reducing worry and rumination before. Without changing this way of responding, it can be hard to make much progress on getting better. For this reason, this therapy will deliberately target worry and rumination because we believe that this is one of the best ways to reduce depression and anxiety. How does that sound to you? Does that strike a chord with you?"

This Therapy Will Coach the Patient in Learning New Approaches

"This therapy will coach you in shifting out of the worry habit into a more useful habit. How does that sound to you?

"We will work together to make these changes. I will act as your coach, giving you advice and support and guiding you on what to do. You will be like the athlete, doing all the hard work to get better. The therapy is like the training—the more you practice, the better you can get. Moreover, you will use your existing skills and abilities to change the habit. You are the expert on you—your knowledge of yourself and your experiences provides us with an amazing resource for what might be helpful for you. Together we will look at the times when you do cope better and see what we can learn from that, so we can make it happen more often, more consistently, and when it is most needed. We will use your own experiences to develop your skills and find alternatives to worry. Does that sound like an approach that might be helpful for you?"

Changing the Rumination Habit Means Becoming Aware of the Triggers to Rumination

"The trick to changing a habit is to become aware of the triggers to the habit and then to repeatedly practice a more helpful response instead of the unwanted habit. Because the habit of worrying sounds quite strong for you, it may take quite a lot of practice to learn a better way of responding. This won't happen overnight, but over time, it can gradually shift."

Following this rationale, it is useful to get feedback from the patient and check on whether there are any doubts, concerns, or questions about what has been discussed. At this stage (typically sessions 1 and 2), it can also be useful to preempt issues that might arise about rumination by working through the different themes that people typically ruminate about.

Discussing this with the patient will help to assure that no major themes have been missed and reassure the patient that the therapist has knowledge, insight, and understanding into his problems and experiences. For example, the therapist might say something like:

"A lot of rumination [replace with word that makes the most sense to patient] is about symptoms and emotional responses—about being sad, not getting better, being angry. It can involve thinking that it is silly or trivial to get upset about something. It is important to remember that emotion is a normal and often helpful response. Does this happen with you? Can you tell me about it?"

It may also be helpful to reflect on the link between rumination and interpersonal relationships, for example:

"A lot of rumination is also about relationships and other people—for example, how will other people think about me? Do you find yourself often running a post-mortem on past events, checking on what you did? Do any of these themes strike a chord with you? Rumination is also associated with avoidance—avoiding people, avoiding jobs, putting things off—what is your experience?"

I recommend discussing with the patient early in therapy that issues with avoidance and rumination are also likely to come up in treatment sessions, so you want to put this on the agenda as soon as possible. It might be useful to say something like:

"Dwelling on things probably happens everywhere in your life to some degree, which makes me think that it is pretty likely it will also happen here, in our therapy sessions. If at any time during our sessions you notice that you are starting to dwell on something or avoiding things, please let me know right away. This is likely to happen. I will try to notice it if I can, but I won't be able to spot it all of the time. So I will ask you if I think you are starting to worry or ruminate, and I would like you to tell me when you notice it happening here. Picking up on this here in the session provides a really good opportunity for you to practice spotting these behaviors and then to learn a new approach to reduce them right here and now."

Socratic questions can be used to explore ideas about how learning new skills can take repeated practice, and how in the course of getting good at something, there may be some blips, mistakes, and periods where things may not appear to be getting better.

For some patients, more specific psychoeducation about particular themes may be useful. Discussion of depression and emotions can be particularly useful.

Depression

With patients who are depressed and ruminate, it is important to clarify their understanding of depression. It needs to be stressed that it is normal to be "depressed about being depressed." Often patients who ruminate ask themselves, "Why am I depressed?"

It is useful to review what we know about depression and potential life events and/or coping strategies that can maintain depression. The BA model of depression can be useful here; this model emphasizes the loss of contact with rewarding events following loss, which is then maintained by further avoidance (Martell et al., 2001). It is useful to stress the particular symptoms of depression (e.g., tiredness, poor concentration) and help patients to see that their reduced performance may be a consequence of the illness, rather than reflecting something about them personally (e.g., "I am lazy or useless"). Some patients ruminate about their own inadequacy and feel anxiety and guilt about not being able to find dramatic reasons for their depression. Because they did not experience serious trauma, they feel there is no good reason for them to be depressed, so they conclude that they are just being self-indulgent. Knowing more about the patients' backgrounds and their beliefs about normality and expressing emotion can be useful here. Providing information about how common depression is may be helpful. Likewise, it is a good idea to explain how people can be vulnerable to depression without experiencing extreme events, particularly for patients with recurrent depression, where subsequent episodes often occur without any major life event. The idea that there may be a genetic vulnerability to depression may help to remove some of the self-criticism from the patient's view of the illness.

It is also useful to review how vulnerability can occur, for example, how learning patterns of responses in childhood and then continuing to apply them later in life might maintain depression. The therapist emphasizes how the patterns of responses may have been useful or functional at the time they were learned (e.g., agreeing with an abusive or aggressive parent to avoid getting into trouble), but that these patterns were overlearned and overgeneralized, so that they continue to be applied to other situations, where they may not be so good a strategy. Therapy is explained as a way of learning to replace these patterns of response.

Emotions

It is also useful to provide psychoeducation about emotions to challenge negative beliefs about emotion (e.g., that emotion is a sign of weakness). It is normal to have sad feelings about being depressed. Sad mood increases our tendency to be negative. Furthermore, emotion is not a sign of weakness, but rather a signal to us of a problem as well as a way of mobilizing resources to help us solve the problem.

Here is an example of how this might be explained:

"Anxiety increases arousal and gets our body all ready for action. Imagine you are walking through the bush and you see a lion—the effects of anxiety will increase your ability to escape. Likewise, sadness tells us we are not making as much progress as we would like on a project or that we have lost something personally important. If we pay attention to those feelings, we can then determine what it is we are losing—and we can stop to think about what to do next. The withdrawal associated with sadness may give us a chance to give up on a goal that is unrealistic and a chance to conserve our energy. There is also a social function—sadness can elicit aid from other people and cause people to become less aggressive toward us."

It can be useful to explore how feeling sad, angry and so on is normal and functional. Rather it is our response to these emotional responses that can be the problem. Rumination and avoidance are good examples of unhelpful responses to emotions. This information can help patients ease off from criticizing themselves.

Goal Setting

Socialization can also be linked to goal setting with the patient. It is important to make the goals as concrete and specific as possible, focusing on short-term (next few weeks), medium-term (next few months), and long-term goals (6 months to 2 years). Goal setting proceeds within the first few sessions following the initial assessment, initial FA, and the provision of the treatment rationale. Goal setting will lay out the main targets and direction of the therapy.

Questions that are helpful for eliciting goals include:

"What goals would you like to work toward in treatment?"

"In what ways would you like things to be different?"

"What would you most like to change about your current circumstances?"

"What things have you stopped doing since you became depressed that you would like to resume?"

"Are there any things you have started doing since you became depressed which you would like to change?"

"What would you be doing differently if you were not depressed?"

Goal Structure

For goal setting, it is useful to fully assess and explore patient's goal structures. Are they realistic, specific, concrete, attainable, time-limited, in harmony, and likely to be beneficial? Focusing on these issues in goal setting is critical for patients with rumination because much of their rumination is about their inability to achieve their goals. So, we don't want to burden patients with even more concerns about goals they are not able to successfully achieve. Rather we want to work with them to restructure their goals in such a way as to maximize their likelihood of achievement, and thus reduce rumination.

When considering goals and plans, it is useful to use and teach patients the mnemonic SMART, which stands for Specific Measurable Achievable Realistic Time-limited.

Specific

The goal or plan is focused and concrete, broken down into small steps, and laid out in terms of how, when, where, with whom it will happen or be achieved.

Measurable

The goal can be described and operationalized in sufficient detail at a behavioral level that it can be assessed and monitored. An important consideration when making goals specific and measurable is to consider whether they are framed as approach goals (pursuing something) or as avoidance goals (trying to avoid something). Many patients with depression and people who ruminate have goals that are focused on avoidance rather than approach. Shifting patients away from avoidance goals to approach goals is another way we target avoidance in RFCBT. When evaluating goals, it can be useful to ask patients, "Are you trying to get what you need or trying to avoid what you fear?"

The evidence suggests that approach goals are more beneficial than avoidance goals, leading to better mood. Furthermore, approach goals are easier to achieve, as there is a clear and specific marker of success, whereas avoidance goals do not have a clearly delineated endpoint to judge when you have been successful, that is, you never get to the end of the path, you can only fail later. Furthermore, avoidance goals make people more focused on where things can go wrong, so they are more sensitive to negative information than positive information. For example, "not to be depressed" is an avoidance goal, as is "to not upset people" or "to not cry so much." It is important to reframe these goals as approach goals, which may involve some changes (e.g., "I want to be happy," which can then be defined in terms of specific activities that the patient would be doing if happy).

Achievable

The goal can be achieved—the desired outcome is available in the environment and world of the patient. It is something that could happen assuming that the patient has the skills and abilities to do the right thing. If the outcome is not likely to occur even if the patient did everything right, then the goal cannot be considered to be achievable. Goals are often not achievable because the goal requires that something out of the patient's control occurs (e.g., for someone else to agree to a request when all the evidence points to the fact that he is not responsive to any requests, whether made reasonably or unreasonably). For example, it would not be achievable to expect an abusive partner to stop being abusive. Whatever the patient does, this situation is highly unlikely to change. In these cases it is useful to recast the goal at the level of what is immediately achievable and within the patient's control. For example, when having difficulties with a person who tends to be selfish and does not listen to others, the goal may be for the patient to make his request, rather than for the other person to agree. Considering this aspect of goals is important because it reminds patients that how plans turn out is not totally dependent upon them, and that even doing the right thing does not always work. It will also be useful because it can help patients to see that they have done everything they can. In situations where one aspect of the environment is unlikely to provide the desired outcome, the goal may be usefully reframed by focusing on either changing the environment (e.g., leaving a relationship) or concentrating on other aspects of the environment (e.g., "Could someone else provide help and support?"). Usually a goal will be more achievable if it focuses on an internal or patient-initiated behavioral change (feeling more confident and ready to handle a job, sending off applications) rather than a change in external circumstances (having a job), which cannot be guaranteed.

Realistic

Can the patient realistically do something to achieve the goal? Is it realistic for the patient to try and solve the goal right now? Assuming that the goal is achievable, does the patient have the skills, abilities, and background to succeed? Ideally a goal should be just ahead of where the patient is now, a small step forward from where she is currently. If the goal is not immediately realistic, look for what stops the goal from being realistic and adjust the goal to deal with the obstacles, or set a new subgoal to build toward that point. If the goal does not seem realistic, look for what stops the goal from being realistic. Is the patient looking for too much too fast?

Time-Limited (Context-Set)

The goal or plan has a time sequence for being achieved and has a time set for when it will be implemented.

This approach to setting goals needs to be explicitly discussed when plans are made at the beginning of therapy. It is also useful for patients to review the SMART mnemonic whenever their plans succeed or fail so that they can learn from their experiences and build on the more useful aspects of the SMART approach for future situations. The handout on goal setting (Handout 3, Goal Setting) provides further detail on this for patients to read as homework.

Goal Conflict

When looking at rumination and looking at how people set their goals, there are a few additional issues that therapists may want to consider. First, once therapists have dealt with all the SMART issues, they need to check that the patient's goals are not in conflict with each other, as this often produces rumination. If there are contradictory goals, patients need to review and prioritize their goals and eliminate or modify goals to remove the conflict. An example of contradictory goals is to want people to do things properly and to want to never disagree with people.

When a list of goals has been drawn up, it is useful to explicitly ask if any of these goals are in conflict with each other and whether they are in conflict with more general values. For example, the therapist could ask:

"Are any of these goals acting in opposite directions to each other?"
"Are any of these goals in conflict with your beliefs or values?"
"Are there any important values that you have not represented by these goals?"

If there are any conflicting goals, the therapist helps the patient to review the importance, realism, achievability, and emotional salience of each goal and then find more balanced, nonconflicting versions. This might involve asking what the advantages and disadvantages of each goal are, whether these goals are achievable, and what more realistic versions of these goals might be.

It is important to ensure that the goals are related to the patient's core values. Values can be assessed by asking questions like:

"What is important to you?"
"What values give your life meaning?"
"What values make activities seem worthwhile?"
"What gives your life purpose? What used to give your life purpose? If you were able to do anything, what would be the thing that would be most meaningful to you?" (These questions may be useful alternatives if people are so depressed that they cannot currently recognize anything of value.)
"Do these goals reflect anyone else's values?"
"Would this goal still be important to you if no one was aware of your success or failure?"
"Are you striving for someone else's approval or working for your own values?"
"Would you be happy if you succeeded at this goal?"
"Would you unhappy if you succeeded at this goal?"
"Would this goal be as important if it did not lead to certain outcomes (e.g., praise, success, promotion, money)?"

Homework

Homework in the initial orienting sessions tends to be relatively simple and focused on further psychoeducation and information gathering, unless a simple and straightforward intervention is immediately suggested by the analysis of the patient's difficulties (see Chapter 7). Common homework plans include:

1. For the patient to read and prepare comments and questions on relevant handouts (e.g., Handout 1, Key Facts about Rumination; Handout 2, Avoidance; and Handout 3, Goal Setting) that reinforce the ideas raised in the session.
2. For the patient to listen to an audio recording of the session to enable further reflection and rehearsal of what was discussed.
3. The completion of a daily record form focused on gathering more information about the nature of rumination (i.e., a form reporting examples of episodes of rumination, their antecedents, and consequences; see Chapters 6 and 7 and Handout 7, Antecedent–Behavior–Consequence [ABC] Form). Such a form logically builds on the detailed analysis of a single episode in the session and supports more detailed FA.

Introducing Self-Monitoring

Warning Signs

Teaching patients to spot the early signs of rumination and avoidance increases their awareness of the behavior and helps them to implement alternative strategies as soon as possible. Awareness of the early signs reduces the habitual nature of rumination and avoidance. Self-monitoring is typically the first homework assignment, along with listening to the audio recordings of the sessions. Patients are usually coached in self-monitoring as the first intervention within the therapy.

The rationale for self-monitoring in rumination is as follows (this rationale could easily be adjusted for dealing with avoidance):

"The longer negative thinking continues, the worse it gets, the harder it is to stop, and the more it becomes automatic. Conversely, the more you can spot the rumination and the more you are aware of it, the less habitual and the weaker it becomes. The earlier you can spot the early signs or triggers for negative dwelling, the earlier you can stop it, and the earlier you can replace the rumination with a different response. The first step in changing any habit is to become more aware of the habit and when it happens: without awareness, it is almost impossible to change.

"Spotting rumination as early as possible and then intervening as quickly as possible has the added benefit of extending the period of time without rumination. Furthermore, if you repeatedly use a different response when the early signs for rumination occur, then these triggers become linked to the positive response instead of to the rumination. Thus, there are many advantages to becoming more aware of the triggers for rumination. Becoming more aware of the early signs will help you to 'nip rumination in the bud.' "

Learning that rumination is associated with particular signs and triggers will help the patient to learn that rumination is a process and does not just come out of the blue. The therapist and patient work together to identify the earliest signs that the patient is about to ruminate. The therapist needs to double-check that an earlier sign cannot be identified. The therapist informs the patient that rumination is triggered by a spiral of interactions between environment, interpersonal responses, thoughts, images, feelings, behaviors, and sensations. The patient needs to monitor all of these triggers, external and internal.

It is useful to use a "treasure hunt" analogy, where the patient is asked to search for signs to rumination and negative thinking. Ask "What new, earlier cues did you discover this week?" Other useful analogies are to a detective looking for clues or a scientist testing out hypotheses and conducting experiments to try and find the earliest warning signs. When reviewing homework at the beginning of each session, the therapist checks whether the patient has noticed any earlier warning signs that week.

The therapist encourages the patient to record signs and triggers as homework over a number of weeks. This homework could involve keeping an expanding list of signs and cues noticed (e.g., a trigger-sign list), or it could involve keeping a rumination diary, in which the patient notes down key episodes of rumination as part of the weekly self-monitoring assessment (Handout 6, Rumination Episode Recording Form). Once self-monitoring has started, it is important to review how it is going at the beginning of the next therapy session and whether any new signs are being observed. This discussion can be supported by Handout 4, Self-Monitoring.

Assessing Rumination

We use two different recording forms to monitor rumination in RFCBT. The first form, Handout 5, Tracking Rumination and Avoidance, assesses the frequency, duration, intensity, and controllability of rumination. This form is helpful in determining if rumination is changing week by week during the therapy, and thereby to evaluate whether interventions are effective. This measure is more sensitive to change than the Response Styles Questionnaire (RSQ), the standard depressive rumination measure, because it evaluates the amount of rumination over the last week, rather than a general trait tendency. Moreover, the RSQ only assesses the frequency of rumination; the

Tracking Rumination and Avoidance form assesses other important dimensions, such as how long the rumination lasts, how disruptive it is, and how much control the patient has over it. This last rating has proved to be useful. Patients often report increasing control over rumination before other dimensions change.

The second form, Handout 6, Rumination Episode Recording Form, captures examples of rumination, just as a thought-monitoring form is designed to capture examples of negative thinking, with a focus on recording antecedents, behavior, and consequences. Figure 5.1 shows the form with sample entries. This form helps the patient to work through an ABC FA and provides further examples to review in the next therapy session.

When patients begin to monitor their rumination, they become more aware of it and often notice that it is happening more often than they had realized. This helps to highlight the value of tackling rumination. Some patients benefit from increasing awareness, as they spontaneously begin to deliberately control the rumination and exert environmental control (see the example of Emily in Chapter 7). Nevertheless, increasing awareness of the frequency and intensity of rumination makes some patients feel worse and becomes a cause of further dwelling ("rumination about rumination," see the example of Anna in Chapter 7, pp. 115–120). It is helpful to anticipate this initial negative response to self-monitoring and to explicitly warn patients that self-monitoring might at first make them feel worse as it makes them more aware of their problems.

As well as the assessment interview, other self-report questionnaires are useful for measuring rumination and how much it changes during therapy. The standard, well-established measures of rumination and worry are the RSQ (Nolen-Hoeksema & Morrow, 1991; Treynor et al., 2003) and the Penn State Worry Questionnaire (PSWQ; Meyer, Miller, Metzger, & Borkovec, 1990).

Date	Time	What happened just before the rumination started?	How did you feel before?	Duration	What were you thinking about?	What were the consequences of rumination—for mood and actions?	What stopped the rumination? What did you try to stop it? Was it useful?
10/5/15	10 p.m.	Went to bed.	Anxious, sad	2 hours	Why do I feel so bad? Why can't I sleep? All the things I didn't do today.	Could not sleep. Felt worse.	Eventually fell asleep after taking sleeping pills.
10/22/15	2 p.m.	Unsuccessful job interview.	Sad	5 hours	I'll never get a job. What am I doing wrong?	Felt very depressed.	Phoned a friend— felt better after talking to him.

FIGURE 5.1. Example of a partially completed Rumination Episode Recording Form.

105

CHAPTER 6

Functional Analysis
of Rumination

Key Steps for Conducting a Functional Analysis of Rumination

Functional analysis (FA) of rumination studies the context and variability of rumination within an individual's personal experience and uses this to guide interventions. Central to this is identifying the antecedents and consequences of rumination, the triggers for rumination, and the formulation of its possible functions as formalized within the ABC analysis described in Chapter 3. In parallel, the CUDOS analysis seeks to determine under what conditions rumination occurs (when, where, how, what, with whom), under what conditions it does not occur, and what conditions influence its differential outcomes (when it is brief vs. long-lasting; when it is helpful versus unhelpful). (See Chapter 3 for the initial description of ABC; Handout 7, Antecedent–Behavior–Consequence (ABC) Form, which supports ABC analysis when completed by either the therapist and/or the patient; and Table 6.1 for a detailed therapist guide to ABC analysis.) Together, ABC and CUDOS provide a framework for the core steps within the FA: the Context and Usefulness components of CUDOS overlap with the ABC analysis in looking at antecedents and consequences, with the other elements of CUDOS looking at changes in circumstances between when rumination does or does not occur.

When conducting FA, the therapist typically starts with a brief general overview of rumination, and when it does and does not happen (see Chapter 4). For example, the therapist asks the patient about when and where the rumination does and does not occur. The next step is to identify and describe several specific recent examples of episodes of rumination. The therapist uses Socratic questioning to map out in specific and concrete detail the sequence and process, including the antecedences and consequences of the rumination moment by moment for each episode, without getting caught up in the content. During this exploration, the therapist looks for common steps, triggers, warning signs, and consequences of the rumination (ABC; see Table 6.1; Handout 7, Antecedent–Behavior–Consequence (ABC) Form; and Figures 6.1 and 6.2 for completed examples) before then examining the situations under which rumination varies and stops (CUDOS; see Table 6.2 for a detailed therapist guide to CUDOS analysis). Throughout this questioning, the therapist models and coaches the patient in the concrete approach by asking active, concrete, experiential, and specific process-focused questions (see the ACES rule in Chapter 3).

The therapist seeks to identify distinct, alternative examples in order to compare variability in rumination and identify its potential moderators. For example, the therapist starts with an example of rumination where the patient got stuck the previous week and maps that out in detail, particularly with respect to antecedents and consequences. The therapist then inquires about and maps out an alternative example in which dwelling on a similar problem was much briefer or had positive consequences, such as effective problem solving, or even a similar situation to that which triggered rumination where the patient coped well without ruminating. Comparing any of these situations to an episode of unhelpful rumination will give clues as to how the environmental context or the patient's own responses influence whether rumination occurs at all, how long it lasts, or whether it is helpful or not.

FA will suggest changes in the environment or in patient behavior that may reduce rumination (see Chapter 7). Plans are then made to implement these changes to test the hypothesized functions and see if the changes produce the desired benefits. Formulations and plans are then updated in light of whether the changes were helpful or not.

The next sections outline in more detail each stage of a comprehensive FA (antecedents and context; consequences and usefulness; development of rumination; alternative options), with examples of useful questions. Although these questions are focused on rumination, exchanging the words referring to rumination with words focusing on avoidance would make these questions suitable for FA of avoidance. Throughout this FA process, it is recommended that the therapist summarize what the patient says and provide good feedback to further engage and socialize the patient into the treatment model.

General Introductory Questions to the Context and Function of Rumination

"What differences do you notice in your thinking patterns when you are having a bad day in comparison to when you are having one of your better days?"

TABLE 6.1. Antecedent–Behavior–Consequence: Therapist Guide

For the therapist, the sequence for an ABC analysis is as follows:

1. Conduct an analysis of antecedents, the behavior, and its consequences in detail.

2. *Formulate a function* for the behavior (i.e., rumination).

3. Collaboratively discuss function with the client and check if plausible.

4. Relate back to overall RFCBT formulation in terms of possible function of the behavior, its antecedents and consequences, and idea of rumination as a habit.

5. Introduce idea of the client using ABC him-or herself.

6. Use shared understanding of function to generate and schedule plans:

   a. Collaboratively generate alternative behaviors to replace unhelpful behavior that meet existing function. If this is difficult, it may be worth repeating ABC for similar antecedent/situation with more positive consequence ("Can you think of a time when you experienced these antecedents and did something else that led to more positive consequences?") This may then lead into an If–Then plan.

   b. Identify environmental factors that precede the target behavior and then remove/increase to reduce/increase the target behavior, with these changes scheduled into activity plans and homework.

"Do you ever ruminate/become preoccupied/seem to get things stuck in your mind and can't get rid of them?"

"What sorts of events or situations trigger this recurrent thinking?"

"What types of things do you become preoccupied with? Can you give me an example?"

"When something gets stuck in your mind what do you do to try and get rid of it?"

"What happens when you become preoccupied and dwell over and over on something? What consequences does it have?"

"What effect, if any, does it have on your mood or your actions?"

"What helps to stop you ruminating/get rid of the preoccupation?"

"Are there any strategies you use to try and avoid ruminating/dwelling on things?"

Examining Antecedents and Context

In this stage of FA, the therapist seeks to determine in what contexts rumination tends to occur and, more specifically, what events, actions, emotions, thoughts, or physical sensations are antecedent cues or triggers to rumination. The therapist wants to specify when, where, what, how, and with whom rumination happens and when, where, what, how, and with whom with rumination does not happen. For this stage of the FA, conducting an ABC analysis overlaps with questions about Context within the CUDOS mnemonic.

Useful questions include:

"What were you doing when you began to start thinking this way?"
"Under what conditions do you ruminate or not?"
"When, where, with whom do you ruminate?"
"What kinds of questions do you ask yourself?"
"What kinds of situations set off your ruminating?"
"What happens when you ruminate?"
"What happened next?"
"What thoughts do you have?"
"What do you do when you have this thought?"

Examining Consequences and Usefulness

The therapist seeks to determine how rumination helps or hinders the patient in getting what she wants. Underlying all of the following questions is an attempt to hypothesize what the function of the rumination (or any target behavior in an FA) might be. The question that underpins the concep-

---

TABLE 6.2. CUDOS: Therapist Guide

A mnemonic to further facilitate and enhance the use of functional analysis:

- The Context that influences the target behavior
  - Specifying what happened and when, where, how and with whom *it happens* and when, where, how and with whom *it does not happen.*
  - What precedes/triggers it?
- The Usefulness/function of the rumination or avoidance
  - What might be the function/purpose/goal of the behavior?
  - What are the consequences/outcomes, pros/cons, or gains of the behavior?
  - What is avoided/reduced/increased?
- The Development of the behavior
  - When did it start?
  - How was it learned? From whom?
  - First memory of the behavior?
  - Was it useful then? What is avoided/reduced/increased?
- Alternative Options or actions
  - What is different between the times when the behavior is prolonged/brief, helpful/unhelpful?
  - What can interrupt or stop the behavior?
  - What happened just before the patient stopped the behavior?
  - Focus on variability.

---

tualization of the rumination is: "What is the function of this behavior?" I recommend that therapists do not directly ask patients this question because that is a somewhat technical approach. Moreover, patients will not always be aware of the effect of their rumination. Rather, the therapist hypothesizes the possible function based on an understanding of antecedents and consequences. For this stage of the FA, conducting an ABC analysis overlaps with asking about Usefulness within the CUDOS mnemonic.

Useful questions include:

"What happens after the rumination?"
"What effect does it have?"
"Let's look at how you are using this?"
"Is rumination useful in any way?"
"What are the consequences of this behavior?"
"What are the pros and cons of doing this?"
"What might you be avoiding?"
"What would you do if you weren't ruminating?"
"What does it stop you from doing?"
"Did you figure anything out?"
"What advantages does rumination have?"
"What disadvantages does rumination have?"
"What do you gain/avoid from dwelling on things like this?"
"What do you think might happen if you did not ruminate?"
"What disadvantages might there be in trying not to ruminate?"
"Could anything bad happen to you if you let yourself ruminate?"
"Could anything bad happen if you gave up rumination?"
"What would be a more useful thing to do?"
"Does this rumination work for you?"

The ABC form (see Handout 7, Antecedent–Behavior–Consequence [ABC] Form) addresses both the antecedent and consequences components of the FA for specific events. When doing an ABC analysis, the therapist can work through the ABC form together with the patient. Alternatively, when mapping out the sequence of a specific episode of rumination in detail, the therapist can prompt to ensure that all the relevant information for the ABC analysis naturally emerges during the flow of questioning. The ABC formulation is then completed afterwards.

Examining the Development of Rumination

In formulating the function of rumination, it is useful to know when it started and whether it followed from particular learning experiences. The therapist is looking to see if there was a particular reinforcing outcome when the patient ruminated in the past that sheds light on its function. The therapist also checks to see if rumination resulted from modeling by a significant family member, for example, the patient copying it from a parent. This developmental background aids the socializing of patients into the idea that the rumination and avoidance are learned behaviors and can be replaced with new habits (see Chapter 5 on the therapy rationale).

Useful questions include:

"When did it start?"
"How long have you had this tendency to ruminate?"
"When did this tendency to ruminate first start?"
"What was happening then?"
"Where or from whom might you have learned this way of responding?"
"What is your first memory of ruminating?"
"What was happening then?"
"Are any of your close family worriers or ruminators?"

Examining Alternative Options

The focus on alternative options is critically important in discriminating what may influence the variability and outcome of rumination. Asking about the patient's options and alternatives, and times when he has successfully managed to control the rumination, guides efforts to develop more effective interventions. Most patients have episodes of rumination that differ in their length and usefulness. Rumination often starts in response to a problematic situation and then sometimes continues unabated for hours while at other times it stops relatively quickly.

Moreover, sometimes dwelling on feelings and problems can be helpful. Because both constructive and unconstructive rumination are initiated as an attempt at problem solving, the ability to discriminate between helpful and unhelpful thinking during rumination (e.g., concrete versus abstract styles), and between soluble problems and unanswerable questions, is critical. Poor discrimination leads to less effective problem solving and results in rumination with positive outcomes reinforcing less adaptive bouts. The more that therapy helps patients to identify, discriminate, and learn from these differences in periods of rumination, the better able they will be to shift to adaptive patterns of thinking. Learning to discriminate when it is and is not helpful to dwell on a problem is thus a useful outcome of FA.

Asking about options and alternatives guides the patient toward a more active, solution-focused approach. A key focus is on identifying and assessing variability (e.g., what is different between the times when rumination is relatively brief versus extended, or results in helpful versus unhelpful consequences?).

It is important for the therapist to examine what is happening just before rumination stops, whether this is due to an external interruption (e.g., a friend calling) or a shift into more helpful thinking (e.g., "I started to think about what I could do next"). Identifying the useful thoughts at the end of a bout of rumination and encouraging their use as an explicit strategy earlier in the ruminative sequence can cut out the unhelpful part of a ruminative bout, considerably shortening its duration.

For this stage of FA, it is helpful to compare multiple episodes of rumination, each with a distinct outcome, and to conduct a detailed microanalysis of each episode. To explore a recent example of rumination, follow the normal CBT procedure of asking moment by moment what happened next in the sequence of thoughts, feelings, and behaviors (see Chapter 4). Having discussed in detail a recent episode of rumination that was prolonged and unhelpful, the therapist asks about a contrasting episode of briefer or helpful rumination after a similar event. A useful guide to this line of questioning is the Being More Effective Form (see Handout 8, Being More Effective, and Handout 9, Being More Effective Form). It compares contrasting and distinct events to explore variability. Typically, the therapist first collaboratively completes the form with the patient during the therapy session. As the patient becomes more familiar with FA, she completes the form herself as part of her homework. Handout 8, Being More Effective, provides psychoeducation about the FA approach.

Useful questions for exploring options include:

"When was your dwelling on things longer (shorter)?"
"What was different when you kept on going over something in your mind for a long time versus a short time?"
"What is different between the times when dwelling on your problems goes round and round over and over without making any progress and the times when it leads to something helpful?"
"Is there a difference in what you are doing?"
"Is there a difference in what you are thinking about?"
"Is there a difference in the way that you are thinking about it?"
"What were you saying to yourself?"
"What were you paying attention to?"
"How were you thinking about this?"

Other useful questions for finding alternatives include:

"What do you do to try and stop ruminating?"
"Where do you focus your attention when ruminating?"
"How do you decide whether to ignore or dwell on a thought?"

"What determines whether you move on to making a plan or keep thinking over and over the same thing?"

"Are there some episodes when the rumination lasts for much longer/shorter periods of time than others?"

"What is different between these times?"

"What can interrupt or break up the rumination?"

"Can you postpone or delay the rumination?"

"How does the rumination come to an endpoint?"

"What happened just before you stopped ruminating?"

"What do you do that influences this process?"

"What are your other options?"

"What could you do instead of dwelling on the problem?"

"How could you solve the problem you are dwelling on?"

"What was different between the times that you quickly reached an endpoint and the times that you did not?"

"What happened just before you reached a conclusion and/or made a plan?"

"What derails you from getting to an intention or plan?"

FA of Avoidance

The approach used to analyze avoidance is the same as that used to examine rumination. Particular questions that are useful for assessing avoidance include:

"In what ways has your behavior changed since you became depressed?"

"Are there activities you have stopped doing since you became depressed?"

"When was the last time you did this? How did you feel then?"

"What are your reasons for not doing x?"

"What enjoyable activities do you do at the moment?"

"What activities did you enjoy before becoming depressed?"

"Are there any activities you have avoided since becoming depressed?"

"Are there any activities you have been putting off?"

"What happens when you avoid doing things? In the short term? In the long term?"

"What happens when you are more active?"

"When do you feel better or worse?"

"If you were to try and do x now, what do you predict would happen?"

"What is the worst thing you could imagine happening?"

"Are there any times of day when activities/tasks are harder or easier?"

"What are the benefits of not doing/avoiding something? What do you get out of it?"

"Are there activities/behaviors you do more since becoming depressed?"

In the same way that weekly monitoring of rumination is helpful, weekly self-monitoring of avoidance helps patients to focus on acting in more productive ways and to determine whether treatment is being effective.

Case Example: Anna

Anna is a 45-year-old divorced woman. She currently lives alone. She works full-time in a shop. She is currently experiencing quite severe depression (Beck Depression Inventory score = 36) characterized by high levels of self-criticism and perfectionism. There is also avoidance of going out and trying new things, and she reports quite high levels of anxiety. She recognizes that she ruminates a lot and that this is a problem.

The initial therapy sessions have led to a collaborative agreement that rumination is a key difficulty and that together Anna and the therapist will work on it. They have also discussed the idea that rumination is a habit. Typical contents of a ruminative bout include "Why can't I feel better?"; "Why is this so difficult?"; "Why can't I stop ruminating?"; "Why do I find this so much harder than other people?"; "Why is everything such a struggle?"

Generally, Anna's rumination is worse when she is at home, in the evening, and on weekends. It is much less when she is at work: she can get absorbed in her work, both talking with customers and working on the shop displays. Common triggers for her rumination include seeing her home messy or thinking about what she has not achieved. Warning signs involve physical sensations like a sinking feeling in her stomach, butterflies, and a sense of feeling drained and lethargic. She often thinks about all the different things she has to do and gets preoccupied trying to decide what to do first, and then gets caught up in ruminating about what to do next. This is particularly bad on the weekend, when she feels bad if she doesn't tidy up and feels guilty if she tries to enjoy herself. She used to enjoy some creative activities like cooking, but does not do so anymore; now she only focuses on the easiest and quickest things to cook. When she tries to do creative activities at home, she has a running commentary about how hard it is and how she should be doing something else.

Her history includes a mother who was always a worrier and spent a lot of time thinking through things, and she describes herself as always being a worrier.

Analyzing a Specific Example of Rumination

The therapist looks for an example of rumination to explore in detail with Anna and notices that she might be ruminating when they review her weekly record. This is used as an opportunity to ask further questions about an episode of rumination.

THERAPIST: What do you notice when you look at the weekly record?

ANNA: I am doing this a lot, nearly all the time. I didn't realize that I was ruminating so much. It is out of control. The rumination is a major problem.

THERAPIST: Does the record give us any clues as to when you ruminate less?

ANNA: (*long pause and silence, looking anxious, inward focus*) It feels like I am doing it all the time.

THERAPIST: Just now as we started to look together at your weekly record of rumination, I wonder if you actually started to ruminate about things. Right now, I am getting the sense that you are a bit preoccupied, anxious, and have turned inward a little. (*Notices that Anna is making less eye contact, looks tense, and has gone quiet.*) Am I picking up on something here or have I got it completely wrong?

ANNA: No, you are right. I am worried about how much I am ruminating. I was surprised at how much it happens.

THERAPIST: That is a pretty common experience when people start monitoring their rumination. Monitoring makes them more consciously aware of it. Becoming more aware of when it happens is the first step to changing it, so it is good to be more aware of your rumination. Obviously being right in the experience isn't very pleasant, but it gives us a good chance to understand and change it. Since it is happening right now, this is an excellent opportunity for us to try and get more of a sense of what happens and look at how we can change it. Are you able to give that a go? What was the first thing that went through your mind as the rumination started?

ANNA: This is only going to get worse.

THERAPIST: What else do you notice as you have the thought that this is only going to get worse, for example, any physical sensations, feelings, or emotions?

ANNA: I am getting a sinking feeling in my stomach, butterflies. I feel my attention narrowing, so I am only thinking about these problems.

THERAPIST: What thoughts followed straight after the thought "This is only going to get worse"?

ANNA: Why do I do this so much? Why can't I stop myself from ruminating? I must be really weak-willed.

THERAPIST: Are these the thoughts still going through your mind now?

ANNA: Yes, I want to know why I ruminate. Why can't I just stop it? Why is this so difficult? Why do I have this difficulty when other people don't? Do you know why I keep doing this?

THERAPIST: These sound like powerful and common thoughts for you that go around and around again and again. We could easily get into a discussion about the meaning and causes of the rumination. I wonder if that kind of discussion would be helpful—after all, thinking about the reasons and meanings of what happens and asking "Why?" is what you are doing all the time, without much success. My sense is that these questions keep coming back without much resolution. Is that right?

ANNA: (*Nods, still looking pensive.*)

THERAPIST: Perhaps it might be helpful to try a different approach. Rather than looking at the reasons why the rumination happens, one alternative is to try and map out the moment-by-moment process of how the rumination happens. We can then look at ways to interrupt this process without necessarily knowing why it happens. Can you stay with your direct experience so we can track the whole sequence of thinking and find ways to step out of it? What do you make of trying this?

ANNA: OK.

THERAPIST: What are you experiencing right now?

ANNA: What does the worry mean about me? Why am I such a bad patient? Why can't I just tell myself to stop? What is it about me that keeps the rumination going?

THERAPIST: I am getting a sense of how insistent and strong the push to worry is for you. This is also giving a clear picture of the way that you dwell on things with lots of thoughts about why is this happening and what this means about you as a person. You are asking yourself lots of questions about your rumination. Do you get an answer to these questions?

ANNA: I keep coming back to it because I am no good.

THERAPIST: How do you feel right now as you have been dwelling on these thoughts?

ANNA: I am getting more and more down and anxious. These problems seem insurmountable.

THERAPIST: OK, so we are seeing how the rumination drives your mood down.

ANNA: I must try harder to stop it.

THERAPIST: What would happen if you didn't think like this?

ANNA: I don't know how to do that. It happens automatically.

THERAPIST: It sounds like part of the answer to why it is so difficult to change the rumination is that it has become a mental habit, which is automatically set off by certain circumstances, such as when you get anxious or expect the worst. Habits go on even when we don't want them to and can be hard to change. To change them, we need to be aware of the habit and its triggers in detail, so we can change the routine. This is why we try and track the sequence of your rumination. Does it feel like a habit to you?

ANNA: Yes, it does. But why do I find it so much harder than other people?

THERAPIST: That's interesting what you just said—do you notice that you just asked another of those "Why is it so difficult?" questions? This illustrates how those questions have become a habit that occurs without you thinking—and how we need to keep our eyes open for the habit. Often habits get strong because our past experience led us to learn the habit or because in some way the habit has an effect that keeps it going, even when it is unhelpful. For example, we can get into bad habits like snacking even when we don't want to, because we get into the routine of eating snacks when feeling bored and because the snacking temporarily distracts us from the boredom. In that situation, someone might feel they would be losing a source of relief or pleasure if they stopped snacking. Would you lose anything if you stopped dwelling on these questions, like "Why can't I stop doing this?"

ANNA: I am not sure.

THERAPIST: What would be the consequences of not focusing on these questions?

ANNA: As I reflect on it, I might not understand what is happening to me. Part of me feels that I wouldn't be taking it seriously if I didn't keep thinking about it.

THERAPIST: Let me summarize this example to see if I have got it all straight in my mind. This rumination started when you realized how much you were ruminating, and you started "ruminating about your ruminating," with lots of questions about "Why do I do this?" and "Why can't I stop?" This fits with the idea that it is an automatic habit that gets applied to whatever comes up. This bout of rumination started with a sinking feeling and a catastrophic thought that it will just get worse, so these may be warning signs for the rumination habit. It made you feel more down and your problems even bigger. There is also a sense that you need to try and understand what is happening and if you didn't dwell on the rumination, you wouldn't be taking it seriously enough. This puts you in the ironic position of trying to reduce rumination by thinking about it even more. Is this an accurate summary? Is there anything I have got wrong?

ANNA: No, that's about right.

THERAPIST: How helpful is it when you ask yourself these questions? Are they useful?

ANNA: Not really. I don't understand things any better.

THERAPIST: In contrast, what effect has it had to step back and track the sequence of rumination in detail?

ANNA: I feel a tiny bit better, but I still worry about how much I am ruminating. Why can't I stop doing this?

THERAPIST: Can you see how once again one of those "why" questions has just come up? That indicates what a strong habit this is. To change the habit, we need to spot when it happens and unpack the sequence of the habit. To do this, let's explore in detail another recent example to see what we can learn and to see if there are any similar patterns to this example. Anna, can you think of another recent time when you found yourself getting caught up in your thoughts over and over again?

ANNA: Yes, I was worried about the how messy the house was on Sunday.

THERAPIST: What was happening just before you started dwelling on things? Where were you? What were you doing?

ANNA: I was sitting in the living room reviewing all the chores that needed doing. I needed to do the laundry, the dishes, some vacuuming, and take care of some paperwork.

THERAPIST: What was going through your mind just then?

ANNA: I am thinking "There is so much to do."; "Where do I start?"

THERAPIST: And how do you feel immediately as you have those thoughts?

ANNA: I feel guilty about not doing the work and begin to feel anxious about getting it done.

THERAPIST: What is the first sign you notice that you are getting anxious?

ANNA: I get a sinking feeling in my stomach.

THERAPIST: And what follows those first thoughts?

ANNA: I start off thinking about trying to prioritize the different jobs, trying to work out where to start.

THERAPIST: And what comes next in that situation?

ANNA: What if I choose the wrong thing to do? What is the right thing to do?

THERAPIST: So you start by thinking about all the chores that need to be done, and then you try and work out where to start, which is followed by questions about what happens if I choose the wrong thing. Is that right?

ANNA: Yes.

THERAPIST: And what comes next as you are continuing to dwell on this?

ANNA: It moves into "Why is this so difficult?"; "Why can't I get started?"; "I should be able to get this done."; "Why am I so lazy?"; "Why am I so weak?"; "I need to try harder."

THERAPIST: How do those thoughts make you feel?

ANNA: Down, tired, and unmotivated.

THERAPIST: And how long did those questions about "Why is it so hard?" and "Why can't I do it?" go on for on Sunday?

ANNA: I stayed sitting in the living room for several hours not doing anything, feeling worse.

THERAPIST: And what effect did it have overall?

ANNA: I felt so tired I went for a nap. I didn't feel like I could do anything.

THERAPIST: What were the consequences of asking these "why" questions?

ANNA: It made it hard for me to do anything.

THERAPIST: And how did the rumination come to an end?

ANNA: Eventually, I was so tired that I fell asleep.

THERAPIST: We can see that there are some clear disadvantages to this worry because it makes you feel down and unmotivated. Looking at the earlier example, do you think that there might be any benefits from ruminating?

ANNA: I'm not sure. I'd like to do it less.

THERAPIST: What would you do if you were not ruminating?

ANNA: I'd probably feel better and get on with more things.

THERAPIST: What would happen if you didn't think like this? Could anything bad happen?

ANNA: I am always concerned that I could get things wrong. I want to feel sure I am doing the right thing before I start and I like to run all the possibilities through my head first.

THERAPIST: So, dwelling on what you could do, the different options, and which chore to start with might be a way to increase your confidence that you are doing it right. And if you didn't dwell on it, you might feel that you hadn't worked out the right way to start and feel less certain about what you are doing. Does that sound about right?

ANNA: Yes.

THERAPIST: What about the other part of the dwelling on things? You had lots of thoughts about "Why am I so weak?"; "Why am so lazy?" I wonder what advantages these thoughts might have. Is there anything bad that could happen if you didn't dwell on these?

ANNA: I don't know. It does feel like I have to ask myself these questions—it is very hard to stop. They keep popping into my head.

THERAPIST: That popping into your head fits the idea that these thoughts are a habit. I wonder if asking yourself these questions might be about avoiding something unwanted. We often find that when people get into repeated habits like this, it is because the habit makes them feel safer. Could that apply to you—that there might be a risk to not asking these questions?

ANNA: I might be even more lazy and weak-willed if I didn't keep thinking about what I need to do. If I didn't dwell on these things, perhaps I would slip even more and just become a complete slob. I need to keep reminding myself of what I have to do.

THERAPIST: That's interesting. It sounds like dwelling on why you can't do things might be an attempt to stop yourself from getting worse, to try and force yourself to do more. Is that right?

ANNA: Yes.

THERAPIST: How well does this rumination work for you? Does it actually make it easier to pursue your tasks, in terms of motivating you to do things?

ANNA: No, I tend to feel worse.

THERAPIST: So, it sounds like this might be a strategy that you have gotten into the habit of using as a means to push yourself to do more, but that it often does not work. Often people give themselves a hard time and point out what they are not doing well as a way to try and improve their performance—but this does not always work, as we can see for you. What might be a more useful thing to do that helps to motivate you?

ANNA: I don't know.

THERAPIST: That's OK. During this therapy, we are going to look at different alternative strategies for you to try. Now that we are beginning to develop some ideas of what might be happening, we can try and find good alternatives.

The information obtained during this FA dialogue between Anna and the therapist can also be written out on an ABC form—see the examples in Figures 6.1 and 6.2 for illustration.

Antecedent	What precedes B? What triggers B: event, feeling, thought, person, place, time, activity? Determine context: where?, when?, who?, what?, how?
	During the therapy, reviewing the weekly record of rumination with the therapist, Anna notices how frequently and commonly she is ruminating. Thoughts like "I am doing this a lot."; "It is out of control."; "This is a major problem." Anxiety response with catastrophic thoughts like "This is only going to get worse."; sinking feeling in stomach; butterflies; attention narrowing.
Behavior	What you did: the target behavior to understand, and increase or decrease. Provide details on how the behavior occurs (e.g., content and style of rumination).
	Rumination about rumination: "Why do I do this so much? Why can't I stop myself from ruminating? I must be really weak-willed. Why do I ruminate? Why can't I just stop it? Why do I have this difficulty when other people don't? What does it mean about me? Why am I such a bad patient? Why can't I just tell myself to stop? I must try harder to stop it." Attention shifts inward and away from the therapist, reduced eye contact, reduced speech.
Consequence	What is the consequence of B—positive/negative, short-term/long-term, for self, for others—on valued goals? What effect does it have? What does it increase/decrease? What are its pros/cons? What does it avoid? What would happen if you didn't do B? What is the effect of not doing B? What would you be doing instead? What has the consequence of B been in the past?
	More depressed and anxious, session less productive, problem feels insurmountable; if did not do it, "Might not understand what is happening to me"; "I wouldn't be taking it seriously"; "I might be even more lazy and weak-willed."

FIGURE 6.1. Example 1 of a completed Antecedent–Behavior–Consequence (ABC) Form for Anna.

Inside the Therapist's Mind 1: Decision Points and Reflections with Anna

The dialogue above illustrates a number of common issues and important principles that occur when starting an FA of rumination. You can see that several examples of rumination appear in the therapeutic session. This is a frequent occurrence and one to be used advantageously, as illustrated here, to come to grips with the rumination. Monitoring of rumination is often a trigger for rumination as patients become aware that they are doing it more than expected. It is a general principle of the RFCBT treatment that when an unwanted behavior such as avoidance or rumination occurs in the session, the therapist spots this behavior, draws the patient's attention to it, and relates it back to the rationale and model shared with the patient. Highlighting the process helps the patient to become more aware of it and to work together with the therapist actively in real time to tackle the problem. Avoidance and rumination are behaviors that can interfere with therapy, so tackling them directly, explicitly, and head on can prevent them from blocking therapy.

Once the target behavior is identified and highlighted, the next step is to consider alternative options, and, where possible, to experiment with trying an alternative response then and there in the session. This allows the therapist to guide the patient directly in trying a new response and to evaluate whether the proposed approach is effective. For example, if a patient was becoming self-conscious and his attention was turning inward during the session, this would limit his focus on the therapy content and impair therapy. Once this ruminative response is identified, a good alternative to practice is for the therapist to encourage the patient to focus his attention externally out into the world, for example, by prompting the patient to listen closely to what the therapist is saying, including the actual words, the tone, pitch, and quality of her voice, and so forth. The therapist can then evaluate the effect of this switch of attention on reducing the patient's rumination and self-consciousness.

Anna provides a good example of "rumination about rumination" and of how patients can get stuck in abstract and evaluative thought. The dialogue also illustrates how she repeatedly wants to discuss this in the session. Holding the ACES principles in mind, the therapist does not want to be drawn into this discussion, and actively steers the discussion to stay on the sequence and experience of the rumination. The dialogue is refocused toward tracking the episode of rumination moment by moment. Because the initial example is so "live" and present for Anna, it is easy to tap into exactly what is happening during the process of rumination, even though she wants to discuss and analyze it. The therapist uses phrases focused on learning, trying things out, and doing something new to shift away from this conceptual response to a more experiential-focused approach.

The dialogue also indicates the value of explaining rumination as a habit. This approach provides a clear account and explanation of the rumination and partially explains why it is hard to change, while enabling the therapist to focus on mapping out the sequence of rumination. The repeated framing of rumination as a habit is used to explain the repeated occurrence of the rumination, to emphasize the value of looking at the antecedents leading up to the rumination and at the sequence of rumination, and later, to justify the repeated practice of alternative strategies.

This dialogue illustrates the use of Socratic questioning, seeking feedback, and working collaboratively to explore and examine the patterns of rumination. The therapist keeps checking in with Anna to make sure that he is understanding what she is saying, to share their growing knowledge, and to shape her toward a more active and experiential approach. When conducting FA, regular summaries and feedback on the emerging ABC and the hypothesized functions are essential to structure the discussion, keep it specific and concrete, and ensure that the therapist has accurately understood the patient and is making sensible and plausible formulations. Sharing the working formulation with the patient provides an opportunity for the patient to disagree and refine the formulation. It also helps to move to the next stage of introducing alternative responses: with joint agreement that the rumination may have particular consequences, both adaptive and maladaptive, the therapist can then start to work with the patient to brainstorm alternatives.

This dialogue also illustrates the value of exploring multiple examples of rumination. This can help to confirm that there are common antecedents and consequences to the rumination and provide convergent evidence to inform the formulation of potential functions of rumination. Throughout the session, the therapist introduces the idea of rumination having triggers and explores possible maintaining consequences. Throughout the dialogue, the therapist asks questions about the consequences of rumination, sometimes in succession, to push for information that can inform the working hypothesis.

Similarly, there is a repeated focus on the therapist examining the utility of the rumination. This is a critical part of the functional-analytic approach underpinning RFCBT. Rather than challenging the accuracy or veridicality of the patient's thoughts as in classical CBT, RFCBT tends to challenge the utility of the patient's thoughts (and other behaviors) by asking if the rumination is helpful. The treatment is focused on helping the patient to become more effective by identifying which strategies work and under which circumstances. Constantly refocusing back to the usefulness of the patient's responses, combined with a close examination of context, is the way to achieve this. We don't prejudge which behavior is good or bad, but take the starting point that this will depend on the environmental context, the patient's mood and internal state, and the patient's approach to the situation. For Anna, the evidence so far suggests that rumination may have both adaptive and maladaptive consequences. A next step might be to help her discriminate when, where, and how it is adaptive versus maladaptive.

During this close examination of two examples of rumination, the therapist works through a detailed ABC and contextual analysis and is able to populate each of the columns in the ABC worksheet. The antecedents for Anna's rumination for both situations appear to be a catastrophic thought about getting it wrong and something getting worse, accompanied by a sinking feeling. This makes it likely that these antecedents may be triggers and warning signs across a number of situations, and thus useful cues for both Anna and the therapist to monitor. The ruminative behavior is strongly characterized by a slew of "Why me?" thoughts focused on asking "Why is this happening?"; "Why can't I do something about it?"; and negative evaluations of herself. The negative consequences of this thinking include feeling more negative, tiredness, and finding problems more insurmountable.

On the other hand, there is a suggestion that without this thinking, things might be worse and that Anna needs to think about these difficulties

Antecedent	What precedes B? What triggers B: event, feeling, thought, person, place, time, activity? Determine context: where?, when?, who?, what?, how?
	Sitting in living room, reviewing all the chores—the laundry, dishes, vacuuming, sorting through papers, "There is so much to do."; "Where do I start?"; feeling guilty about not doing work, feeling anxious about getting it done, a sinking feeling in the stomach.
Behavior	What you did: the target behavior to understand, and increase or decrease. Provide details on how the behavior occurs (e.g., content and style of rumination).
	Starts off thinking about trying to prioritize the different jobs, thoughts about how big a job it is, leads into "What if I choose the wrong thing to do?"; "What is the right thing to do?," which moves into "Why is this so difficult? Why can't I get started? I should be able to get this done, Why am I so lazy? Why am I so weak? I need to try harder."
Consequence	What is the consequence of B—positive/negative, short-term/long-term, for self, for others—on valued goals? What effect does it have? What does it increase/decrease? What are its pros/cons? What does it avoid? What would happen if you didn't do B? What is the effect of not doing B? What would you be doing instead? What has the consequence of B been in the past?
	Stays sitting and ruminates for several hours, feels down, tired, and unmotivated, takes a nap, does not feel like doing anything. Excuses herself from doing anything. "I want to feel sure I am doing the right thing before I start. I want to feel confident about what I am doing."

FIGURE 6.2. Example 2 of a completed Antecedent–Behavior–Consequence (ABC) Form for Anna.

in order to take them seriously and to tackle them. Together these ABCs suggest several working models as to the potential overlapping functions of Anna's rumination: the therapist hypothesizes that her rumination may be intended to seek understanding (for example, her thoughts like "Why do I keep ruminating?") in order to reduce this unwanted behavior; reduce risk by ensuring confidence and certainty in decisions; and self-motivate to avoid an unwanted self (push herself into activity to avoid being lazy by reminding herself of what she has not achieved). These functions are not always effective given the consequences of her rumination, but either a past history of these functions being reinforced or current perceived benefit could maintain the rumination.

At this stage, because the most reliable warning signs for rumination appear to be internal (sinking feeling; catastrophic predictions), the therapist may be leaning toward developing If–Then contingency plans. However, there may also be environmental cues to internal responses that occur earlier in the etiological chain, such as a messy house, which could be removed through behavioral plans (e.g., activity scheduling to tidy up the house). Such simple behavioral interventions can often be powerful, and it is important not to overlook them. One of my most effective interventions was for a patient whose rumination was triggered by noises from outside (neighbors, dogs, cats, etc.) at night, which fed into ruminations about not being able to sleep. The whole cycle of rumination associated insomnia and tiredness was removed by a simple expedient—the behavioral experiment of the patient trying out earplugs.

Before selecting a potential intervention, it is useful to complete a thorough FA. When training therapists, I have observed that there is often a tendency to want to jump quickly into suggesting alternative behaviors for the patient to try, before working through the detailed FA. It is worth resisting this temptation because the final plans are much more likely to be effective and helpful if there is a deeper and more elaborated understanding of an individual's rumination.

Moreover, the dialogue with Anna above has mainly focused on the ABC, context, and consequences of her rumination, addressing the Context (in part) and Usefulness elements of the FA (from CUDOS). The Development part of the analysis has already been addressed in the initial assessment, with the therapist learning that Anna learned to ruminate from an early age as her mother was a worrier. However, the Options element of the FA, which is focused on variability, remains to be completed to get a sense of what influences the rumination, which is critical in informing potential interventions. The close examination of situations that differ in their extent or quality of rumination is critical to determine the Context that may underpin the rumination: if we only examined situations where the person ruminated, we would not know what environments, situations, or behaviors are specifically contingent with rumination, but know only that certain situations or behaviors are associated with it. To be more confident that these factors are contingent with and potentially influence rumination, we want to know that they are only present when rumination is present and only absent when rumination is absent. To ascertain this, we also need to look at when rumination does not occur. The next vignette therefore explores an alternative situation similar to the one just discussed, but one where Anna was not ruminating. The therapist and Anna will look for what might differ between the times that she ruminates more versus less.

As noted earlier, other comparisons could be between times when rumination had a positive versus negative outcome or between longer versus shorter bouts of rumination. Comparison can also focus on sections within the same bout of rumination by discriminating what was unhelpful and helpful in the same episode. The dialogue immediately below follows from the previous dialogue within the same treatment session.

Example of Variability in Duration and Outcome of Rumination

THERAPIST: Anna, we have just talked about several examples of when you got caught up in dwelling about difficulties, each of which lasted several hours and made you feel worse. The first example was when you realized how much you were ruminating. The second example we discussed was triggered when you thought about all the chores you had to do. It would be useful to also look at times when you cope better and ruminate less so that we can learn from your own experience about what helps you to be more effective. To achieve this, it would be good to talk through in detail a situation that is potentially stressful like the ones we just discussed but where the outcome was different and things turned out OK, for example, when you were able to get on with doing things or when the rumination was relatively brief and not so intense. Can you think of a recent example when you faced such a situation and you didn't ruminate as much, for example, having chores to do and starting to feel anxious?

ANNA: Yes, I can think of another time when I had chores to do but I was able to get on with it much more easily.

THERAPIST: That sounds like a good example. When was that?

ANNA: Sunday morning a few weeks ago.

THERAPIST: What time was it?

ANNA: About 10 A.M.

THERAPIST: Where were you?

ANNA: I was in the kitchen.

THERAPIST: What were you doing?

ANNA: I was looking at all the chores that needed doing, the cleaning, ironing, all of that.

THERAPIST: You said that you were looking at all the chores to do. Can you describe in a bit more detail how you were doing that?

ANNA: I was sitting at the kitchen table, thinking through all the things I needed to do.

THERAPIST: Getting a vivid picture of what happened will really help me to understand what was happening. Can you describe as concretely as possible to me what you could see and hear at that moment in time?

ANNA: I can see my kitchen, the kitchen table, the view through the window into the street.

THERAPIST: To help me get a sense of your surroundings and this context, can you describe your kitchen in more detail, so I can get a picture of it in my mind? For example, tell me the about the layout, the colors, the fittings.

ANNA: It is a small kitchen with one side having a counter with cupboards underneath and the adjoining wall having the stove and an old fridge, and the washing machine. The walls are painted white, and there is a tiled floor. There is a small round wooden table with four chairs in the middle of the kitchen. There is a pile of dirty dishes in the sink, and the breakfast things are still on the table. The ironing board is standing in the corner with a basket of laundry.

THERAPIST: That's great—that is a really good specific and concrete description. I can really picture it now. And was anyone else there?

ANNA: No, I was on my own.

THERAPIST: And how were you at that point? What was your state of mind?

ANNA: I felt a little apprehensive and tired.

THERAPIST: What were you focusing your attention on?

ANNA: I was looking at the list of things to do I had in front of me.

THERAPIST: What did you notice immediately after focusing on the list?

ANNA: I felt tense and anxious.

THERAPIST: What exactly was the first thing you spotted as you got tense and anxious?

ANNA: I felt a sinking feeling and butterflies in my stomach, my stomach churning.

THERAPIST: OK, so that sounds like a very similar feeling to that we observed came before the other times you ruminated, is that right?

ANNA: Yes.

THERAPIST: What happened next immediately as you spotted the sinking feeling?

ANNA: I started to think about what to do first. I wondered where I should start. I began to ruminate about how difficult it was to decide what to do, and how it was all too much. I kept dwelling on what I should start with, would I get that wrong, and then why is this so difficult for me. I kept ruminating about this for a while, but then after about 20 minutes, I stopped worrying and got going on tidying up the kitchen.

THERAPIST: OK, this sounds like a really good example of when you could have gotten stuck in rumination, but something different happened. Let's look at this in detail to see what we can learn from your own experience that helped you to step out of the rumination. How did the rumination come to an end?

ANNA: After a while I just stopped ruminating and started on the task in front of me and began to clean up the kitchen table, and go about my chores. I cleaned the table and washed the dishes.

THERAPIST: It sounds like just then you moved a little away from describing the specific details of the experience second by second and instead summarized the overall experience, compressing quite a few minutes into a few sentences. It is helpful to stay with the experience as it unfolded moment by moment as best you can. Let's try and slow that period down and take it moment by moment. Recall what was happening there as if playing a film in slow motion. Let's rewind the film a bit and then run it forward nice and slow. Let's look at what was happening toward the end of the rumination. Can you get yourself back in that moment, imagining it as vividly as possible?

ANNA: (Nods.)

THERAPIST: What were you thinking just before the rumination stopped?

ANNA: Why is it so difficult for me to do even easy things that everyone else can do?

THERAPIST: What did you say to yourself just after asking that?

ANNA: I remember thinking I have had enough of feeling fed up.

THERAPIST: What happened immediately after having that thought?

ANNA: I asked myself "What can I do now?"; "How can I get started?"

THERAPIST: What was the effect of asking those questions?

ANNA: I started to make a plan in my head and I looked around looking around for something to do.

THERAPIST: Any other effects you noticed?

ANNA: I felt a little bit energetic and motivated.

THERAPIST: And what did you do then?

ANNA: I started washing and drying the dishes.

THERAPIST: What was the effect of getting started on the dishes?

ANNA: I felt a bit more positive.

THERAPIST: What happened to the rumination?

ANNA: It had gone away.

THERAPIST: OK, let me check that I have followed the sequence properly. You were sitting in the kitchen looking at the list of things to do and you started to notice that sinking feeling and begin to ruminate, asking the "why" questions about why this was so difficult, but after 20 minutes, you thought, "I've had enough of this" and instead asked yourself, "What can I do?" and "How can I get started?" and then you focused on what you could do that was right in front of you, and you got started on the dishes. Is that right?

ANNA: Yes.

THERAPIST: What do you think you can learn from this situation?

ANNA: I am not sure.

THERAPIST: I wonder if it gives us any clues as to what might help you to move away from rumination. For example, what can you learn about the effects of the questions you ask yourself?

ANNA: I think I see what you mean. When I get stuck dwelling on things, I keep asking "Why?" and "Why is this so difficult?" but this time I asked something different, about what I could do and this seemed to help.

THERAPIST: I agree. It looks as if the questions you ask yourself when faced with a problem or a chore might have a big impact. Asking "What can I do?" and "How can I start?" moves you to thinking about action and into making plans, whereas asking "Why is it so difficult?" appears to make it harder to do things and pulls you down. It looks as if sometimes when you ruminate, you start off by thinking about what you can do to tackle a problem, trying to choose what job to start with, but then you get hijacked by thinking about the causes and meanings of what is happening—asking those abstract "why" questions. I wonder what would happen if you could ask the useful questions from this recent example earlier in a bout of rumination. Imagine asking them right at the beginning of the rumination, when you first notice the sinking feeling. This might cut out all of that negative and demotivating rumination. What do you make of that idea?

Inside the Therapist's Mind 2: Decision Points and Reflections with Anna

You can see from the previous dialogue that the therapist is working hard with Anna to get details about this alternative time when she did not ruminate as much, in order to identify possible moderators of the rumination. The first thing to notice is the way that the therapist sets up the search for an example that can introduce variability with respect to the outcomes of rumination. The most useful comparison is one that matches closely existing examples of rumination in terms of the initiating context and level of stress and difficulty, but which differs on outcome. It would be trivial and uninformative to simply compare a time when the patient got good news versus a time the patient got bad news or an easy success versus failure on something difficult. The comparisons need to relate to situations when the rumination could occur and where there is some commonality.

The best starting point is to ask the patient to recall a memory that is as close as possible in terms of situation to a recent example of rumination but that had a different outcome, such as less rumination or a positive consequence. This is the approach the therapist takes here. Notice that this is done as specifically and concretely as possible, with the therapist describing the context of the situation in detail ("having chores to do and starting to feel anxious, when you didn't ruminate as much"). Such specific prompting should help the patient to identify another specific memory. If the patient is unable to identify an alternative memory, perhaps because the request is too narrow, then follow-up questions can move to more general descriptions (e.g., another time that was about as difficult and stressful as the recent ones where you ruminated, but where things went well).

The therapist needs to be prepared to try different versions of the question about variability until one is found that resonates with the patient. Nearly every patient will be able to identify times when the rumination changes to some degree, but the therapist may need to persevere to identify one at first. Remember that the variability could be in terms of whether rumination occurs or does not occur, is helpful or unhelpful, is longer or shorter, or is more intense or less distressing, and whether the patient copes well or badly with a situation. It makes sense to start with the more categorical differences (e.g., helpful versus unhelpful) when searching for alternatives, and to then move to the dimensional differences if these examples are hard for the patient to find (e.g., longer or shorter duration of episodes of rumination). This comparison of variability can be recorded in Handout 9 (Being More Effective Form). Figure 6.3 is a filled-in version of the Being More Effective Form that demonstrates how the therapist or Anna could complete it to summarize the sample situations discussed in the two preceding dialogues about having chores to do.

The early part of the interview is a good example of the therapist working hard to establish context and detail. Notice how the therapist works through the "what," "where," "how," "when," and "who" questions early when discussing the memory. This is a good example of how to do this for any memory that is being discussed. It helps give the therapist details on the context that may be relevant for the FA. The therapist is also prompting Anna to be more concrete and specific throughout the dialogue. The therapist focuses on getting Anna to imagine and describe the setting for the memory to enhance the recall of detail, as well as to shape and coach Anna into being more concrete and specific (the ACES principle). Doing this early in the exploration of a memory will pay dividends later, as more detail and greater richness of information typically follow.

The language used by the therapist also bears close observation. You might notice particular questions like "What were you focusing your attention on?" or "What did you say to yourself just after asking that?" These questions treat the patient's thinking as a behavior, and, more specifically, as a behavior that the patient may be able to control. This is consistent with the functional-contextual approach of RFCBT, in which we view thinking as another behavior that we examine in terms of antecedents and consequences. Furthermore, because both attention and inner speech are under deliberative and voluntary control, the therapist's language explores where the patient may be influencing what happens in a situation. This language also prepares the way for later interventions in which the therapist may manipulate the focus of attention or what Anna says to herself as a means to influence her rumination. Focus of attention, a particularly important element, is discussed in more detail in Chapter 10.

You may also notice how the therapist is asking questions that structure and shape Anna's responses and try to keep the focus of the discussion tight and discrete. Questions tend to refer to what has just happened and ask about what immediately follows in order to fix Anna to her immediate and direct experience and to reduce the likelihood of her moving to a more abstract, implicational, or interpretative response. The frequent summaries and checking in with Anna serve the same purpose of keeping the discussion tight, specific, and on track.

The dialogue also illustrates a common problem and one way of responding to it. Patients will frequently find it hard to stay in the moment-by-moment experiential detail of what is happening when imagining or remembering a situation. Instead, there is a natural tendency for ruminating patients to produce abstract summaries and decontextualized generalizations that report the gist of what happened, rather than the details. This can take the form of compressing minutes or hours of behavior, such as a bout of rumination, into a sentence or two. This abstract way of describing events loses much detail and context that may be useful for identifying

Detailed questions	Current situation[a] (success/failure) (e.g., intended to do something and did it)	Similar situation with opposite outcome[b] (failure/success) (e.g., intended to do something and did not do it)
What? Include goal, events, actions, feelings, physical state, outcome	Looking at the mess, thinking, "There is so much to do.", "Where do I start?"; feeling guilty, anxious, feeling tired and unmotivated, sinking feeling, "butterflies"	Thinking through all the things that need doing, dirty dishes in sink, basket of laundry to be done, feeling apprehensive and tired, looking at list of things to do, sinking feeling, "butterflies"
Where? Location, setting, state	Sitting in living room at home	Sitting at kitchen table at home
When? Time, day, what preceded the situation	Sunday morning, poor night's sleep the night before	Sunday morning, 10 A.M., several weeks ago
How? Step by step how the event unfolded, your approach during the situation	Try to prioritize what to do, then think "What if I choose the wrong thing to do?" then think "why is this so difficult? Why can't I get started?"; felt less motivated, sat there for several hours, eventually fell asleep	Thought about what to do first, thought about how difficult it was to decide, would I get it wrong? Then thought "I've had enough of feeling fed up," then asked "what can I do now?"; "How can I get started?" Made a plan, then cleared off table and washed dishes
Who?	Alone	Alone

[a]What was unique about this situation? Describe in detail the context of the event in response to each question. Was the event a success or failure?

[b]Describe a similar situation or task that had a different outcome (e.g., success or failure), and that happened either this week or earlier. How do the situations differ? What can you learn from this?

Plan/decision for the future: *When I get stuck, ask myself, "What can I do now?"; "How can I get started?" not "why" questions.*

FIGURE 6.3. Example of a completed Being More Effective Form for Anna.

antecedents or moderators of rumination. This abstraction can also take the form of interpretations and analyses about what happened, rather than describing the actual behavior (e.g., "He insulted me"; "I was useless"). In these situations, the therapist needs to deliberately and explicitly highlight this shift into abstraction and refocus back into experiential detail. In this dialogue, Anna initially encapsulates the twenty minutes of rumination and its termination into a few sentences that are vague about what actually happened. This is a critical juncture that the therapist needs to understand in detail. You can see how the therapist draws attention to Anna's moving away from the details of the situation and asks her to move back to those details. A number of ploys are used to facilitate this shift in focus, including asking her to imagine the situation and to look at it in slow motion. The therapist makes the decision to examine in detail the period when the rumination comes to an end, and to leave the early sequence of the rumination less explored. This is a pragmatic decision because finding out more about what might impact the reduction of rumination is the priority and there is not sufficient time to track the full episode in detail before the end of the session.

The therapist asks a series of questions to get a detailed sense of what may have contributed to the end of the rumination. Asking what happened just before a bout of rumination ended can be very informative, as it is here with Anna.

This dialogue suggests potential points for intervention. The most obvious intervention is to develop a contingency If–Then plan (see Chapter 7) in which Anna's warning signs of a sinking feeling and/or asking "why" questions are paired to her practicing the alternative response of asking herself more helpful questions like "What can I do?"; "How can I start?" This would be a sensible plan that has the benefit of naturally emerging from Anna's own experience and would reflect an attempt at taking a helpful response already in her repertoire and getting her to apply it more consistently and systematically. The final summary at the end of the dialogue is intended to set the scene for such an intervention. The FA could therefore lead directly into a behavioral plan.

CHAPTER 7

Choosing
Treatment Interventions

Core Interventions

The core interventions in RFCBT—self-monitoring, directly altering environmental contingencies, and developing contingency If–Then plans—are derived from FA and used with all patients.

Self-Monitoring

All patients are encouraged to monitor their rumination and avoidance. Increased awareness of a habit is critical to changing that habit. Furthermore, for many patients, becoming more aware of what they are doing is in itself sufficient for them to shift out of rumination. Awareness of warning signs provides an opportunity to "nip rumination in the bud."

Directly Altering Environmental Contingencies

For many patients, FA will reveal aspects of their environment that increase the likelihood of rumination. Simple homework exercises set up as behavioral experiments can be tried from as early as the first or second session to influence rumination.

Developing Contingency If–Then Plans in Response to Warning Signs

These contingency If–Then plans involve strategies to break up the rumination and functionally replace it. These new strategies are repeatedly practiced in response to the cues that trigger the ruminative habit to countercondition an incompatible response, thus weakening the ruminative habit. Typical alternative strategies include applied relaxation, visualization exercises, shifting processing style, assertiveness, experimenting in the real world, and approach behaviors. The development of If–Then plans starts early in treatment and continues to be consolidated and practiced throughout the course of the treatment.

It is important to start working on making changes from the first session to counter any hopelessness the patient has and to increase the momentum of the therapy. Relatively brief interventions can be quite productive in the first two or three sessions. Having completed the initial formal FA and provided a convincing rationale for therapy, the first interventions need to build rapid changes from these assessments.

Initiating Interventions

I recommend a three-step process for initiating interventions with patients. First, a possible moderator of rumination (or any target behavior) is identified by examining the patient's own experience in the FA. Second, the therapist tries out this moderator in the session, using a behavioral experiment to confirm that changing this aspect of behavior directly and positively influences the patient's experience. Third, after confirming the usefulness of this manipulation in the session, the therapist and patient make plans for the patient to repeatedly practice this strategy in daily life, usually in response to a warning sign, as part of their homework. This three-step approach maximizes the likelihood that the therapist has identified a genuinely useful intervention before the patient tries it out in her daily life. It also increases the patient's engagement and motivation: successful experience in-session with the behavioral experiment makes it more likely that the strategy will be used outside the session. For example, for Anna, it might be useful to try an in-session behavioral experiment in which she imagines a difficult situation, such as being faced with chores, and then compares the effect of asking herself the "why" and "how" questions identified in the prior FA with Anna (see Chapter 6). (See the Why–How experiment in Chapter 9 for detailed exposition of this approach.)

The early interventions for the first few sessions are based on what has been learned in the FA: interventions will be chosen on the basis of contexts and strategies known to influence rumination and based on the hypothesized functions of the rumination for each patient. Thus, if rumination serves the function of reducing hostile feelings to other people, an alternative strategy may involve teaching anger management techniques.

Altering Environmental Contingencies: Interrupting Cues to the Habit

FA may reveal aspects of the wider context that are associated with the onset of rumination, whether aspects of the external environment (people, places, times of day, objects), aspects of behavior and routines (sequences of actions performed by the patient), or internal states (mood, physical sensations, thoughts). Those aspects of the environment that increase or decrease the likelihood of the target behavior will be targeted in behavioral treatment plans, because controlling the environment controls the rumination. In particular, the therapist looks for those cues or warning signs that are repeatedly associated with the start of rumination and automatically trigger the habit. Reducing or removing these cues is a relatively easy way to reduce the overall frequency of rumination. This is easier for aspects of the external environment and behavioral routines than for internal states.

It is less straightforward to directly prevent or remove the feelings, sensations, or thoughts that trigger habitual rumination. When an internal cue triggers rumination, the treatment options are to either identify potential environmental cues earlier in the antecedent chain that trigger this internal response (e.g., a physical reminder that sets off an upsetting memory) or to countercondition an alternative response to this internal cue. RFCBT tends to focus on the latter, with a strong emphasis on the patient learning new helpful habitual responses to the cues of low mood, anxiety, or stress arousal.

If possible, simple homework exercises are set up as behavioral experiments to change external environment in the first few sessions in order to provide an early positive experience for the patient and a "quick win" in reducing rumination. If possible, the therapist introduces these changes as behavioral experiments within the first few sessions. The therapist asks the patient to predict what he expects to happen if the suggested intervention is implemented. In the next session the accuracy of this prediction is evaluated.

In general, increasing structure, activity, and routine reduces rumination. Once a potential cue or trigger to habitual rumination is identified, behavioral experiments are used to examine the consequences of addressing the environment. FA is likely to suggest particular aspects of context that are associated with rumination and avoidance.

Key aspects of the environment to consider during FA and when thinking about how to alter the environment to reduce rumination and avoidance include:

1. *The richness of the environment.* A rather uninteresting environment lacking much in the way of diverting sensory stimuli may be associated with more rumination.

2. *The time of the day.* Rumination is typically more frequent first thing in the morning and when going to bed at night.

3. *Solitude.* Rumination is often associated with being alone.

4. *Rituals and routine.* Increased rumination occurs during regular routines and becomes associated with those routines (e.g., sitting down to have a coffee and cigarette in a particular chair after getting back from work and reflecting on the day).

5. *Mood triggers.* Unsurprisingly, rumination is often associated with events that can change mood (e.g., criticism, losses, threats). It is also set off by triggers over which patients may have more voluntary control (e.g., listening to sad music).

6. *News signals.* Events that herald new information that patients expect to be negative are often triggers of rumination. For example, the telephone ringing or the arrival of the mail can be sufficient to start rumination about what bad news might be received and what it might mean.

7. *Evaluating self, plans, and outcomes.* Rumination is often triggered when people start to consider what they need to do or what they have just been doing, or start making comparisons between themselves and other people. Thus, times when an individual is involved in planning or reviewing progress can trigger rumination, as can impending situations that are perceived to involve some measure of self-ability (e.g., presentations, tests, interviews), potential tests of a person's worth, or activities that induce social comparisons (e.g., meeting new people, exposure to highly evaluative family members, hearing about a friend's success, or seeing an attractive person).

8. *Reminders of upsetting or traumatic events.* Rumination often starts in response to the involuntary and intrusive recall of an upsetting or distressing memory. The patient may recollect this upsetting event and begin to reexperience the associated negative emotions, but then often begins to analyze the event and to consider its causes, meaning, and implications (e.g., "Why me?"; "Why did this happen to me?"; "Why couldn't I have stopped it?"). This rumination can then be quite prolonged. Abstract rumination distances the patient from close and direct experience of the event, its context, and full emotional experience, preventing habituation and any coming to terms with the upsetting event. While it is not always possible to identify the environmental trigger to the initial intrusive memory, exposure to both semantic information and sensory–perceptual details associated with the upsetting event probably increase the likelihood of the memory entering consciousness. For example, for a patient who experienced a painful and difficult divorce, television programs and newspaper articles that mentioned divorce or featured arguing couples set off her memories of the divorce,

leading to bouts of rumination. The anniversary dates of these upsetting events can also act to trigger rumination.

For each of these possible triggers of rumination or avoidance, the therapist needs to consider what aspect of the situation is most likely to be responsible for the initiation of rumination and to use this formulation to design the change in environment. Thought experiments can be useful here to determine which aspect of the situation is most important. For example, many patients report that being alone triggers rumination. The therapist can usefully consider which aspect of being alone triggers the rumination. Is it feeling lonely? Is it lacking someone to encourage the patient to do things? Is it not doing things because they don't feel worth doing alone (e.g., cooking, going to the movies)? Is it lacking the structure an interaction might produce? Is it lacking an external distraction from negative thoughts? Identifying which aspect of being alone matters will influence what change to implement.

Questions to help clarify this include:

"What aspect of being alone do you find most difficult?"
"What do you really value about being with someone else?"

Likewise, the therapist checks with the patient to determine whether the situation would be so difficult if particular dimensions were different. For example, the therapist asks the patient:

"Assuming that you were doing something interesting on your own, would you be bothered about being alone?"
"How likely is this to activate rumination?"

Breaking down which aspect of the context is important allows the therapy to make more effective alterations in the environment. If the patient feels lonely, then thinking about ways to get in contact with people will be helpful. Phoning people, arranging to meet friends, even writing a letter to a close friend might increase a feeling of contact. Alternatively, if the problem with being alone is a lack of structure, then the therapy needs to focus on teaching the patient to structure his or her own time. Again, it is advisable to set up these interventions as behavioral experiments so that we are able to refine our hypothesis and intervention if it is not successful at first.

Simple, easily accomplished interventions can have quite far-reaching effects. For a rather impoverished environment, introducing new elements in the external world that give the patient something to pay attention to can be an effective intervention (e.g., playing music, turning on the radio, putting nice-smelling essential oils on the pillow). One patient reported that she tended to start ruminating when driving in the car alone on the way to work. When asked in more detail, she reported that she tended to listen to slow, rather sad classical music in the car, which seemed to be associated with the start of her negative thoughts. As a behavioral experiment, she replaced the sad music with more upbeat folk-rock music that she also enjoyed. This simple change of music reduced her rumination at the beginning of the day. Because rumination is often self-fulfilling and can persist later into the day (e.g., patients think that the day has started badly so it will continue to go badly, leading to further rumination), a small but significant decrease in rumination at the start of the day can have positive repercussions for the rest of the day.

Patients often report that the rumination starts first thing in the morning when they wake up. The FA needs to consider what the precise trigger to the rumination could be. Is it there first thing when the patient awakes or does it follow from some other action? For example, starting to think about what needs to be done that day, or reviewing the day before, or thinking about how he has nothing planned for the day, or noticing how tired he feels could all trigger rumination.

Different triggers require different interventions. For example, if rumination in the morning is related to physical feelings, it may be that doing something physically active first thing in the morning is helpful. Getting up and out of bed and becoming more active may reduce the opportunity for rumination. If rumination is related to thinking about what needs to be done, making a list of what needs to be done the day before and then focusing only on the top item on the list would reduce rumination. When lying in bed, attention may be focused inward on internal sensations of tiredness and sleepiness. In this instance, listening to the radio in the morning to shift attention away from the feelings of tiredness and toward the external world is useful. Changing the waking and getting up routine is a useful experiment, as rumination is often associated with particular aspects of the routine, and altering them will reduce its automatic triggering.

Often rumination also occurs at the end of the day, when the person is lying in bed trying to get to sleep. As in the morning, this situation is conducive to rumination because the person has fewer external stimuli to focus on, making it more likely that he will turn inwards to rumination. He may also be reviewing what happened that day or reflecting on what is coming tomorrow. This rumination at night commonly contributes to insomnia. Again, changes in the routine before going to bed and when in bed can disrupt this rumination. If the patient is unable to sleep, getting out of bed to do something else is a useful change, if only to reduce the association between being in bed and ruminating. Rumination has become a habit triggered by aspects of the routine, and therefore changing the routine interrupts the rumination, making it less frequent.

Patients sometimes report particular places as being associated with their rumination. A number of patients have associated rumination with their housing, for example, when they live in a rundown apartment, which they perceive, probably accurately, as being uncomfortable (e.g., noisy and aggressive neighbors, dampness in the walls, poorly decorated, or too small). In this situation, it is useful to determine what aspect of the apartment the patient ruminates about and whether there is any variation within the apartment (e.g., are some rooms worse than others?). Furthermore, it may be that there are aspects of the apartment that can be altered to reduce rumination (e.g., decorating or tidying it up). Making small changes to an environment such as tidying up a room can remove some of the cues to the rumination. Being able to go to other places that do not trigger the rumination can be a simple way to produce some respite early in therapy.

More general aspects of a patient's environment and lifestyle also contribute to the onset of rumination. Many patients report feeling under pressure, in a hurry, in a rush, and having to juggle many different activities and tasks, whether at home or at work. This situation is conducive to rumination as it tends to generate stress and increases the likelihood of making mistakes and not meeting deadlines. Moreover, patients often try to do multiple things at once and switch between tasks. This can make it hard for them to be absorbed in what they are doing, which also increases the likelihood of rumination. I have found it generally useful to encourage patients to focus on only doing one thing at a time, to pace themselves, to give them some space to calm down and to slow things down.

The other way that a patient's general environment and lifestyle may encourage rumination is if there is an imbalance between the patient's routine chores and obligations and those activities that she finds enjoyable, interesting, and self-fulfilling. In the RFCBT trial for patients with residual depression, patients often had given up doing the activities that they found most interesting and enjoyable. Because they had reduced energy and found doing things hard work, they tried to conserve resources and prioritized activities they judged to be essential such as daily chores, work, and obligations to others. While these activities were undoubtedly important, they tended to be boring and tiring and were often accompanied by a sense of reluctance and resignation. With the lack of absorbing and enthusing activities, patients became more prone to rumination. Rumination will be more frequent when activities are not engaging and are done because of a sense of obligation. In this context, thoughts often focus on "Why am I doing this?"; "Why is this so tedious?"; "Why am I so tired?," and so forth. These are the kinds of tasks that require an effort to complete and can be quite fatiguing. Moreover, by dropping engaging and pleasurable activities, the patient misses an opportunity to improve her mood and energy. Therefore, in RFCBT, the therapist explains the importance of shifting the balance of activity from routine chores and obligations toward self-fulfilling activities. The therapist explores with the patient how such activities are valuable because they can recharge her batteries as well as give her mental space away from ruminating.

An Example of FA Leading to Environmental/Behavioral Change: Emily

Before looking at the next transcript, let's introduce Emily, a patient with a long-standing history of major depression, as well as comorbid GAD, PTSD, and bulimia. Her rumination is often very self-critical and focused on judging and evaluating herself as lazy, arrogant, and selfish. She has a difficult relationship with her mother, whom she experiences as insensitive, domineering, critical, and opinionated. She has just had a difficult breakup.

The following dialogue occurred in the third session with Emily. Together, Emily and the therapist have already spotted some warning signs, and she has become more aware of the rumination habit. They have discussed the idea that Emily does not need to automatically go into rumination but can learn to do something different instead. The therapist starts off by following up on the previous self-monitoring homework (using Handout 6, Rumination Episode Recording Form) and then examines some recent situations to learn what might influence her rumination.

THERAPIST: How did you get on with spotting your early warning signs this week? Did you come up with any new ones?

EMILY: No, not any more this week, although I am beginning to notice them faster.

THERAPIST: That's great. What are the good ones that you are noticing?

EMILY: My heartbeat speeding up, my posture changing and getting all tense, feeling hot.

THERAPIST: What can you do differently at this point to interrupt the rumination?

EMILY: I can stop and think, "Hang on a minute, it does not have to be like this." I can ask, "How can I deal with this?" and instead of blaming myself I can try and do something to make myself feel better.

THERAPIST: That sounds like a good way to step back from the rumination. Were you able to do that last week at all?

EMILY: I was able to step back from the rumination a couple of times during the week, but there were lots of times when even though I noticed the warning signs I could not stop it. Sometimes I found myself dwelling on things without being aware of how it started.

THERAPIST: Most people have that experience when they first start to try and change the rumination—this is exactly what we would expect from a strong habit. To start with, a strong habit will keep occurring most of the time, but gradually as you become more aware of it and keep doing something different instead of ruminating, this will get easier and the habit will get less. Did anything help you to stop ruminating when you noticed the warning signs?

EMILY: It helped when I was able to change my surroundings—once or twice I stood up and went out into the garden when I noticed I was getting irritated and this helped to calm me down. But there were quite a few times last week when I couldn't do that. The worse one was when I had to go to my ex's to collect some stuff—that was really stressful and set off a really bad bout of rumination.

THERAPIST: I can see that you wrote that situation down in the monitoring form. It looks as if it was a particularly upsetting situation for you. It says here on the form that you ruminated for 5 hours afterwards and that there were lots of negative thoughts during the rumination like "I'm not good enough" and "he hates me," and it made you feel worse. Is that right?

EMILY: Yes, it was the worst point of the week.

THERAPIST: Then would it be worth looking at this situation in more detail? I wonder if it might help to look at this situation and try and learn from it, perhaps also by comparing it with another situation. Shall we try that?

EMILY: Yes, that could be helpful.

THERAPIST: Tell me a bit more about this stressful situation with your ex.

EMILY: I had to go over to his apartment to pick up my stuff. While I was collecting my stuff, he came in and started going on about things, and it got really stressful. We both got really angry and reacted badly. We were both worked up. I got really upset and stormed out and spent the rest of the day ruminating about it.

THERAPIST: OK, it sounds like there is a lot going on here and you have sped through a number of things there. Can you recognize that you are summarizing in a general and abstract way what happened and are moving away from the exact details of what happened? Remember that we talked about how it is easy to shift back into this habit of being abstract. It may be helpful to really slow this down and go through step by step. Can you try and do that?

EMILY: Yes, although it is hard.

THERAPIST: Not to worry—this is not something we usually do, so it feels a bit unnatural and takes a bit of effort at first. Let's try it out and see if it is helpful. Let's go back to the beginning. What was happening before you went to your ex-partner's?

EMILY: I was at home doing some chores.

THERAPIST: How were you feeling then?

EMILY: I was a little tense and apprehensive about going to see him. I also felt a bit rushed and hurried because I was trying to get a few chores done before going.

THERAPIST: OK, and what happened next?

EMILY: I drove to the apartment after breakfast.

THERAPIST: What happened next?

EMILY: Well, it was a bad drive—the traffic was terrible, it was rush hour, there was a long traffic jam and it was quite a stressful drive.

THERAPIST: What was the effect of the trip?

EMILY: It made me more stressed and wound up because I was in a rush and had agreed to be there early before going to work.

THERAPIST: OK, and what happened when you got to your ex-partner's?

EMILY: I started going through the stuff in the apartment to work out what to take. I was still feeling stressed because I wasn't sure what to take or leave and felt I had to get it figured out quickly. I was worried about getting it wrong. I also was concerned about how my ex would respond.

THERAPIST: So in summary, you were already feeling pretty stressed and worked up because of hurrying, the chores, and the drive, and so on, while you were sorting through things in the apartment. Is that right?

EMILY: Yes.

THERAPIST: How did you notice the stress?

EMILY: I noticed that my heartbeat was speeding up and I was feeling hot, my thinking was a bit messy and muddled. It was making it hard to work out what to do and how to pack things up.

THERAPIST: Were you ruminating at that point?

EMILY: No, I was just managing to focus on what I was doing, but I really lost it when my ex started up.

THERAPIST: OK, tell me exactly what happened then, keeping it nice and slow, second by second. What did he say and do?

EMILY: He came into the room and looked at what I had sorted out—I was starting to pile up things to take and leave on separate sides of the floor—and he said something like "Is that all you've done?"; "You need to get a move on, I don't have all day."

THERAPIST: How did he say that?

EMILY: He had an irritated, impatient, contemptuous tone of voice.

THERAPIST: How did he look?

EMILY: He looked annoyed and angry.

THERAPIST: And how did you respond mentally and emotionally just as he said that?

EMILY: I felt deflated and really put down. I thought, "Oh no here we go again."

THERAPIST: And what did you do just then?

EMILY: I tried to explain to him that I wanted to check with him first before I took things.

THERAPIST: Can you remember exactly what you said and how you said it?

EMILY: Something like "It is hard to work out what to take, and I wanted to be sure you were happy with my choices, and it isn't made any easier by having you get on my case." I may have sounded a bit irritated and edgy.

THERAPIST: What happened right after that?

EMILY: He responded by saying that this should be easy and that I was always making things more complicated than they need to be. He started rehashing all the things that led up to our breakup. He said it was typical of me to make a mountain out of a molehill, and why can't I just be more efficient.

THERAPIST: And what effect did that have on you?

EMILY: It just brought up all the memories of arguments and feelings of being criticized throughout the relationship. Why do I find it so difficult?

THERAPIST: Is it about now that the rumination really kicked in?

EMILY: Yes, I got more and more irritated. I started shouting at him, "Why do you always do this?"; "Why do you always put me down?"

THERAPIST: And what happened next?

EMILY: He starts to raise his voice back at me, and we are both getting worked up reliving our past history and pointing out each other's bad points. Why do you always do this? Why do you always do that? I am shaking with anger and he gets more and more sarcastic, pointing out how thoughtless and selfish I am.

THERAPIST: How long does this argument last?

EMILY: We are going at each other for about 5 minutes, and then I can't take it anymore and I leave the room and walk out of the house and out to car. After a few minutes I drive off.

THERAPIST: And what are you focusing your mind on?

EMILY: I am ruminating over and over again.

THERAPIST: What are the thoughts and the questions you are saying to yourself over and over again just then?

EMILY: Why is this so difficult? He despises me—lots of extreme thoughts, I can't stand this type of thought.

THERAPIST: What is the effect of these thoughts?

EMILY: They make me sad and angry.

THERAPIST: What comes into your mind after those angry thoughts?

EMILY: Then I start to doubt myself and wonder "Why am I so irritable?"; "Why am I so selfish?" Perhaps this happens because I am not very nice and I am not good enough. I feel really down.

THERAPIST: How long did this rumination go on?

EMILY: It went on all afternoon and late into the night. I couldn't sleep.

THERAPIST: What kept it going so long? What happened with the sequence of your rumination? I wonder if it followed any of the patterns we identified before and mapped out for your rumination?

EMILY: Yes, I would dwell on why does he do this and feel angry, and then after a while I would start to blame myself and wonder why I keep causing these situations and why am I so useless, and feel down, and then this would switch back to the anger.

THERAPIST: OK, so the rumination followed the sequence of switching back and forwards between anger and self-blame.

EMILY: Yes.

THERAPIST: How did it end?

EMILY: Eventually I was so exhausted and worn out that I fell asleep.

THERAPIST: Thank you for staying with that situation longer and in more detail. I can see that it was a very difficult and stressful situation for you. What was your experience of staying with this situation and breaking it down into detail just now?

EMILY: It is hard and it is bringing back some of the feeling—I feel a bit stressed, but it is helpful to see what happened and share it with someone else. I can see there is a definite pattern here.

THERAPIST: That's good. If we look at this and try and learn from it, it looks like one thing to recognize is that you were stressed already and nervous before meeting with your ex-partner. We can learn even more if we can look at a time when you were able to step away from ruminating in a similar situation and notice any differences between that time and this time when you got stuck in rumination. There are advantages to spotting a time when your strategies work and one when they don't. Is there another time, perhaps when you had to meet with your ex, when things went differently and you did not get caught up in rumination?

EMILY: Yes, I had to go and see him again later in the week to finish packing things up, and this time I coped much better, even though he was still difficult.

THERAPIST: That sounds like an excellent example to look at in detail. What happened that time?

EMILY: I went to his apartment on Sunday to collect some furniture and other stuff. I was in the apartment again, looking at what was there. He started up again, saying I needed to get things sorted out quickly and picking on me again about the other day. However, this time, I was a bit calmer and managed to stay calmer even though I was a bit stressed and just go with things, and with making the decisions. It was difficult but I coped.

THERAPIST: How did you feel in that situation?

EMILY: I was getting a little tense, hot, heart beating faster—all the signs that I am getting irritable and anxious—but I was able to keep my thinking clear.

THERAPIST: What did you do that helped you to keep your thinking clear?

EMILY: I decided that I was just going to try and focus on getting the job done, and I kept reminding myself that all I needed to do was to work down my list.

THERAPIST: What list?

EMILY: Oh, before I went to my ex's, I sat and wrote down a list of what I wanted to collect and marked down which ones I wanted and could fit in the car in one trip, so I was prepared for the trip.

THERAPIST: That sounds like a good plan. Was there anything else that was different about what happened before going to see your ex this time?

EMILY: I arranged to meet him in the afternoon, and before going I went to spend the morning with my friend Joy, which helped me to feel calm and serene.

THERAPIST: What about your travel there?

EMILY: I wasn't in such a rush and the traffic was much quieter, so it was a more relaxing journey.

THERAPIST: OK, so it sounds like you were feeling a lot calmer before you went there this second time, and that might have helped you to cope with the situation. As well as that, you were better prepared with a list to help keep your mind focused and clear. Is that right?

EMILY: Yes, I was much less stressed the second time, and in a better place to cope with my ex.

THERAPIST: It sounds like you coped better in the heat of the moment the second time. What exactly did you focus on and say to yourself in that situation?

EMILY: After keeping the daily monitoring form, I had seen how unhelpful it was the previous time when I had let him get to me, and how it had only fed the situation. So this time I resolved that I was not going to respond, and I had some ground rules in my head about what I would do and say, for example to keep my answers as short and straightforward as possible, just yes and no answers, and to only focus on the task at hand. I figured I could worry about all the difficulties about our relationship another time.

THERAPIST: And how did that work?

EMILY: It helped me stay focused and leave quicker. I was still stressed and I don't know if I could have kept it up much longer—and I doubt if I could do it all of the time or even some of the time with my ex, but I was able to do it the other day.

THERAPIST: OK, so it sounds like the second time you went to see your ex you didn't just repeat what happened the first time, but having recorded the first time in your diary, you had made some changes in your environment and response to cope better. What can you learn from comparing these two situations?

EMILY: It was helpful to be prepared in advance, to have a list of what I was going to do, and to have thought through a plan of what I was going to do in response to my ex. It was helpful to be calmer before meeting him.

THERAPIST: What did you do to ensure you were calmer before going to meet him?

EMILY: I was in less of a rush and less of a hurry so I didn't feel under pressure to get there. I spent time with a good friend before going, which put me in a good mood before I saw him.

THERAPIST: So it sounds like the second time you set things up so that you were calmer before meeting your ex, giving you a bit of a buffer from getting wound up, making it easier to manage those situations. Coupled with your preparations—and in particular having very concrete and detailed plans for what to do and say—this made the second situation easier to cope with and stopped you from having an argument and getting caught up in rumination. Is that a fair summary?

EMILY: Yes. Hearing it like this, it sounds obvious what I could do to cope better. It is embarrassing and stupid that I hadn't done it before.

THERAPIST: The good news is that this suggests there may be simple things you can do that could help in the future, such as making time, doing something relaxing, and preparing in detail, before similar stressful situations. I don't think there is any need to be down on yourself about this. After all, you came up with and put all these plans into action, indicating you know how to do this. Most people aren't great about doing these simple and sometimes fairly obvious things, because they don't always pay attention to what they are doing in as much detail as we have just been doing. Moreover, we have talked about getting stuck in an unhelpful way of thinking and of it being a habit. That explains why you don't always do the most helpful things. Lots of very clever people get stuck in doing unhelpful things again and again because they have become a habit. These habits often start young and develop when we are children and adolescents. They reflect what we learned over time. Comparing these two situations suggests ways you can change these patterns of behavior to move forward—and the first step to changing the habit is becoming aware of what works and what doesn't work, which is what we have just done.

EMILY: I guess these patterns are old-fashioned reactions that were formed when I was young and not my fault. I need to stop and consciously see them to alter them.

THERAPIST: That's right. Does this approach seem like it might help to do that?

EMILY: Never been able to it before but this has helped. Having talked it through today, I can see it is in the detail and the breaking down, going over what happened. This is more of a challenge than just getting sympathy.

THERAPIST: Reflecting on what we have done, what do you think you could do in the future when faced with a difficult situation?

EMILY: It looks like it would be helpful to manage my time and organize my schedule so that if I know I have to do something stressful later, then beforehand I am not in a rush and do something relaxing to get myself in a good state of mind for it. It would also be helpful to prepare a concrete plan.

Inside the Therapist's Mind: Decision Points and Reflections with Emily

The vignette above illustrates again the value of asking in detail about context and using questions that seek more specific detail about what is happening to make the discussion of the ruminative events as rich as possible. It also shows the value of comparing two distinct events directly against each other to look for differences that could account for the variability in the rumination (see Chapter 6).

The discussion with Emily highlights that what happens before an episode of rumination can be important, and that this is potentially under environmental and behavioral control. Simple planning and contingency management such as making more time, building in breaks, or scheduling relaxing activities before and after anticipated difficult or stressful tasks shifts the context in a constructive way to limit rumination. This example indicates how changing environmental contingencies also includes changes in patterns of behavior and time management. It also demonstrates how concrete and focused preparation can be useful for difficult situations.

As is often the case, these environmental and behavioral changes are simple, straightforward, and, perhaps, even obvious. These approaches are usually easy to implement with a good chance of success. On the downside, patients often criticize themselves for not doing these things already. It is important for the therapist to normalize this and to note that while these changes can be easy to see once you look for them (and in hindsight), most of the time we are not looking for them. It also takes a concerted effort to put them into place, especially against habitual ways of behaving.

Reflect on your own personal experience. My guess is that some of these principles about organizing time, such as having a calm space before an anticipated difficult event, apply to your own life. I wonder how much you actually put them into action on a regular basis. I know that I don't always succeed in putting these principles into action myself. Many of us are aware of simple and sensible things we could do to improve our quality of life, without necessarily having implemented them. This dialogue illustrates how the therapist tackles this directly with Emily.

The dialogue also highlights the focus of Socratic questioning in RFCBT. Questions are focused on the utility of what Emily is doing, on highlighting what she can learn and what she can do next. In this discussion, possible changes in Emily's behavior that could make her more effective are identified by comparing events with different outcomes and summarized by the therapist, who then asks Emily to summarize them back to check what she has learned. Finally, the therapist asks her to think about how she could use them in the future. The questions serve to highlight new ways of doing things and to tie them closely to actions and plans.

Counterconditioning the Ruminative Habit: Generating If–Then Plans

Once patients have identified warning signs for rumination, a key step in RFCBT is to generate explicit If–Then plans to use when they notice these signs in order to interrupt and cut off rumination, and replace it with a more helpful strategy. Repeated practice of these plans is aimed at developing a new helpful habit instead of the rumination by counterconditioning an alternative response incompatible with rumination to the same cue.

These plans are called If–Then plans or contingency plans because they link the occurrence of one event (the warning sign or cue) with the enacting of a new behavior. These behaviors are simply explained to patients as If–Then plans because this describes the structure of the plan: "If I notice this warning sign, then I perform this alternative response instead of rumination." By spelling out the trigger and response, the If–Then plan makes the response clear and increases the likelihood of its being implemented. The logic of linking a planned action to the identified warning sign is that it helps the response to stick in the patient's mind and to be recalled in daily life. This approach draws on the experimental literature on implementation intentions (Gollwitzer, 1999; Gollwitzer & Sheeran, 2006; Holland, Aarts, & Langendam, 2006).

Goals and plans are much more likely to be implemented when they have an intention implementation, that is, an explicit statement that "I will do this at a specific time and place" (Gollwitzer, 1999; Gollwitzer & Sheeran, 2006; Holland et al., 2006). Such an explicit commitment with a clear time course reduces the risk of putting it off (e.g., "I will do it tomorrow") and reduces the risk that the plan will only be implemented when "I feel like it, or when I feel well enough to do it." When setting an action implementation intention, patients need to specify the how, when, whom, and where of responses leading to goal attainment. Thus, the patient links steps for goals and plans to environmental cues, rather than to feelings. This approach is particularly useful in reducing procrastination and the tendency for depressed patients to only do things when they feel well enough. This approach takes the initiation of a plan away from feelings and links it to more stable factors, such as completing another task, a particular place, or a particular time.

For example, patients can be encouraged to make plans that take the form "If situation X is encountered, then I will perform behavior Y." By making plans linked to the environment, patients become more consistent, and they begin to assert some control over what they do, rather than letting feelings dictate. Furthermore, there is evidence that making the If–Then plan can increase automaticity and reduce the mental effort required to implement the plan (Gollwitzer, 1999; Gollwitzer & Sheeran, 2006; Holland et al., 2006). For all these reasons, RFCBT uses If–Then plans as the simplest and most memorable way to make contingency plans to replace rumination. Implementation intentions lead to better action initiation (Brandstätter, Lengfelder, & Gollwitzer, 2001).

As well as directly stating how, when, and where plans will be executed, it can also be useful for patients to be coached to ask themselves "How will

I get started?" and "How will I stay on task?" Once the concept of action planning is introduced, it should be linked up to other aspects of therapy, especially homework.

These contingency plans are similar to and parallel the approach within BA (Addis & Martell, 2004; Martell et al., 2001), which refers to identifying TRAPS (Trigger Response Avoidance Patterns) and shifting out of these traps to get back on TRAC (Trigger Response Alternative Coping). Both RFCBT and BA share the idea of spotting a warning sign or trigger—the antecedent—to the unwanted target behavior, which then produces a response (e.g., sad mood), which is then followed by an avoidant response (e.g., withdrawal, rumination). Both BA and RFCBT share the idea of replacing the avoidant response with a functional and adaptive alternative behavior. In this way, If–Then plans and going from TRAP to TRAC are conceptually equivalent. Both can be used with patients to explain the process. The main difference between RFCBT and BA is that RFCBT emphasizes that the unwanted rumination and avoidance are a habit, the associated importance of the cue as automatically triggering the rumination, and the need for repeated practice of the alternative incompatible response to produce lasting change. RFCBT has also framed these contingency plans as If–Then plans to garner the evidence-based benefit of implementation intentions.

These plans need to be drawn up in concrete detail using the SMART mnemonic. Plans will work best if they build from the FA; alternative strategies that in the patient's own experience have shifted rumination into more adaptive thinking or shortened the duration of rumination are good for If–Then plans. In this way, contingency plans build on the patient's own experience and make his or her own strategies more effective and more systematic.

An experimental approach is also taken to the generation of contingency If–Then plans: each strategy is tried out to test how helpful it is. The recommended steps are to review what is learned from the FA, try out new strategies in the session as behavioral experiments, and then build these strategies into plans to be followed each week. A contingency plan may have several steps, including environmental changes, behavioral changes, and cognitive changes.

The most commonly used interventions within contingency plans are (1) applied relaxation, (2) problem solving, (3) visualizations and imagery including absorption and compassion, (4) shifting thinking styles, most typically becoming more concrete, and (5) approach behaviors. For example, contingency plans can involve using absorption-process-focused imagery to counteract the rumination. Each of these interventions will be reviewed in more detail in this chapter or in the following chapters on concreteness training (Chapter 9), absorption training (Chapter 10), or compassion training (Chapter 11). It is important to recognize that many of these approaches overlap, which suggests that we can intervene at multiple points with a single intervention.

Contingency plans draw on what the FA suggests will be most helpful for any individual patient. Hence, the alternative response to be used will be completely idiosyncratic from patient to patient. There is no standard correct alternative behavior. Contingency plans can be as simple as "When I notice the warning signs for rumination, I will phone my friend John or my friend Sue for a chat." Furthermore, the plans are adjusted in the light of empirical testing and experience. One set of strategies may work very well for one patient but not for another. If a strategy is routinely implemented for several weeks without any change in rumination or mood, a new strategy may be required.

Plans are drawn up explicitly and concretely with patients. The logic of the plan is shared with the patient as it is set up. This follows naturally from the FA. In effect, through FA, the therapist discusses with the patient that there are particular antecedents to his unhelpful behavior, and identifies potential helpful alternatives. The If–Then plan constitutes the formal planning for how to systematically use an identified alternative in response to the warning sign.

For example, for Emily, the therapist might say something like:

"We have learned from talking through several examples that your rumination is often triggered when you get tense and irritable and notice yourself getting hot. You also talk about your mind going foggy. It sounds like finding a way to reduce that tension and helping to keep your mind clear might be a useful first step to manage things better. Looking back, we can see that you coped better at times when you were less stressed. On this basis, practicing techniques that reduce tension and stress might be a good way to reduce your rumination. Progressive muscle relaxation is a good way to do that. It will be particularly useful if you can pair in your mind experiencing the feeling of tension with then performing the relaxation exercise. To achieve this, we make an If–Then plan, which is a verbal way of making the link 'If I notice I am getting tense, then I will listen to my relaxation exercise.' What do you think?"

Practice, Practice, Practice!

Because the contingency plan is designed as an alternative to replace an unhelpful habit, it will require many rehearsals and much repeated practice to become fully established and to have its maximum effect. The therapist stresses the importance of repeated practice to patients, linking this to the development of a habit. It helps to note that it is normal to not be able to practice the new response every single time because the old habit is well established, but that every time the new response is practiced, it strengthens the new habit.

It is good to practice the new approach or technique in the therapy session to check that the patient knows how to do it. Audio-recording the exercise so that the patient has a structured and guided version of the technique to practice again and again for homework also helps. I recommend practicing the new approach daily, and whenever the linked warning sign occurs.

It is also useful to directly practice in session the use of the contingency plan in response to the warning sign to strengthen this association, make it more likely that the alternative response will be cued by the warning sign, and improve the generalizability of the plan into the real world. This is best done by exposing the patient to the identified cue, either in vivo or in imagery. For example, if the warning sign for rumination is beginning to get irritated, the therapist asks the patient to recall as vividly as possible a recent memory of feeling irritated to induce irritation and bring some of that experience "live" into the session. Once the patient is in touch with that experience and reporting and displaying some irritation, then the new alternative response is practiced. In this way, the patient directly and experientially learns to do something different in response to the warning sign. Multiple practices of this pairing are a good idea, working up through an exposure hierarchy starting with situations that induce mild irritation and are less serious, and, with each success, moving to the next level of the hierarchy. It is possible to practice several repetitions in a single therapy session this way.

How to Choose the Target Trigger: The "If"

There is no hard-and-fast rule to choosing the antecedent or warning sign for the contingency plan. FA will reveal one or more cues that are hypothesized to trigger the rumination (or any target behavior) such as emotions, thoughts, memories, or physical sensations. Any cue frequently associated with rumination and found to be contingent with it (i.e., not occurring when rumination does not occur; occurring only when rumination tends to occur) is a good selection for the warning sign, the "If" in the If–Then plan. Of course, there may be several steps in the antecedent chain with several possible antecedents following each other in a sequence. For example, a patient sees a photograph, which reminds her of a sad memory, which makes her feel sad, which is followed by thinking "Why me?"—all coming before the bout of rumination. It is good practice when identifying antecedents to try and track back early in the chain because it will be easier to block and interrupt the rumination the earlier the sequence is broken. On the other hand, events earlier in the chain may be harder for the patient to spot, as they may be more subtle and less directly linked to the rumination. Moreover, earlier steps may not occur frequently or not always be linked with rumination, whereas steps later in the chain may be more closely linked to rumination and occur more frequently. It is useful to look for antecedents that are part of a "final common pathway" into the target behavior such as rumination. For example, whereas seeing an upsetting picture does not always trigger rumination, thinking "Why me?" probably does. Furthermore, a range of other situations may set off the "Why me?" response. Pragmatically, the best antecedent is easily noticed by the patient and is reasonably frequent. In sum, the therapist looks for an antecedent that comes early enough to easily break the sequence, is late enough to be a frequent event, is easily noticed by the patient, and is part of a final common pathway. Whatever it is, the warning sign needs to be specified in as much concrete detail as possible.

How to Select the Alternative Behavior for the Contingency: The "Then"

Almost any behavior within the cognitive-behavioral repertoire is a potential alternative behavior to use for the "Then" part of the If–Then plan. The selection of the behavior reflects the FA and the formulation that arises from the FA. The chosen behavior is selected to be incompatible with rumination and to address its hypothesized function. It needs to be useful in shifting away from rumination and moving to a constructive outcome. When selecting a possible alternative behavior, we look for the "path of least resistance"—an alternative behavior that is going to be incompatible with rumination and has the greatest chance of sticking as a habit in response to the warning sign. It is of no value to choose a new behavior that does not counter the rumination or itself acts as a form of unhelpful avoidance, hence the importance of examining the utility and function of the alternative response. Equally, it is of no value to choose a behavior that strongly interrupts or counters rumination but that the patient cannot use repeatedly in daily life and that cannot easily become a habit.

There are a number of principles that help to select a particular technique to use.

Function and Formulation

We want to select an approach that is consistent with the formulation of the rumination and that acts counter to the rumination. Where possible, we also want the alternative behavior to serve the same positive functions as the rumination so that we can replace rumination with a more helpful behavior that performs the same function. Such functional equivalence makes it more likely that the new behavior will stick, be repeated, and become maintained. The patient is more likely to engage in the behavior if she feels that it addresses an important personal concern. Moreover, if the identified function was reinforcing the rumination, any alternative behavior needs to be reinforced at least as much in order to replace the rumination, even when the patient is not consciously aware of the function of rumination. For example, if rumination appears to reduce anger and this seems to be reinforcing the rumination, and controlling anger is important to the patient, giving the patient an alternative to rumination that does not address anger is unlikely to generate much enthusiasm or practice. In this situation, an alternative action that helps to reduce anger, such as relaxation or compassion, is indicated, and is more likely to provide a viable alternative to rumination.

Experiential Evidence

Is there evidence for the usefulness of the strategy from the patient's own experience? Ideally, we want to use a treatment approach that fits with what the patient has already reported in the FA and one for which the patient's own experience offers evidence that it works. If we have tried a behavioral experiment or an experiential exercise and it has confirmed that the strategy is useful, this is even better. The more evidence and pilot data we have of the usefulness of this approach for the particular patient, the more confident we are in selecting this strategy. We want a patient to be positive and motivated to try a new approach. This is best accomplished when the patient has already tried the approach and found it to be beneficial in the treatment session. Such a positive experience makes it more likely that the patient will implement the approach and gain benefit from it. It also means that we know this approach has the potential to work. For this reason, a common sequence in RFCBT is to (1) identify a possible treatment approach from reviewing the patient's experience; (2) try out the suggested technique as an experiment or experiential exercise together in the session; and (3) if it is successful, plan for the patient to practice it further in daily life as part of his homework.

Repertoire

Is the behavior required for the technique already in the patient's repertoire? We want the behavior to be adopted easily. Selecting behavior that the patient can already do and that does not require new learning helps with this. If it is already in her repertoire, we know that she can do it, and we don't need to do much further training. It also helps to validate and engage the patient.

Practical and Easy

Is the treatment strategy practical and easy to use? We want to make sure that any intervention fits the circumstances of the patient and there are not practical hurdles to its delivery. For example, we want to make sure that a planned activity is not too expensive or time-consuming, and this it is possible on a practical level (e.g., not beyond the patient's physical ability). We want the new alternative behavior to be as easy to perform as possible. Simpler plans are better than complex plans. Likewise, the more the alternative response can be spelled out in concrete and specific terms (what, where, when, how, who) and broken down into smaller steps the better. Is the response one that can be repeated again and again? To successfully train a new habit, the alternative response will need to repeated and rehearsed many times. If the chosen response is hard to repeat because it is too tiring, too long, or only usable in a limited set of circumstances, it won't be a good alternative.

Closeness to the Warning Sign

The goal is for the new response to be closely paired to the existing cues for rumination. This will be easier if the alternative response occurs naturally after the warning sign itself or is a response that has some ecological closeness and association with the warning sign. This will make it easier to learn the association. Completely arbitrary alternatives will be harder to learn. For example, if the warning sign is an internal physical sensation such as tension, then an alternative response that involves awareness and focus on such physical sensations, such as relaxation, will have a natural linkage. If the warning sign is a cognitive response such as a "why" question, then another cognitive response, for example, a "how" question, provides a more natural fit.

Some Common Alternative Behaviors for Contingency Plans

Applied Relaxation

An important early intervention in some treatments for worry (Borkovec & Newman, 1998) is teaching applied relaxation, which patients use with self-monitoring as a strategy to disrupt the loop of worrisome thinking. Relaxation has the advantage of reducing tension and anxiety, which are often found in these patients. Furthermore, it is easily learned, so that relaxation has the potential to provide an early positive experience of successfully coping with difficulties and reducing symptoms. Since anxiety and physiological arousal tend to feed into more worry and rumination, reducing tension and anxiety can reduce worry and rumination. Furthermore, by encouraging patients to focus on physical sensations and by using imagery techniques, relaxation acts as a counter to rumination and breaks the loop of rumination. Relaxation is also used to facilitate imagery work, so learning to relax may support later elements of RFCBT. We have encouraging evidence that teaching patients with depression to relax in response to their warning signs is an effective treatment for depression symptoms in its own right (Watkins et al., 2012). It is stressed that the applied relaxation needs to be practiced regularly (twice-daily practice of progressive relaxation/breathing) so that patients can learn to become faster and more efficient at relaxation.

The form of applied relaxation used is progressive muscle relaxation, with slowed breathing and some use of relaxing imagery (for a detailed script, see the section on applied relaxation in Hawton, Salkovskis, Kirk, & Clark, 1989). This approach involves the patient paying attention to different muscles through the body, working down from the head to the feet, deliberately tensing and holding tight each muscle and then releasing and relaxing it, with instructions from the therapist or an audio-recorded exercise. The instructions emphasize that the patient is becoming calmer and more relaxed as he or she completes the exercise. The exercise involves slowing down breathing, breathing deeply from the diaphragm, and having longer exhales than inhales. All of these physical actions serve to reduce tension and physiological arousal in the body, slowing breathing and heart rate. Thus, relaxation can be a useful alternative response when the warning sign of rumination is tension or stress, and a good functional substitute for rumination designed to control feelings.

It is useful to practice relaxation in a therapy session and then for patients to practice at home using a recording of the session. For further practice, a brief 5-minute relaxation could be used at the beginning of each session. As patients become better at relaxing, the therapist can make an analogy between letting go of tension and letting go of thoughts and feelings. Relaxation is then used as a model for a wider strategy to let go of concerns and worries. Once the patient has become good at inducing a state of relaxation, he or she can then practice more regularly using the relaxation in response to the warning signs for rumination.

Problem Solving

Rumination often starts as an attempt at problem solving, which is hijacked by thoughts about the causes and consequences of problems. Thus, teaching patients more explicit problem-solving strategies is often useful. The concreteness training approach improves problem solving and includes a problem-solving element (see Chapter 9).

In addition, the therapist can use the explicit problem-solving therapy format of D'Zurilla and Nezu (1999), which features the following steps:

1. Assess and improve problem orientation.
2. Assess and improve problem definition.

3. Assess and improve generation of alternatives.
4. Assess and improve solution implementation.

Problem orientation refers to the attitude the patient has to solving a problem—whether he has an optimistic or pessimistic approach to solving the problem and whether he believes solving the problem is within his ability or not. Problem definition refers to how the problem is described and conceptualized. Generation of alternatives refers to the ability to think of different ways of tackling the solution. Solution implementation is the putting into action of any plans and then evaluating and refining them in the light of what happens.

Problem-solving therapy provides training in whichever of these areas may be deficient. The therapist adapts this approach to fit with FA by using the ABC and CUDOS analyses to look at the patient's attempts at problem solving and determine where they become hijacked by rumination. Detailed analysis of attempts at problem solving, comparing successful attempts versus attempts that became stuck in rumination, will help to indicate where the process is going wrong.

For many depressed ruminators, the impairments in problem solving are a consequence of their overgeneralization and unhelpful abstract thinking style (e.g., asking, "Why did this happen to me?" or "What does this mean?" rather than asking, "How can I do something about this?"; "What can I do now to make things better?"). This style of thinking often manifests itself in difficulties with problem definition. The problem ends up being defined too abstractly, with a focus on evaluations and comparisons. Such an abstract, overly general style of thinking is also likely to cause difficulties in generating alternative plans of action. For this reason, concreteness training is often a useful alternative if the rumination appears to be thwarted problem solving.

For negative problem orientation, the therapist can use visualization of success and positive self-talk to increase positive orientation (see imagery rehearsal of plans in Chapter 9). For poor problem definition, the therapist trains the patient to ask "What is the problem?" and to seek all the facts. Problem definition strongly overlaps with goal setting: in both, patients need to learn to identify obstacles and to set realistic goals for problem definition. Thus, the section on SMART goal setting (see Chapter 5) is relevant to problem definition. Shifts to more helpful styles of thinking (e.g., "how" versus "why" thinking) can also help (see Chapter 9).

For poor generation of alternatives, the therapist coaches the patient in brainstorming and deferment of judgment. For example, patients are encouraged to think of as many uses for a brick as possible and told not to rule out any possibilities and not to judge any options they generate. FA, in which effective versus ineffective attempts at problem solving are compared, helps to generate possible alternatives.

For poor decision making, the therapist teaches patients to use likelihood estimates and cost–benefit analysis to improve their decisions. For example, patients are encouraged to look at the potential advantages and disadvantages, both short-term and long-term, to themselves and to others, for each potential solution, as well as the likelihood of the solution working successfully. This approach naturally builds from the functional philosophy of RFCBT.

Replacing Avoidance Behaviors with Approach Behaviors

When the formulation suggests that the function of rumination is to avoid an undesired outcome, avoid an unwanted self, or motivate the self, planning an approach behavior is often an effective alternative and counter to rumination (see Table 7.1. for common avoidance behaviors). The goal served by the rumination is recast and reframed collaboratively with the patient to change it from one of avoidance ("to avoid being selfish," "to prevent bad things from happening") to one of approach and promotion ("to become a more thoughtful person," "to promote good things"). This switch is helpful in reducing avoidance and increases the likelihood of the patient being in contact with reward and positive reinforcement. It also brings the patient more into contact with the world, improving his or her chances of learning new things. Furthermore, progress on approach goals is typically easier to notice than on avoidance goals (see Table 7.2 for common approach behaviors).

This reframing suggests alternative behaviors for the patient to try, for example:

"Rather than trying to prevent yourself from being arrogant by beating yourself up over and over again in your ruminations, I wonder if an alternative way to achieve the same goal is to work on how you can be a nicer person. What could you do to develop as a nicer person? What would you be doing differently?"

When planning and increasing approach behaviors, the therapist explicitly discusses and frames the approach behavior as an alternative to the rumination and avoidance, so that the patient is encouraged to use the approach behavior as an alternative strategy when faced with problems or when exposed to the triggers for rumination. In this way, increasing approach behavior is tied in with self-monitoring and the FA approach. Approach behaviors are best introduced as behavioral experiments, as ways of testing things out directly rather than trying to work things out in the head. Predictions can be explicitly set up and then tested out (e.g., "What do you think will happen when you try this?"; "How can we define what you think will happen?").

TABLE 7.1. Common Avoidance Behaviors

- Rumination
- Staying in bed
- Staying at home
- Putting off jobs
- Avoiding people
- Avoiding promotion at work
- Avoiding evaluation, judgment by others (e.g., tests, exams, interviews)
- Cognitive avoidance, including abstract thinking
- Avoiding conflict
- Avoiding risk, challenge, and responsibility
- Distraction
- Analyzing events over and over for certainty and control
- Reassurance seeking
- Complaining
- Emotional avoidance (blocking, suppressing)

The approach behavior is more likely to be successful if it is a genuine functional alternative to the unwanted rumination or avoidance and addresses the same concerns. For example, a patient who ruminated to avoid getting angry may learn relaxation to control physiological arousal, followed by graded exposure with other people to practice not losing his temper. An alternative approach behavior here is assertiveness.

Make behavioral plans as specific and concrete as possible (using SMART again). It is essential to specify the number of times each week, the specific times for the plan, and any possible obstacles, as well as to rehearse ways around these obstacles.

An important aspect of approach behaviors is encouraging patients to attend to experience. The therapist instructs the patient to focus on and be aware of all sensations (colors, shapes, sounds, smells, textures) during an activity, such as going for a walk or doing a chore, as a means to temporarily reduce rumination. Asking patients how much they can remember of the

TABLE 7.2. Common Approach Behaviors

- Direct action
- Asking people for help and support
- Being assertive
- Taking risks
- Trying new things
- Making decisions and plans
- Taking responsibility
- Expressing feelings to others
- Social contact
- Activity scheduling—pleasure and mastery
- Testing things out by trial and error in the world
- Problem solving
- Learning and developing skills
- Allowing oneself to experience feelings
- Staying with details of memories

sights, sounds, smells, and other sensory experience will provide clues as to how much they were really involved in what they were doing. An alternative is to ask patients to spend a few minutes trying to notice all the different shapes and shades of color in the environment or to notice how many different sounds they can hear. Patients can use these questions on their own as a way to engage with external stimuli during rumination. This approach is further developed and elaborated in Chapter 10.

When increasing activities, it is useful to focus on positive, enjoyable activities and on keeping plans simple. Look out for task-interfering thoughts and the consequences of these thoughts; explicitly identify negative predictions and test them out.

Since a patient who ruminates is likely to be concerned about evaluating her performance and how she is coming across, the therapist can usefully point out that any plans are not about testing her and not about seeing what she can do, but are rather further opportunities to see what happens when she does things differently. For example, the therapist can say, "It's not a test of you; it's a test of the activity and whether or not it will prove helpful in managing your depression."

Approach behaviors can also be part of an If–Then plan or integrated into managing environmental and behavioral contingencies. For example, building in more absorbing activities may be one way to reduce the general likelihood of rumination. For Ruth, the quiet time in the evening after she has put her children to bed was identified as a risk period for rumination. Scheduling in different approach activities here changes the environment to reduce rumination.

CHAPTER 8

Practice at Developing Interventions

Addressing Difficulties and Hurdles

To provide practice at developing interventions from FA, this chapter provides a new case summary (Peter) and examples from completed Antecedent–Behavior–Consequence (ABC) Forms. This provides the background for thinking through the formulation for Peter and considering alternative treatment possibilities. Alternative options for formulation and treatment are summarized at the end of the chapter. Common difficulties and ways to address them are then reviewed.

Working through an RFCBT Formulation

Case Example: Peter

Peter is a 35-year-old married man with no children. He works full-time in an office as a public service administrator. His relationship with his wife is good. He reports a long history of chronic depression and anxiety. Current symptoms are moderately high (BDI = 30). He recognizes that he ruminates a lot and that this is a problem. He talks about always analyzing what he is doing and how he finds himself easily getting stuck in overthinking. In the initial therapy sessions, Peter and his therapist reached a collaborative agreement that rumination is a key difficulty and a habit, and they agreed to work on it.

Typical contents of Peter's ruminative bouts include "Why are people acting like this?"; "What does this mean?"; "Why did they do that?"; "Why do I feel like that?"; "What did he/she mean by that?"; "What will he/she do next?"; "Why did he/she say that?"; "Why did that difficult thing happen?"; "Why do I have thoughts like this?"

His rumination is often triggered by interactions with other people, particularly when there is some ambiguity and uncertainty about what the other person does or means, for example, when a person says something ambiguous, when he reads an e-mail and isn't sure about the tone, or when he is summoned to a meeting. Rumination increases before and after such interactions. He also ruminates a lot about past difficulties, such as the ends of relationships or things he regrets. He is often tired at work and feels he is often putting on a front with people.

Warning signs for his rumination involve physical sensations like feeling tense or hot, feeling self-conscious, and a narrowing of his attention to focus on his concerns. Peter describes himself as someone who is very rational and logical, who likes to understand and make sense of things. He considers himself to be a scientific and analytical kind of person who is good at working things out. He used to be involved in more physical and social activities when he felt better—he enjoyed cross-country running and kayaking with friends in the countryside. He has stopped doing these activities since his depression has become worse.

His past history includes a period of bullying at school, when he became quite self-conscious. He started thinking a lot about how he was coming across to other people and trying to work out what might set off the bullying and how to avoid being bullied. He described himself as quite an academic boy who focused on his studies.

In the early treatment sessions, the therapist reviewed several examples of rumination with Peter, which are summarized in two Antecedent–Behavior–Consequence (ABC) Forms (see Figures 8.1 and 8.2). Together, Peter and the therapist also reviewed a situation when he didn't ruminate as badly, summarized in Table 8.1. See the box on page 166 for guidance on how to formulate Peter's case and develop treatment plans, and then compare them with the discussion that follows.

Antecedent	What precedes B? What triggers B: event, feeling, thought, person, place, time, activity? Determine context: where?, when?, who?, what?, how?
	An open-plan office, sitting at desk, e-mail appears from boss setting a meeting for next day, initial thoughts include "I wonder what this meeting is about."; "What could my boss want?"; mild anxiety and apprehension, tension.
Behavior	What you did: the target behavior to understand, and increase or decrease. Provide details on how the behavior occurs (e.g., content and style of rumination).
	Starts off thinking about the meeting: "What could the meeting be about? What does my boss want? What does this mean? Have I done anything wrong? What if I am in trouble? What if I make a fool of myself in the meeting? Why has he called a meeting? What will happen in the meeting? Why does he want to see me? Why is he acting like this? What is he thinking?" Reviewing recent meetings and imagining different outcomes.
Consequence	What is the consequence of B—positive/negative, short-term/long-term, for self, for others—on valued goals? What effect does it have? What does it increase/decrease? What are its pros/cons? What does it avoid? What would happen if you didn't do B? What is the effect of not doing B? What would you be doing instead? What has the consequence of B been in the past?
	Hard to concentrate on other tasks, ruminates for several hours, anxious but a bit better prepared for the meeting. Response to "What does this avoid?"; "What would happen if I didn't think like this?" is "I need to understand what is going on and other people, I want to feel prepared to make sure it goes well."

FIGURE 8.1. Example 1 of a completed Antecedent–Behavior–Consequence (ABC) form for Peter.

Antecedent	What precedes B? What triggers B: event, feeling, thought, person, place, time, activity? Determine context: where?, when?, who?, what?, how?
	A bit tense waiting for meeting with boss and wondering what will happen, watching TV in lounge at home, program on place I went on vacation with ex-girlfriend before I got married, brings up memories of that vacation, which leads to memories of end of relationship. Attention narrowing inward.
Behavior	What you did: the target behavior to understand, and increase or decrease. Provide details on how the behavior occurs (e.g., content and style of rumination).
	Rumination about end of relationship, intrusive memories about final days and upsetting memory of when girlfriend said it was over. "Why did this relationship end?"; "Why did she end it?"; "What does this mean about me?"; "Why didn't it work out?" These thoughts make me anxious and tense, but then lead into other thoughts like "Why am I thinking about this now?"
Consequence	What is the consequence of B—positive/negative, short-term/long-term, for self, for others—on valued goals? What effect does it have? What does it increase/decrease? What are its pros/cons? What does it avoid? What would happen if you didn't do B? What is the effect of not doing B? What would you be doing instead? What has the consequence of B been in the past?
	Feels anxious, feels guilty and ashamed. If I didn't think it through and work out what happened, I might repeat same mistakes again. In past, sometimes this kind of thinking has made me feel like it prevents bad things from happening.

FIGURE 8.2. Example 2 of a completed Antecedent–Behavior–Consequence (ABC) form for Peter.

TABLE 8.1. Comparing Variability in the Duration and Outcome of Peter's Responses

What: E-mail circulated from colleagues that was a somewhat ambiguous review with judgments on prior jobs, including those Peter was involved in. Did not ruminate and felt more positive.

Where: At work.

When: First thing in the morning.

How: Wondered what it might mean with some initial anxiety, but then reminded self of recent positive feedback from colleagues and clients. Another colleague involved was in the office, and Peter asked him what he made of it, and he expressed the view that it was not important.

Who: Another colleague present.

Self-Test: Planning Treatment Options for Peter

Look at the information in Figures 8.1 and 8.2 and Table 8.1 and begin to map out a formulation and potential treatment interventions for Peter. The following questions are useful to guide your formulation and treatment planning as a therapist:

- What comes before Peter's rumination?
- What are common and frequent antecedents to the rumination?
- Does this suggest possible changes in environment or patient behavior to reduce cueing of rumination?
- What follows the rumination?
- What are its short-term effects and consequences?
- What are its longer-term effects and consequences?
- How might the rumination have developed?
- How might this knowledge contribute to the rationale given to Peter?
- What does this suggest about possible functions of the rumination?
- How can I further test this working hypothesis?
- What other information do I need?
- What do I need to check in more detail when discussing specific examples?
- What are possible external environmental moderators that influence the frequency, duration, or usefulness of Peter's rumination?
- What are possible behavioral or mental state moderators within Peter that influence the frequency, duration, or usefulness of his rumination?
- What might be informative and therapeutically useful behavioral experiments to do in session?
- What next steps might be possibilities for interventions?
- What monitoring might be useful for Peter?
- What changes in environment and routines might interrupt the cues to rumination?
- What might be good alternative behaviors for Peter to practice within an If–Then plan?

Reflections on Peter: Considering the Formulation and Possible Treatment Options

• *What comes before the rumination? What are common and frequent antecedents to his rumination?* Feeling tense, attention narrowing, asking "why" questions, situations where Peter is concerned about what other people might think about him; uncertainty and ambiguity, particularly in social situations.

• *Does this suggest possible changes in environment or patient behavior to reduce cueing of rumination?* There are no obvious environmental cues to remove that would not be counterproductive. We would not want to reduce rumination by having him avoid all situations. It may be possible to remove reminders to some past upsetting events, although these may not be prominent. There may be scope for Peter to manage his contingencies better with respect to stress, for example, building in times to calm down and relax, which would reduce his tension and thereby reduce rumination.

• *What follows the rumination? What are its short-term effects and consequences?* Poor concentration, sometimes more anxiety, sometimes less anxiety, feels more prepared for situations. Peter wants to understand and feel ready for situations. He feels guilty and ashamed. Sometimes it feels as if thinking things through helps to prevent bad things from happening.

• *What are its longer-term effects and consequences?* His depression has gotten worse over time and he is doing less and less (i.e., reducing physical and social activity).

• *How might the rumination have developed?* It may have developed as a consequence of childhood bullying and his attempt to understand what was happening and to prevent it by thinking about it over and over.

• *How might this knowledge contribute to the rationale given to Peter?* It helps to give a reason why his tendency to dwell on ambiguity and uncertainty has developed. This made sense when he was being bullied to help him try and stay out of trouble, and it was overlearned so it is now a habit that occurs in a range of situations. Peter may also have learned that logical analysis was successful in addressing academic problems, developing a habit for thinking things through, but without realizing that such abstract thinking may not work so well for emotional difficulties.

• *What does this suggest about possible functions of the rumination?* There are several possible functions that are not mutually exclusive:

1. Trying to understand why unwanted events happen and why people act the way they do, in order to better understand and avoid problems and to avoid making mistakes again. This is consistent with the high frequency of questions focused on causes and meanings ("why?"). These questions may be asked again and again even when

they fail to derive a conclusive answer. Indeed, if gaining understanding is very important, Peter may redouble his attempts at asking himself these questions because they are not working ("I am not getting an answer, so I need to try harder").

2. Preparation for situations so that he is not caught off guard when they happen and is ready for negative events. This is a form of preempting what could happen by anticipating it.

3. Underpinning (1) there may also be a function of trying to be certain about things before doing them to avoid things going wrong.

4. There is a lot of thinking in his head rather than doing in the world, so there may be a function of avoiding getting into trouble with other people by not interacting with them.

• *How can I further test these working hypotheses?* These hypotheses can be tested by looking at further examples and seeing if the same patterns emerge, sharing the working formulation with Peter and checking it with him, and by relevant behavioral experiments. In particular, the therapist could ask about examples of situations where he felt he lacked understanding or preparation for events to see if this was associated with increased rumination. In contrast, it would be useful to see if when he gained understanding or a sense of preparation, this reduced rumination. Comparing such situations may suggest environmental and behavioral factors that influence how much he gains understanding or becomes prepared, which could feed into improved plans.

• *What other information do I need?* It would be helpful to determine whether his current strategies work well in terms of gaining understanding and becoming prepared. How well does rumination work to gain understanding of his emotions or other people's responses? This raises the possibility that this strategy is not that successful, leading the therapist and Peter to consider alternatives that may work better. The therapist could also examine the goals that underlie Peter's need for understanding and preparedness. What would happen if Peter could not understand something? What would happen if he were able to understand something? What would he do then? For example, the therapist might ask, "If you were able to understand everything about why this happened, what would it allow you to do?" or "What could you do if you understood things better than you do now?" or "How would gaining understanding improve this situation for you?" With these questions, the therapist explores the potential underlying function behind Peter's seeking understanding or being prepared. One hypothesis is that this is about gaining certainty or control. There may be a hierarchy of functions, and the therapist wants to establish which function is critical. This clarification will improve the formulation. It also provides a point of leverage for later change. If Peter's search for understanding is about gaining control, then therapy can target gaining control without necessarily increasing understanding. Interventions can work to improve Peter's control without addressing greater understanding. For example, the therapist can say, "Peter, we have seen that your attempts at gaining understanding sometimes get you into distressing rumination and don't always result in answering your questions. Do you need better understanding to gain more control over a situation? What can you do to fix a situation without understanding it fully?" This line of inquiry leads into more direct engagement with the world and turns Peter toward approach behaviors.

Similarly, the therapist can examine the value of trying to gain understanding, control, and certainty, and what is a useful and adaptive goal to seek on these dimensions. For example, having more understanding, control, and certainty will probably increase safety and reduce the risk of bad things happening. However, it is not possible to achieve perfect understanding, control, and certainty, and in some situations, it may not even be possible to achieve high levels of understanding, control, and certainty. Moreover, there may be a point of diminishing returns where increasing understanding or increasing control (or attempts to do so) do not actually lead to better plans, reduced risk, or increased safety. Having realistic expectations of the ability to gain these outcomes is adaptive.

It would be helpful to determine Peter's views on these issues, and to explore the idea that there may only be a limited amount of understanding, control, and certainty that can be achieved. His personal experience can be reviewed to examine what level of understanding, control, and certainty is realistic and useful to aspire to, that is to analyze the functional utility of continuing to seek understanding. This is where the concept of having a "good enough" outcome, such as a reasonable level of understanding or control, is helpful. This can be compared to needing to meet a 100% or perfect standard. The relative advantages and disadvantages (i.e., usefulness) of different standards can be reviewed. Peter might find it helpful to recognize that when he keeps trying to get more and more understanding, there comes a point when he is putting in a lot of time and energy without gaining any further incremental advantage. Looking at rules of thumb to decide whether his repeated thinking helps can be an effective approach, such as asking whether this continued thinking is adding value, whether Peter is asking unanswerable questions, and asking whether the thinking is leading to plans or actions.

• *What do I need to check in more detail when discussing specific examples?* It would be useful to explore the issues noted above. We don't have much sense of the environmental moderators of his rumination, so it would be good to ask more about this external context in relation to his rumination.

• *What are possible external environmental moderators that influence the frequency, duration, or usefulness of his rumination?* We have not learned much about environmental moderators that influence Peter's rumination, other than to see that ambiguous and uncertain situations increase rumination, while resolution of that uncertainty reduces rumination, for example, when a colleague said that a message was not important. It is possible that Peter could change his behavioral approaches to reduce the likelihood of uncertainty, for example, by engaging more with people rather than thinking things through on his own.

• *What are possible behavioral or mental state moderators within Peter that influence the frequency, duration, or usefulness of his rumination?* Talking to other people about a situation rather than rehashing it in his head seems useful to reduce rumination. Reminding himself of times when things went well seems useful when faced with ambiguity. There seems to be value in shifting his focus of attention externally to gather new information rather than trying to analyze the same information internally.

• *What might be informative and therapeutically useful behavioral experiments to do in session?* One option is to test in a behavioral experiment the idea of asking questions of others rather than of himself, although this may work better out of session, for example, by setting up an experiment for him to compare the two approaches (asking himself vs. asking others) and test their different consequences in everyday settings. A behavioral experiment to examine whether it is possible to respond usefully to a difficult situation by moving directly to plans without seeking understanding may be useful (e.g., by comparing problem solving to analyzing the situation to understand its causes, or by comparing "how" versus "why" manipulations). Because Peter's warning signs include increased tension and attention narrowing, the therapist and Peter could experiment to see if relaxation is a useful coping strategy that reduces his tension and makes him feel more in control.

• *What monitoring might be useful for Peter?* It might be helpful for Peter to monitor ratings of understanding, preparedness, certainty, and control as part of a diary form linked to rumination to generate more detailed information and examine the relationships between these states and rumination. This could establish whether understanding and control improve following rumination, testing its possible functions. The therapist could encourage him to play closer attention to his tension response to determine the earliest possible warning sign.

• *What changes in environment and routines might interrupt the cues to rumination?* The therapist needs to determine if there are particular places and times where Peter tends to ruminate when he is reflecting on what has happened. If there are particular patterns, these provide routines that can be interrupted. Looking at pacing his daily activities, doing one thing at a time, and building in times to relax may improve his routines to reduce rumination.

- *What might be good alternative behaviors for him to practice within an If–Then plan?* There are multiple options for If–Then plans:

1. There could be an If–Then plan linking the warning sign of tension to the alternative response of relaxation. Relaxation is a straight-forward and easy alternative that matches well with feeling tense. However, it is not clear that relaxation addresses the potential functions maintaining Peter's rumination.

2. The therapist could encourage Peter to shift away from thinking about the causes and meanings of events toward finding ways to address them. This may emerge as a good choice if the discussion of understanding indicates that always seeking understanding is not the most helpful approach, and if an experiential exercise in session indicates the value of asking concrete "how?" questions instead of abstract "why" questions (see Chapter 9). The If–Then plan could then be "If I notice I am beginning to ask 'why' questions, I will shift to asking more helpful 'how' questions."

3. Building on the comparison of a situation where Peter responded better to an ambiguous situation by recalling a positive memory, the therapist and Peter could collaboratively develop a plan in which Peter looks out for warning signs of feeling uncertain and then deliberately reminds himself of similar situations that have turned out OK. To do this, Peter and the therapist will need to operationalize his warning signs for uncertainty so that Peter can clearly and precisely spot them. The therapist may also work with Peter to identify specific positive memories in advance for Peter to focus on in detail, to make it easier for him to implement this strategy.

4. Peter spends a lot of time analyzing situations and asking himself questions about what happened to try and make sense of these situations. It is easy for him to get stuck in this thinking. In one example, he found that asking someone else about the situation helped to resolve it. A sensible plan might then involve moving from rumina-tive avoidance to approach behavior focused on testing things out in the real world. More specifically, Peter could practice switching from asking himself questions to asking other people questions. The If–Then plan here could be "If I notice that I am asking myself ques-tions to understand why something happened or what something means, then I will ask someone else's opinion." Practicing the exact wording of these questions for a range of situations, perhaps in role plays with Peter, would help to consolidate the plan in his mind, ensure that useful questions were being asked, and steer him away from insensitive or counterproductive questions.

5. It appears that one function of Peter's rumination is to avoid making

mistakes and to prevent bad things from happening. For example, he ruminated about problems in his relationships with his ex-girlfriend and with his wife to try to prevent difficulties recurring. Rather than focusing on preventing bad things from happening, Peter could be encouraged to shift to more constructive approach behavior, such as focusing on how he could promote and improve his relationship with his wife. The therapist could usefully ask what Peter could do to strengthen his relationship without needing to understand what happened in the past. This focus on promotion rather than avoidance could be part of an If–Then plan, or it could feed into general changes in his behavioral routine.

The selection of which plan to apply with Peter will be based on (1) which emerges naturally from reviewing his recent examples, (2) which is most consistent with the FA, and (3) a collaborative discussion with him. The principles for selecting an alternative behavior listed in Chapter 7 (function and formulation; experiential evidence; repertoire; practical and easy; closeness to the warning sign) should determine which option looks like it has the greatest chance of success. The plan is then tried out and reviewed, and refined or changed in the light of the observed outcomes.

Addressing Difficulties in Implementing Plans

The patient will not always be able to implement the If–Then contingency plan consistently. Sometimes he or she tries the plan and finds that it did not stop rumination or improve mood. What does the therapist do in these situations?

The first step for dealing with these difficulties (as with most difficulties that come up in therapy) is to return to the basic therapy principles (see Chapter 3). It may be that the plans need to be more concrete, detailed, and specific, and broken down into smaller steps (Principle 3: Encourage active, concrete, experiential, and specific behavior; Principle 7: Shift to an adaptive style of thinking). It is often useful to reiterate the idea that rumination is a habit and to review with the patient that habits take time and repetition to change, and that because habits are highly learned responses, they will keep coming back even when the patient does not want them to, until a new habit is learned (Principle 1: Normalize the patient's experience of rumination). The conceptualization of rumination as a habit takes the blame off the patient for not succeeding, normalizes the fact that interventions only work some of the time, and encourages the patient to keep repeating the response (Principle 5: Link behaviors to triggers and warning signs; Principle 6: Emphasize the importance of repetition and practice). Further FA may be warranted to check that the formulation is accurate or to directly tackle the difficulties in completing homework or other forms of avoidance (Principle 4: Take a functional-analytic approach). More practice in session and between sessions may be required.

For patients with depression, a common problem is low motivation and difficulties in getting started on new behaviors. RFCBT is designed to overcome this low motivation. The rationale and socialization into the treatment model is aimed to be relevant and engaging for the patient, while giving hope that this approach may be of value. We emphasize the use of experiential exercises in therapy sessions to give patients positive experiences and the sense that new strategies help to increase engagement and motivation. We directly tackle avoidance by identifying it in FA, collaboratively reviewing its consequences and usefulness with the patient, explicitly naming it when it occurs during therapy, and looking for alternatives.

Another helpful approach developed within BA (Martell et al., 2001), which is consistent with RFCBT, is to encourage change from the "outside in" by changing behavior without waiting for any internal change (change from the "inside out"). This approach overlaps with the idea of linking responses to warning signs in the contingency plans. Patients are encouraged to act according to their goals rather than their feelings. The idea is to divorce the patient's action from mood dependence or state dependence. The patient is encouraged to act while acknowledging that they didn't feel like acting at that moment. This is usually done as a behavioral experiment, focusing on the patients taking a small step first. Patients can be asked which is more helpful—to act in line with their goals despite how they feel or to wait until they feel in the right mood or frame of mind before acting.

Previous personal evidence can be used to link increased activity to feeling better. Patients can be asked which they have more control of: their feelings or their behavior, and, therefore, which strategy is better to improve mood: to do it from the inside out (waiting to feel better before acting) or from the outside in (acting to feel better). Furthermore, the therapist asks patients to consider the longer-term implications of each alternative:

"What happens if you only follow through with plans when you feel OK? What consequences does this have for you over time? Conversely, what happens if you do something despite how you are feeling? If you do this repeatedly what effect does it have?"

Patients may recognize that over time they are learning to be in more control despite their feelings. It is also useful for therapists to encourage patients to review how accurate their feelings are as a sign of their ability to do a task, for example:

"Can you think of times when you felt tired or low and then you did something—what happened then? Are there times when you did something despite these feelings? What was the outcome? What can you learn from this?"

Another important way to encourage behavioral change is to review the advantages and disadvantages of the original rumination or avoidance behavior and of the potential new approach behavior. This is a more detailed way of considering the function and usefulness of behaviors. It can be particularly useful to look at how helpful the rumination is by asking questions like "Can you work it out in your head?"; "Do you figure anything out?" The therapist explicitly discusses the pros and cons of doing something versus thinking about it. In this way, patients may begin to recognize that many things in life are not logical, not linear, not straightforward, and in fact a bit "messy." This particularly applies to other people and to relationships with them. Thus, guided discovery can explore how working things out logically may not be effective for these situations. For some situations, it may be more effective to work things out by trial and error, experimentation, and by building up a feel for what happens from direct experience. In the same way, it can be adaptive to look at doing things as a way to gain more knowledge, to refine performance, and to make judgments more accurate. There is value in reviewing whether logical conceptual analysis is a good strategy for all situations. Intuition may work as well as if not better than conceptual and abstract analysis for complex, dynamic, unknowable systems, such as our own emotions and other people. In such systems, we never have all the relevant information, and, even if we did have it, we wouldn't know what information to prioritize, and it would be too much to compute and process. Moreover, the system is always changing in response to what just happened.

Some patients use rumination to try and understand their problems, which leads them to keep running over things in their heads. This effectively involves asking themselves questions (e.g., "Why did this happen?"), while rehashing the same information over and over. The therapist can note that this approach does not generate new information. This leads to the consideration of alternative approaches, such as asking other people questions (i.e., seeking information from the external world) as a way to introduce new information.

This examination of advantages and disadvantages supports the use of FA to explore under what contexts a particular response is helpful versus unhelpful. Logical analysis and abstract thinking can be helpful in some circumstances, for example, when working on a practical, physical problem or when thinking through long-term life decisions. However, it tends to be less useful for dealing with difficulties, emotions, and other people. One goal of the FA is to improve the patient's discrimination of when, where, under what circumstances, with whom, and how a particular strategy works or does not work. In RFCBT, FA is used as a form of discrimination training. Increasing discrimination for the use of different strategies within the patient's repertoire is a useful outcome of thinking through the pros and cons of different behaviors.

FA and Therapeutic Hurdles

Whenever you encounter a hurdle or difficulty in therapy, it is worth considering whether further FA might be helpful. It often will be. For example, if a patient is not completing homework exercises, then FA can be used to examine the contexts in which homework is completed or not completed, or times when similar plans have been completed. This then suggests ways to increase the likelihood of the homework plans being implemented. When difficulties come up, the standard approach is to explicitly point them out to the patient and relate them back to the principles and model of therapy.

FA is particularly valuable to address behaviors that interfere with therapy. These behaviors will often have an avoidant function, for example, not completing homework, not attending sessions, shutting off from emotion, talking in an abstract way, changing the topic or switching across topics within the session, seeking reassurance, or turning attention inward onto personal preoccupations and away from the therapist. These avoidant functions are negatively reinforced by removing short-term distress. If a patient engages in a behavior that is disruptive of therapy, such as avoiding staying on topic and switching topics in the therapy session, then this is explicitly highlighted by the therapist and examined under the FA microscope, its functions considered, moderators identified, and plans then implemented to tackle the behavior. For example, if one of the imagery and visualization exercises, such as absorption and compassion, does not work consistently for a patient, then FA is used to examine the circumstances under which the exercise worked versus when it did not, and to inform plans to increase the likelihood of the exercise being effective.

When addressing such therapy-interfering behaviors with a patient, the first step is to identify the problem behavior and to formulate its potential function (Principle 4: Take a functional-analytic approach). For example, if a patient is always generating "Yes, but" responses when new solutions or experiments are suggested, the therapist observes the antecedents to and consequences of this behavior to garner a sense of what its function may be. For example, therapy-interfering behaviors may have become habitual for the patient and may function to help him avoid discomfort and distress and make him feel safe by defending him from exposing himself to difficulties. Repeated and lengthy talking about difficulties and problems may serve a similar function of providing justification for not doing anything, as well as seeking support and reassurance for the patient's difficulties.

The second step is to explicitly point out the behavior to the patient and relate it back to the treatment model (Principle 1: Normalize the patient's experience of rumination; Principle 2: Make rumination an explicit target of therapy; Principle 8: Focus on nonspecific factors). This is best done in an exploratory and collaborative way, relating it back to the ideas of habits and avoidance and asking about its usefulness, while still validating and supporting the patient. For example, for the patient who keeps saying "Yes, but," the therapist might note that she has noticed this response keeps coming up and wonders if this might be a habit for the patient, for example:

"I have noticed that every time we begin to consider trying something new for you to do, you come up with a list of obstacles and difficulties, saying things like 'Yes, but.' What is your experience of this?"

The therapist asks what the effects of saying "Yes, but" are on the patient, his feelings, and his behavior, as well as on other people. This involves asking about the utility of this behavior (i.e., "Is it helpful to do this?"). This provides an opportunity to collaboratively explore whether it might be a form of avoidance, and whether it might have short-term gain but cause longer-term problems.

The response can be explored while still validating the patient by noting that it makes sense within the patient's context and life history and normalizing it as much as possible. For example, for the patient who keeps bringing up and wanting to share new problems, it is useful to acknowledge the importance of these difficulties for the patient, how they must be hard to deal with, how it is natural to want to talk about these difficulties and express these feelings, and to feel supported. During this validation, where possible, the therapist responds to the possible constructive functions of the patient's behavior. For example, a patient who keeps bringing up and wanting to discuss problems may be seeking someone to take her problems seriously and to contain her emotional upset. It is important to do this by acknowledging and validating her response, while at the same time linking it into the RFCBT formulation. For example, the therapist explicitly links the patient's response to particular antecedents or triggers and notes that her response is a natural one to these triggers, thus simultaneously explaining the RFCBT model and validating her experience (Principle 5: Link behaviors to triggers and warning signs).

A similar thing can be done when looking at the consequences of the behavior. The therapist continues to take a patient's difficulties seriously and acknowledge that she does have many real problems, while asking about how focusing on these difficulties in this way makes her feel and how it influences what she does, as a means to link into consequences. Exploring whether the patient's responses are helpful both long-term and short-term is critical (Principle 4: Take a functional-analytic approach; Principle 8: Focus on nonspecific factors).

An important part of this process is collaboratively and explicitly sharing the working formulation of the function of the patient's behavior. The formulation can be shared in a tentative way, as a hypothesis for the patient and therapist to consider together, for example:

> "I am not sure about this, but I wonder if it might be that whenever I raise something different to try, you find reasons not to do it because that feels safer. I wonder if trying new things feels risky because it puts you on the line and has the potential for failure, whereas being negative about things not working out, at least short-term, means you don't have to take those risks. Wanting to feel safe is a very strong and natural human motivation, and I can really see how you would do anything you can to feel safe, especially given some of the bad things that happened to you in the past. If I were in your shoes and had gone through what you had, I would really prize my safety too and do whatever I could to feel safe. What is your experience of this? How does this fit or not fit with you?"

This enables the therapist to move on and consider how well this approach is working, for example:

> "I wonder what effect finding reasons not to do things has for you in the long-term."

There is scope here to review the patient's history and the development of his emotional difficulties, for example, to see whether his problems in general have been getting better or worse over time as he practices these strategies. Often, patients find that these avoidant strategies have at best not improved matters, and often made things worse, as problems remain unresolved and as their lives get more and more closed down. The therapist can usefully reflect that the current approach does not seem to be working and that it may be worth considering an alternative.

For example, for the patient who in every session wants to talk through and emote about new sets of difficulties and constantly seeks support and reassurance, the therapist validates her experience and desire for support, while noting that this approach alone has not helped her get better:

> "I looks to me as if you are going back into the habit of wanting to talk about all the difficulties you have, your feelings, and what it means for you. I can really understand that—these are real problems for you and they bring up strong feelings. It is normal and natural to want to share those feelings and get support for these difficulties and to feel that some-

one else cares about you and takes your problems seriously. You are in a tough place and deserve support. Together we will look at your problems and work to move forward. I wonder if just thinking about and talking about your feelings and difficulties and what they mean is enough to help you feel better. After all, this is what you have been doing again and again for a number of years now, and it sounds as if you still feel stuck. This wanting to share your distress can easily become unhelpful rumination. It looks like this approach isn't working and you need to try something different. What can we do together that takes your very real problems seriously, supports you, and at the same time helps to move things forward?"

This is a useful place to refer back to elements already covered in the therapy. For example, if a patient is being very abstract in the session, the therapist points out that the pattern of abstract responding seems to be occurring again, reviews whether it is helpful, and looks at other options (Principle 3: Encourage active, concrete, experiential, and specific behavior—the ACES rule; Principle 7: Shift to an adaptive style of thinking). Once the therapist has named and labeled an unhelpful pattern of responding, it is easier to refer to it again in therapy. This requires persistence on the part of the therapist (Principle 8: Focus on nonspecific factors). Because these unwanted responses are often habits, they will keep reoccurring, and the therapist needs to keep pointing them out and naming them to the patient. Each time the behavior is named and an alternative response tried, the therapist increases the patient's awareness of the habit and strengthens an alternative response (Principle 6: Emphasize the importance of repetition and practice).

The third step is to consider what a useful alternative behavior might be. This could involve experimenting with an alternative response right then and there in the therapy session (Principle 3: Encourage active, concrete, experiential, and specific behavior—the ACES rule). Suggesting or prompting an alternative for the patient and getting him to try it immediately in the session can be a powerful way to shift modes and gather more information. For example, for the patient who says, "Yes, but," the therapist asks him to experiment with saying something more neutral instead, such as "This might or might not work. I don't know. Perhaps I can try it out and see," and observe his experience of doing that. With a patient who turns inward and becomes preoccupied in rumination, the therapist prompts her to focus her attention externally and listen carefully to the therapist's voice. For a patient who wants to talk at length about different difficulties and emotions, the therapist seeks agreement on one problem to focus on, enabling a more detailed focus, using this as an example of the approach. A behavioral experiment is tried in session in which the therapist and patient spend 10 minutes talking about the feelings and meanings of the situation versus spending 10 minutes working on problem solving and making a contingency plan. The effects of these distinct approaches can then be compared. These alternative behaviors are then built into an If–Then plan to practice in daily life, including the therapy itself (Principle 6: Emphasize the importance of repetition and practice).

This same approach and sequence of steps are used to directly address emotion when it comes up in therapy. It is not unusual for discussion of difficult subjects or the memories that occur during imagery and experiential exercises to bring up strong emotions, for example, causing patients to become tearful and cry, or to become irritated. This is an opportunity to practice using the techniques when they are most needed, that is, in response to challenging moods. The therapist validates and normalizes the patient's emotion and provides empathy and sympathy for her experience, while concurrently linking the emotion into an ABC FA and exploring its function and utility. When a patient becomes emotional in a session, the therapist determines what caused or triggered the emotion (what was the antecedent?) by asking what happened just before the emotion came on, and reviewing with the patient what made her feel this way. The trigger is then explicitly discussed, while noting that it makes sense that the patient has this emotional response to this trigger.

It is useful to keep an open mind about the emotional experience of the patient because the emotion itself could be adaptive or maladaptive. Often the emotion will be a normal and helpful response to the trigger. It is important to acknowledge this to the patient and to stress that emotions can be good, rather than something to judge or fear (Principle 1: Normalize the patient's experience of rumination; Principle 8: Focus on nonspecific factors). For example, the therapist can say:

> "It sounds like this discussion has brought back memories of this upsetting event. This was a big loss for you and it is normal to feel sadness following a big loss. Indeed, feeling sad can be helpful in this situation because it communicates to others that you have experienced a loss and need support, and because it signals to you that there has been this big change that you need to resolve."

The responses that follow the emotion are particularly important because this is where unhelpful avoidant responses, such as rumination, emotional numbing, distraction, or withdrawal, may be triggered by the emotion and lead to more negative consequences. Tracking through the ABC analysis determines the consequences of the emotion and of the responses to the emotion. If the patient has a tendency to avoid the emotion, then this provides an opportunity to try something different in the session, for example, by asking her to stay with the feelings.

CHAPTER 9

Shifting Processing Style

Becoming Concrete and Specific

$\mathbf{A}$ core element within the RFCBT approach is identifying unhelpful styles of thinking during rumination about difficulties and then helping the patient to shift into a more constructive and helpful style of thinking. Chapter 2 summarized the experimental evidence for distinct styles of processing in rumination and highlighted the evidence that concrete processing is more helpful than abstract processing. A key principle within RFCBT is to guide patients toward active, concrete, experiential, and specific ways of responding (ACES; Principle 3, Chapter 3) as a deliberate means to shift patients who ruminate away from their default tendency of abstract, evaluative, comparative, conceptual, and passive ways of responding.

Ruminative thinking tends to be focused on causes, consequences, and meanings rather than on how to solve problems. The style of ruminative thinking tends to be abstract, extreme, and overgeneral, and to be concerned with evaluations and not linked to the details of what happened. This more abstract and extreme style makes it harder for patients to solve problems and tends to make situations seem worse, as patients tend to see things in a context-free way (e.g., "I am always getting it wrong"), rather than in a context-rich way (e.g., "I made a mistake at a particular thing, when I felt a particular way, in a particular place at a particular time, with a particular person"). The more specific and discriminative the patient's descriptions are, the more helpful they will be at guiding actions and the less likely it is that the description will set off a general theme of similar memories (e.g., "other times I failed"), which is typical of rumination. The more any thought is tied down to the specific contingencies of a situation, the less extreme it is likely to be.

This chapter provides a detailed description of how to identify abstract thinking and of different approaches for shifting patients into more adaptive, concrete processing. Within RFCBT, the focus is on training patients to spot their abstract style of thinking and then to change their style of thinking, as an alternative to challenging the content of each individual negative thought. By shifting the whole style of thinking, we hope to shift people out of the unhelpful depressive ruminative mode.

It is important to keep this approach simple by focusing on one or two strategies. The strategies that are most easily explained and that seem most helpful to patients include:

1. Replacing unhelpful "why" questions with helpful "how" questions (see Chapter 2 for background and evidence).
2. Training patients to use a specific, discriminative, and concrete style of thinking focused on the context and sequence of what is happening. For example, patients are asked to practice generating highly specific and detailed memories and concrete descriptions of current situations. (The combination of these first two strategies forms the concreteness training package explicitly tested as an individual treatment with encouraging preliminary results [Watkins et al., 2009, 2012].)
3. Training patients in self-implemented FA, where they learn to identify when their own thinking is helpful (and typically characterized by concrete thinking) and when it is less helpful and typically more abstract.
4. Using visualization and imagery exercises that shift patients into a more process-focused and less outcome-evaluated mode as described in Chapter 10.

Identifying the Patient's Style of Thinking

The first step is to determine if a patient's thinking is abstract, and if so, to help the patient recognize this pattern of thinking. There are several ways to do this. All involve drawing attention to a particular aspect of abstract thinking and then looking at the consequences of that way of thinking.

"Why"–Type Questions

One way to identify abstract thinking is to look for the spontaneous utterances of "why"-type questions within the treatment session when patients describe their rumination or their responses to problems. By "why"-type questions, we mean questions focusing on the causes, consequences, and meanings of events, typified by questions like "Why did this happen to me?"; "Why can't I do this?"; "Why me?"; "Why did they do that?"

It is useful to note down these questions when patients use them and to build up a list. After a session or two, the therapist can review them with the patient and ask what he makes of the fact that he is asking himself all of these questions. These questions are easily spotted when exploring a recent episode of rumination and tracking the sequence of thoughts moment by moment in detail. The therapist asks, "What happens when you ask yourself these questions? Do they help you to reach any useful conclusions?"

The therapist also explores what alternative questions the patient might ask himself in the same situation and what effect this might have. Patients often spontaneously recognize that they could ask how to solve the problem or what to do next. However, if the patient does not recognize this spontaneously, the therapist can note:

"It is interesting that for all these situations, you keep asking 'Why did this happen to me? What does this mean about me?' etcetera, but you don't ask 'How can I do something about this? What do you make of this? What might happen if you asked 'How can I do something?'"

This approach helps patients to recognize that the types of question they ask themselves may be unhelpful and unbalanced. We can then explore the benefits and disadvantages of asking different types of questions (see Why–How behavioral experiment later in the chapter).

Abstract Descriptions

Another way to help patients recognize that they are using abstract and evaluative thinking is to notice and point out every time they describe a thought or a situation in an abstract, overgeneral, or extreme way. For example, a patient might report an abstract and overgeneral thought such as "I can't cope." This thought is abstract because it is not specific to a particular situation and has no details about the circumstances in which the coping does not occur. Thus, every time the patient describes a situation or makes a judgment that lacks detailed discriminative information about *with whom, when, where, under what circumstances,* and *how* the event occurs, the therapist stops and notes that thought and then collaboratively reviews this with the patient. It is essential to keep a nonjudgmental and curious attitude when doing this, for example:, "It is interesting that you describe it like that. Are there any other ways you might describe it?"

For example, if a patient says, "I am a failure. Nothing I do seems to work" when describing not completing her homework, the therapist could note that this comment seems to be missing a lot of potentially relevant information and is quite abstract. Taking a guided discovery approach, the therapist can ask:

"Does this way of describing the situation leave any information out? How would you describe this thought—how detailed is it? How rich in information is it? How vague is it?"

If the therapist has already explained the difference between abstract and concrete styles of thinking (see the section below on explaining this distinction), she might ask, "Could this be an example of being too abstract?"

As noted in Chapter 3, it is often necessary to ask further questions, seeking more detail and information, until you have a detailed, specific, and concrete answer. Questions like "What exactly did he do?"; "What were the exact words?" and "What physical sensations do you notice when you are angry?" achieve greater specificity and concreteness. The therapist also explores with the patient the value of describing the actual behavior that occurred in a situation—what was said and done by whom—because this clarifies what happened and shows ways to learn from or resolve a situation.

It is useful to consider whether a description involves some level of interpretation rather than directly describing what happened. As discussed in Chapter 3, if a patient reported that a friend snubbed her, you don't know exactly what happened because this description involves an interpretative verb that is ambiguous. The therapist highlights such descriptions and points out how they are distanced from the direct experience of what happened and instead summarize and interpret the experience. The therapist then explains how this is a good example of describing an event in an abstract way, and that it is useful to practice describing the event in terms of more concrete, detailed, and specific behaviors and circumstances. A more behavior-based description of what happened may suggest a different interpretation and help the patient to gain perspective on the situation.

Similarly, we want to look out for descriptions of events and situations that use adjectives, particularly those that relate to personality and character traits, as another sign of abstract thinking. If the patient describes himself as stupid or another person as untrustworthy, these are examples of abstract representations, which would be useful to then explore, asking the patient to describe the events more specifically and relate them to particular contexts.

Once a patient is aware of the different styles of thinking and their effects on mood and rumination, the therapist then explicitly trains him out of the less helpful style into a more helpful style. For example, the therapist says:

"It looks like you are spending a lot of time evaluating things around you and thinking about things in quite an overgeneral way—summarizing across lots of different situations and not considering the unique details of each individual situation. We know that this style of thinking is unhelpful. Would you like to work on ways of training yourself to think in more helpful ways?"

If examples of abstract, evaluative thinking do not come up spontaneously (don't worry—they most probably will!), they can be sought by asking patients to describe what they were thinking during a recent problematic situation or by asking them to keep a thought record. The therapist also checks to see whether this way of thinking occurs quite often. Is it a frequent style of the patient? Recognizing that it is a general style helps to emphasize the importance of trying to change this style of thinking.

The Why–How Behavioral Experiment

A behavioral experiment that helps to encourage concrete thinking is the Why–How experiment. The therapist works with the patient to identify a current concern or problem. The patient then compares the effects of spending several minutes thinking about this difficulty using "why"-type questions with spending several minutes thinking about the problem with a series of "how"-type questions. The "why"-type questions are based on the questions the patient naturally uses, which the therapist has noted during the first few sessions. The patient is encouraged to rate her mood before and after using each set of questions (e.g., how sad, tense, focused, or confident she feels on a scale of 0–10). It is useful to get the patient to rate how manageable she feels the problems are after each set of questions and whether she came up with any solutions to the problem. I typically find that the majority of patients report their mood and confidence in their problem-solving abilities are worse following the "why"-type questions compared to the "how"-type questions. Thus, this experiment usefully reinforces the idea that "why"-type questions may not be helpful and introduces a more adaptive alternative in the form of "how"-type questions. Each experiment is focused on a recent problem associated with rumination that the patient brings up in the treatment session.

Some patients believe that these "why" questions are essential and useful, reflecting perceived functions of rumination such as gaining understanding and insight into problems. This behavioral experiment provides a powerful means to disconfirm these beliefs. An alternative or follow-up experiment is for patients to compare how they feel and how they cope with things when they spend alternate days asking themselves a list of "why"-type questions compared to a list of "how"-type questions.

The following is an example of a Why–How behavioral experiment, which follows a patient describing a recent bout of rumination that occurred when she was waiting in a café for a friend. When the friend did not turn up on time, the patient began to ruminate more and more about the situation. The therapist first explores this situation in some detail with the patient and identifies the abstract questions being asked. The therapist is then well positioned to prompt the patient to imagine herself back in the situation again. The therapist then prompts the patient with her own "why"-type questions. The therapist uses details from discussion of the recent episode to prompt recall of the scene and to make it as vivid as possible.

The therapist initiates the first part of the experiment as follows:

"OK, now close your eyes and imagine that you are back in the café, waiting for your friend to turn up. As best you can, imagine that you are there right now, looking out through your eyes on the scene in front of you. Create an image of this situation that is detailed and vivid . . . feel your seat behind you and your cup in your hand . . . see the café clock on the wall in front of you . . . hear the clock ticking above the murmur of the other customers around you . . . visualize the hands on the clock shift to 10:00 . . . and see the café door in front of you ease open . . . but it's a stranger . . . your friend has not shown up on time . . . As vividly as possible imagine yourself in the café, waiting for this person when he hasn't shown up . . . and ask yourself the following questions:

'Why is this happening to me?' . . . [pause for about 3 seconds between questions]
'What does this mean about me?' . . . [3-second pause]
'What will the consequences be?' . . . [3-second pause]
'Why does this keep happening to me?' . . . [3-second pause]
'Why me?' . . . [3-second pause]
'Why is this always happening to me?' . . . [3-second pause]
'Why did he treat me like this?' . . . [3-second pause]

"Notice what thoughts you have now. Note what feelings you have—how intense are they. Notice any physical sensations. Notice what thoughts, feelings, and sensations you are experiencing as you experience being in the café, your friend not showing up, and ask yourself these questions. Make a mental note of what you are experiencing and hold on to it for later."

The therapist then pauses to reflect with the patient on the effect of reimagining this situation while asking these more abstract "why"-type questions. This includes exploring the effect of recalling this situation on how the patient feels and on other aspects of her experience. As well as taking quick 0–10 ratings of mood and relevant symptoms (sadness, tension, anxiety, confidence, tiredness), the therapist might also ask:

"What is your experience of asking yourself these more abstract questions focused on causes, meanings, and implications? What do you notice? Is this typical of the thinking that you do some of the time?"

The therapist then explores the patient's response to imagining the same situation while asking more helpful concrete "how" questions:

"Let's return to the image that you created before and try thinking more about this situation again . . . close your eyes and once again, and as vividly as you can, imagine that you are waiting in the café to meet this friend, for this meeting that means a lot to you, and that he is already late. As best you can, imagine that you are there right now, looking out through your eyes. Create an image of this situation that is detailed and vivid . . . imagine your seat back behind you and your cup in your hand . . . see the café clock on the wall in front of you . . . hear the clock ticking above the murmur of the other customers around you . . . visualize the hands on the clock shift to 10:00 . . . and see the café door in front of you ease open . . . but it's a stranger . . . the person you are expecting has not shown up . . .

"As vividly as possible, imagine that you are in the café and that your friend has not shown up, and ask yourself the following questions:

'What details do I notice when I concentrate on my experience in the café?' . . . [3-second pause]
'What is the sequence of events that led up to our arranging to meet?' . . . [3-second pause]
'How is this situation different from other times when I have met people as planned?' . . . [3-second pause]
'What might be the sequence of events leading up to the person not showing up?' . . . [3 seconds]
'How would things be different if I moved forward or dealt with this problem?' . . . [3-second pause]
'What first step can I take to move toward my goal?' " . . . [3-second pause]

"Notice what thoughts, feelings, and sensations you are experiencing as you are in the café, your friend has not shown up, and you are asking yourself these questions. Make a mental note of what you are experiencing and hold on to it for later."

As with all cognitive therapy questions, it is good to find versions of "how"-type questions that are most meaningful to patients and reflect their own words. Here are some useful illustrative examples:

"How did this event happen?"
"What was the sequence of events leading up to this event?"
"How can I learn from this?"
"How do I get to a useful endpoint—an intention or a plan—from here?"
"How do I solve this problem?"
"How do I start to approach this problem?"
"What is the first or next step I can take that is most likely to produce the best outcome for me?"
"How do I decide what to do next?"
"How do I make a decision?"
"How useful is this thought to me?"
"What is helpful to me?"
"What is most likely to get me what I want?"
"Is this the best way to get what I want?"
"What can I do to maximize my likelihood of getting what I want?"
"How can I maximize my chances of getting what I want?"

Furthermore, any "why"-type questions used by the patient can be reframed into "how"-type questions by refocusing the question from understanding the situation and reflecting about the meaning of the situation to how the patient can do something about the situation and on the specific contextual details of the situation. For example, "Why can't things be easier?" can be reframed as "How can I make things easier?"

The therapist briefly reviews the experience of asking these "how"-type questions when dwelling on the same difficult situation that had previously led to rumination. He or she then pauses to reflect with the patient on the effect of reimagining the situation while asking these more concrete "how"-type questions, repeating the same questions and ratings as asked after the "why"-type questions. The responses to the two versions of imagining the same situation are then compared to examine whether the different styles of processing had different effects.

The therapist looks for examples of a more positive response to the same situation when the patient is asking the "how"-type questions rather than the "why"-type questions. Among the benefits we often notice for "how"-type questions relative to "why"-type questions, patients report feeling calmer, more positive, more energetic, more confident or more active in problem solving. The abstract condition is often accompanied by feeling worse, down, more anxious, more tired, and stressed. We also sometimes observe that patients find it easier to make constructive plans when asking the "how"-type questions. Furthermore, one effect of thinking abstractly can be to cause individuals to overgeneralize beyond the specifics of the particular situation and begin to remember or imagine other similar situations (e.g., other times the patient has been stood up; other times she feels she has been let down). The therapist can therefore usefully check whether the concrete questions help to keep difficult events in perspective and prevent such overgeneralization. The benefits of being more concrete can be simply summarized to patients as becoming more action oriented, putting problems into perspective, and improving problem solving. The concrete "how"-type questions may still be accompanied by some upset and stress, but I have found that many patients experience a much more positive result than when asking their default "why"-type questions.

As throughout all of the RFCBT treatment, we seek to facilitate the comparison between abstract and concrete situations through Socratic questions. For example, the therapist says something along the lines of "By comparing the two times you imagined the person not showing up we can compare the two ways of thinking. What did you notice, how would you sum up the differences?"

Once the therapist has reviewed the effects of the two different ways of thinking and highlighted any differences, he or she summarizes their different effects and explains the difference between abstract versus concrete thinking (see the next section). The final step may then be setting a homework plan in which the patient practices looking for unhelpful questions and replacing them with helpful questions.

Explaining the Distinction between
Abstract and Concrete Processing Styles

I recommend explaining to patients the relative advantages and disadvantages of abstract versus concrete processing. Key messages to convey are that both abstract and concrete ways of thinking are normal and that each can be helpful or unhelpful depending on the situation and context. It's important to normalize the tendency to be abstract (Principle 1: Normalize the patient's experience of rumination) while pointing out the value of looking at problems in a more concrete way. For example, the therapist may say, "Everyone does it, and you can't stop doing it and would not want to—however, too much of it can make it hard to sort problems out."

Here is an illustrative script that captures many of the key messages for the therapist to impart, which can be adapted and edited down as required:

"Both abstract and concrete ways of thinking are normal and helpful ways of thinking when used appropriately. There are some key differences between them. Abstract thinking tends to be general and global, asks 'why' questions, and is focused on the gist that is common across many situations. It has an emphasis on the meanings and implications of events and asks 'Why did this happen? Why me? What does this mean about me?' Abstract thinking is focused on evaluating the reasons, meanings, consequences, and implications of behaviors and events. It tends to be more outcome focused, more analytical, and more conceptual. We often find that this way of thinking is common when people are ruminating and caught up in depression.

"In contrast, concrete thinking tends to be more specific, local, asks 'how' questions and is focused on the circumstances and context and sensory details of a particular situation. Concrete thinking is concentrated on the means and methods of events and actions—how did the event happen, how is it done, including the process and sequence of an action or an event. It involves more directly experiencing the situation and being in the situation, rather than thinking about the situation. That is, using all of our senses to become aware of the specific details that make a situation distinctive and unique. Importantly, this includes noticing the process by which events and behaviors unfold and the particular situation and circumstances of an event, and being aware of the sequence of events: what comes before, and what follows after each action. It includes asking 'How did this happen?' and 'How can I do something about it?'

"An abstract way of thinking about brushing your teeth is to focus on its purpose, namely, to improve dental hygiene, whereas a concrete way of thinking about brushing your teeth is to focus on how to do the action, namely by moving a toothbrush across your teeth.

"We all use both styles of thinking, they are part of everyone's mental toolbox, and we regularly move between them. However, it is important to have balance and flexibility in using these different ways of thinking, and to be able to shift the way we think depending on our circumstances.

"Both types of thinking are useful. Abstract descriptions help us to make general evaluations, learn across situations, and be consistent in our goals, but aren't very good for directing action. Because of its emphasis on wider issues, abstract thinking such as asking 'What does this mean to me?' and 'What are the implications of this?' can help us to keep track of what is important to us, our longer-term goals and ambitions. Abstract thinking is also invaluable in enabling us to transfer our learning from one situation to another, by seeing what is general and common across situations.

"However, as you learned in our previous experiment [refer back to the Why–How experiment, if conducted], abstract thinking can also be unhelpful when used for difficult or stressful events. Remember the . . . [example from Why–How experiment]. In these circumstances, abstract thinking contributes to some of the problems found in depression such as rumination, overgeneralization, and reduced activity.

"Concrete descriptions don't give us a wider overview but help us to make plans. We tend to move down to more concrete descriptions when we get stuck, and move back up to more abstract levels when things go well, as we consider the implications of our actions. In depression and rumination, this balance often gets disturbed, with a tendency for more abstract thinking and less concrete thinking. This disturbance in the balance of thinking can then influence problem solving and negatively influence thinking. We are going to practice different ways to redress this imbalance.

"Rumination occurs when thinking about problems gets stuck, goes on too long, and does not seem to reach any kind of solution. This is more likely to occur when someone is being abstract, thinking about the meanings and implications of the problem. This is because abstract thinking moves away from the specific details of the situation and does not give clues as to what to do next. Moreover, abstract thinking about meanings and implications is the kind of thinking that leads to more thinking, rather than the kind of thinking that leads to plans and actions. Rumination occurs when thinking leads to more thinking rather than leading to plans and actions.

"Overgeneralization is the tendency to jump to broad conclusions, to lose perspective, to get things out of proportion, and for thinking to spiral out from one situation to encompass many other situations. For example, when dropping a plate leads to thinking 'I'm always making a mess of everything,' which leads to believing 'I'm a klutz, I can't be trusted to do anything.' Overgeneralization involves abstract thinking that looks at what is common across different situations and looks for general features across situations, rather than staying with the specific details of the particular situation.

"Reduced activity can also result from too much abstract thinking. Thinking more abstractly makes it harder to get started on doing things because it does not involve thinking about how to put plans into action. Moreover, more abstract thinking involves focusing on the bigger picture and on a task or goal in its entirety, rather than on the smaller steps within the task. This abstract thinking can make an activity seem bigger and harder to do, even overwhelming. When you can't break a task down into smaller steps, the overall job may appear too huge and difficult to do, which can lead to putting it off.

"In contrast, concrete thinking asks 'How did this happen?' and 'What can I do about it?' This can be helpful when thinking about difficulties or stressors in a number of ways. Concrete thinking keeps things in perspective so that we don't jump to conclusions about ourselves, don't lump things together, and don't generalize from one event to many other situations. Being aware of the specific sensory details and circumstances of an event helps us to spot the differences between this event and other situations, preventing overgeneralized conclusions. For example, after not being successful at a task, it is more useful to think 'I failed because I was tired and unprepared' than to think 'I am a complete failure'—it keeps it in proportion, and gives clues as to what to do next time to get a better result.

"Concrete thinking helps us to learn. By thinking about the sequence that led to an event, we can begin to notice what factors influenced the outcomes, whether there were any warning signs or clues as to what was going to happen, and whether and where the outcome could have been influenced by doing something different. Noticing that the details were different between two situations can help you in learning what factors influence success or failure.

"Concrete thinking is more action oriented and puts us in a better position to ask 'How will I move on from here?' Imagining the details of an event and what you might do next helps to generate possible alternative courses of action, which improves problem solving. Furthermore, being more concrete helps us by breaking the problem down into smaller, more manageable steps, so that it does not seem so overwhelming, so huge. You are more likely to get started on the garden if you're keeping it in perspective and seeing it as a series of small tasks; weed one bed at a time, prune the fruit tree, and so on, with breaks in between.

"Every action occurs in a different context—a unique combination of what you do, how you do it, when you do it, where you do it, why you do it, who else is involved, your physical and mental state, and the conditions under which you do it. Having a good awareness of all these elements is essential to learning what factors influence outcome for better or worse. Thinking in a more concrete way can help you to become more aware of this context and how it influences what happens.

"A good way to tell whether your thinking styles are in balance is to consider the relationship between thinking and action: if thinking about a problem only leads to more thinking, your thinking is probably too abstract, feeding off itself, spiraling out to rumination, overgeneralization, and inactivity. If thinking about a problem leads to a plan, a decision, and to some kind of action to deal with it, you are probably thinking concretely. This is exactly what you need to do when faced with difficulties or stressful events."

Setting Up a Homework Plan

A helpful experiment in the session provides a strong rationale for the patient to continue with more concrete thinking in daily life. The experience of improving mood and confidence after only a few minutes of thinking differently can demonstrate convincingly the difference between the different modes of processing and motivate the patient to try this approach. The experiment often convinces the patient that the abstract style is unhelpful and suggests that there is a viable, feasible, and useful alternative. At this point, the therapist encourages the patient to build the "how"-type thinking into a contingency If–Then plan (as discussed in Chapter 7). For example, on noticing early warning signs for rumination, including "why"-type questions, the patient instead practices "how"-type questions. An audio recording of the behavioral experiment to guide further practice outside of the therapy session is helpful. We encourage patients to first practice by listening to the exercise conducted in the session over and over to familiarize themselves with the way of thinking and then to build this into how they respond in daily life.

I recommend trying to adapt the "why"-type questions into "how"-type questions that are personally relevant. It is also important to encourage patients to think through a "how"-type question and then act on their answers to it (i.e., use the question to initiate problem solving and action planning). "How"-type questions are particularly useful when combined with training in problem solving, since these questions remind patients to practice problem solving rather than rumination and help them keep on track (i.e., not go off on a tangent when problem solving). Furthermore, these questions emphasize taking an approach based on skillfulness and effectiveness. They have the advantage of focusing patients on making decisions and plans and in this way can help them to break out of the ruminative loop. Patients report these questions as useful when they are able to stop and use them in a difficult situation.

An important issue is ensuring that patients are able to use these questions when they are most needed—that is, when stressed and experiencing difficult emotions (Principle 5: Link behaviors to triggers and warning signs). Several steps can be taken to facilitate this. First, as mentioned above, these functional questions can be directly built into patients' If–Then plans. Second, some patients find it helpful to prepare small portable flashcards on which they write their most useful questions. Carrying these memory aids in handbags or wallets where they are handy can help remind patients to use this technique in daily life. Third, imaginal rehearsal can be useful. Repeatedly imagining difficult and upsetting situations and then rehearsing this strategy can consolidate this alternative response (e.g., imagining being in a problematic situation and imagining spotting "why"-type questions and replacing them with "how"-type questions). The more this imagery work induces and includes real-world warning signs to rumination for the patient, the more helpful it will be because it directly associates the new coping response with the existing cue, making it more likely that the more adaptive response will be used when really needed.

The sequence just described illustrates a common and important pattern of steps used within RFCBT:

First, we seek to explore the patient's own experience (e.g., identify the "why"-type questions) (Principle 1: Normalize the patient's experience of rumination; Principle 4: Take a functional-analytic approach).

Second, we experiment directly with an alternative approach to give the patient a different and hopefully more positive experience (e.g., the Why–How experiment) (Principle 3: Encourage active, concrete, experiential, and specific behavior—the ACES rule; Principle 7: Shift to an adaptive style of thinking).

Third, if the experiment is successful, we establish the new approach as a regular exercise that the patient repeatedly practices in his or her daily life (i.e., by listening to a recording of the session daily and making it part of an If–Then plan) (Principle 5: Link behaviors to triggers and warning signs; Principle 6: Emphasize the importance of repetition and practice).

The mnemonic for this approach is six E's or E^6 (Explore Experience, Experiment with Experience, Exercise and Engage). The threefold logic behind this approach is to keep the focus of the treatment on shifting experience (Principle 3: Encourage active, concrete, experiential, and specific behavior—the ACES rule), to work on repeated practice that links into daily life (to better target habits, see Chapter 2; Principle 5: Link behaviors to triggers and warning signs; Principle 6: Emphasize the importance of repetition and practice), and to build up the positive expectations and hopes of the patient by giving him positive experiences in the session and building new behaviors on these experiences (Principle 8: Focus on nonspecific factors).

Concreteness Training

I have developed a training task in which people repeatedly practice generating concrete representations of various situations and have found that repeated practice on this task can reduce rumination and depression (Watkins et al., 2009, 2012; see Chapters 1 and 2 for further details). Within RFCBT, the concreteness training approach builds from a successful Why–How experiment, providing patients with ways to shift their thinking style.

The key steps each patient practices during the training are summarized below. The instructions are applied either to a recent upsetting event, where the patient recalls the event as vividly as possible and works through the steps, or to a current problem as it is happening. The therapy session in which the concreteness exercises are practiced is audio-recorded, and the recording given to the patient so that he or she can repeatedly practice the exercise as homework.

Principal Instructions and Core Elements of Concreteness Training

Focus on Sensory Details and Notice What Is Specific and Distinctive

- "Notice what you are experiencing in the moment. Focus your attention on the specific details of the situation: sights, sounds, tastes, smells, textures, when and where it occurs, who is there, what happens, the sensations you feel in your body."
- "Notice what makes an event different from other similar occasions. Notice what marks an event as distinct in time, place, setting or circumstances."

Notice the Process by Which Events and Behaviors Unfold

- "Be aware of how situations occur. Be aware of the sequence of events— what comes before, and what follows after each action and event. Notice the series of steps or actions that lead up to an event."
- "Look out for clues or warning signs. Notice indicators that suggest a difficulty may be coming."
- "Look out for turning points. Notice any points or steps where a different decision, action, or circumstance might change what happens."

Focus on How You Can Move Forward

- "Be specific about how you want things to change. Imagine how things would be different if you dealt with a given difficulty. Be specific and realistic."
- "Plan. Ask yourself how you can break things down into discrete, manageable steps that you can take to move forward into helpful action."
- "Act. Take the first step in the chain of actions (whether mental or physical) that you can do to deal with a given difficulty and then follow the sequence, step by step, dealing with new difficulties as they arise and acknowledging your own progress when things go well!"
- "To make the most of every experience, make a mental note of what you learn from dealing with each difficulty, how you can use this learning in the future, and any plans you might make as a result."

Once you have explained the difference between concrete and abstract processing (as described above), concreteness techniques can then be introduced and practiced in the therapy session, as discussed in Watkins et al. (2012). Guidance for the therapist is in parentheses throughout the following script:

"To help you think more concretely, I would like you to practice a set of special thinking exercises. These are designed to reduce the problems of rumination, overgeneralization, and inactivity, which we know contribute to depression. The main set of exercises involves learning to be more concrete when faced with problems, difficulties, or stressful events. This is what we will practice today. Research studies have shown that 30 minutes of daily practice on these training exercises substantially reduced symptoms of depression, so we know that this training can help.

"To help you concentrate during these exercises, I will ask you to close your eyes or to look at the floor, wall, or ceiling—something dull that won't grab your attention. Settle into a comfortable position with your feet on the floor. If you find your mind wondering at any time, don't worry, just gently move your attention back to focus on what I'm saying. And if at any time you feel uncomfortable, please let me know. OK?

"We'll practice thinking in a concrete way with a number of different stressful and difficult events. Repeated practice at concrete thinking for stressful events will allow you to strengthen your ability to move into the concrete way of thinking, making it more of an automatic habit . . . so you can find it easier and more natural to use . . . so you can use it to be more effective, when you most need it . . . naturally and instinctively . . . when faced with difficulties or stress day to day.

"Let's start by practicing a past example from your own life in detail to illustrate how to think concretely. Earlier you mentioned a situation where there was a difficulty with rumination [or overgeneralization or inactivity]."

The therapist refers back to a previous example the patient has mentioned of ruminating or overgeneralizing. It is useful to choose an example that is likely to be amenable to the training: where there is scope to discriminate the event in more detail and where the event is not too difficult or too emotionally challenging for the patient. It is best to start practicing with a mildly to moderately upsetting event rather than a more severe event.

"Do you feel OK talking this event through? Good, I'll give you quite a lot of guidance on this first one to help you come to grips with the exercise.

"Let's start by setting the scene. Tell me briefly about the event and what happened."

The therapist prompts for more detail about the event as necessary by asking "Where did it happen?"; "When was it [day, time]?"; "Who was there?"; "What was happening?"; "How did it happen?"; "What was your response?"; "What did he/she do?" The therapist prompts until there are enough details to vividly imagine the scene and to get a sense of the situation's tractability.

> "Because this event has already happened, to be able to think concretely about it, you need to first mentally re-create it and get immersed in it, as if you're there right now, looking out of your eyes, within your body, reliving the event. By doing this, you are already starting to practice the first stage of being concrete—focusing on sensory details in the moment and noticing what is specific and distinctive. Seeing things from your own perspective in this way is very important because it makes the experience more real, connects you to your direct experience, and encourages a more active role. In depression, people often imagine events from a 'fly on the wall' perspective, observing themselves within the scene, which makes them feel disconnected or distanced, leading to a passive, unengaged approach that doesn't help them get on with their lives.
>
> "Now, as best you can, just concentrate on following my instructions—keep focusing on what I am saying and on what you are imagining—until I ask you to tell me what you are experiencing. [This instruction is useful in the training, as some participants keep interrupting to explain what they are doing halfway through instructions.]
>
> "OK, I'd like you to imagine, as vividly and concretely as possible, being in this situation [give reminder if necessary] . . . as if you are there right now . . . seeing through your own eyes, in your own body . . . [2-second pause] . . . Focus your attention on the specific details which make your experience distinctive . . . stand out . . . [2-second pause] . . . Notice what you are experiencing in the moment . . . See the situation from your own viewpoint, as if you are looking out on the scene. . . . Build a clear image of where you are, of your surroundings as [fill in from brief account] . . . Notice the specific [fill in from brief account relevant sights, sounds, etc.] . . . Be aware of the sensations you feel in your body . . . Notice the specific details that make this situation distinctive and unique . . . [5-second pause] . . .
>
> "Tell me briefly, what do you notice about this situation? Tell me what you can see in the scene?"

The therapist checks and probes for concrete details (e.g., facial expression, tone of voice, sensory information). The therapist gives feedback, examples, encouragement, guidance, rationale, and further prompts if necessary to shape the patient toward more concrete descriptions. The therapist needs to check that there is detailed and specific imagery and that the patient is using a field perspective, for example, "As you imagine the scene, are you looking out through your own eyes or do you see yourself in the scene?"

"What makes this event different from other times like this? What marks it out from other similar situations in time . . . place . . . setting . . . circumstances? What helps you to locate this event at a particular place and time? What makes this event distinctive? . . . "

The therapist gives feedback, examples, encouragement, guidance, rationale, and further prompts if necessary.

"Next, while continuing to practice imagining being in your body, looking out on the scene, we will practice another element of concrete thinking: noticing the process by which events and behaviors unfold, becoming aware of the sequence of events, what comes before and what follows after each action and event. This helps you to see how one thing leads to another, helping you to learn from events, predict what might happen next, and see how you can act to change things.

"So, still seeing through your own eyes . . . focus your attention on how this event occurred . . . focus on the sequence of events leading up to this event . . . As vividly and as concretely as possible imagine the series of steps, of actions and events, that led up to this [insert brief description of scenario], still looking out from your own eyes, in your own body . . .

"Just like you can replay a film at different speeds, for example in slow motion to capture key events, when you imagine what happened, you can control how fast or slowly you experience the sequence of events to capture the key steps and moments leading up to the event. These might last seconds, minutes, hours, days, or weeks. Often it's helpful to imagine the event very slowly, to experience what happens second by second, as if experiencing things frame by frame . . . all the time seeing the sequence unfold from your own perspective as if you are there right now, looking out from your eyes . . . Notice what process, what sequence of events led to this event . . . [5-second pause] . . .

"With your eyes remaining closed, talk me through the series of steps that led to this event."

The therapist checks and probes for concrete information and gives feedback, examples, encouragement, guidance, rationale, and further prompts, if necessary. Once it is clear that a suitably detailed sequence of steps is imagined, the therapist asks questions about warning signs and contingencies:

"As you imagine the sequence of events that led up to this difficult situation, can you spot any clues or warning signs that indicated this difficulty was coming? Tell me what signals and cues you can spot. Are there any earlier cues?

"As you imagine the sequence, do you notice any points where a different decision or action or different circumstances might have changed what happened? How could you have influenced what happened for better or for worse? Tell me what could have influenced what happened.

"Great, so now that you have achieved a clear grasp of the details of the specific situation you are in and how you came to be in this situation, you are in a good position to practice another element of concrete thinking: focusing on the detailed steps of how you can move forward from here, the means by which you can do something about the problem. [The therapist specifies the problem to the participant.]

"First, consider briefly, as concretely as possible, how things would change, how things would be different, if you moved forward from this difficulty . . . dealt with this problem . . . What would you be doing differently? . . . [2-second pause]

"With your eyes remaining closed, tell me how would things be different if you moved forward from this difficulty and dealt with this problem? What would you be doing differently?"

The therapist checks and probes for a realistic goal, described in terms of specific changes in behavior or environment and gives feedback, examples, encouragement, guidance, rationale, and further prompts as necessary.

"Next focus your attention on how you can move forward from here . . . the initial steps you can take to move forward . . . how you can make a plan, how you can move forward into helpful action . . . Remember that the steps you take could include both physical and mental 'actions,' like the act of 'walking away' or the act of 'making a decision' or 'saying something to someone' or 'telling yourself something different' [or an action that previous sections suggest might be useful for person].

"Now imagine that you proceed, still looking out from your own eyes, in your own body . . . Imagine as best you can, as vividly and concretely as possible, what you do next to deal with your situation . . . Again imagine the steps you take across the most helpful time frame— these steps might take seconds, minutes, or they may occur over the next days, weeks, or months . . . the important thing is that you imagine breaking the task down into discrete, manageable steps, as concretely as possible. See the first step in the chain of actions that you can take to deal with this difficult event . . . and then follow the sequence of how one step leads to another . . . imagining it as vividly as possible . . . [5-second pause] . . .

"Tell me what was the first step you took toward your goal and then how did you proceed?"

The therapist checks and probes for the discrete steps taken, reflecting a sense of sequence and contingency, that seems helpful.

> "Tell me what you have learned and how you can use this in your life now and in the future. Make a mental note of what actions you plan to do next. What have you learned that might be useful to you in the future?"

The therapist checks and probes for learning with respect to particular contexts and circumstances that influence outcomes. Which particular behaviors increase the chance for success and for a clear plan of action that could be implemented either then or now?

> "What was your experience of thinking about this difficult event more concretely?"

The therapist checks for any experienced benefit, corrects any confusion and uncertainty, and reviews if there are changes in rumination and overgeneralization.

> "So you've just thought through a difficult, stressful situation in a concrete way . . . using all of your senses to become aware of the specific details that make the situation distinctive and unique . . . focused on noticing how things happen . . . keeping things in perspective . . . putting you in a better position to see how you can move forward . . . problem-solve . . . helping you to make plans and to notice what influences your progress so you can be more aware of what is important in the future.
>
> "Good, we have now practiced thinking more concretely about a past personal stressful event. Any questions?"

After practicing on a past event and establishing that the patient understands the exercise, the exercise is then repeated in the session, either with another past event or with an ongoing difficulty of the patient, working through the identical instructions. It is important to ensure repeated practice of the exercise in the session. Consistent with the view of rumination as a habit, the therapist emphasizes the importance of repeated daily practice of the concreteness exercise, initially by the patient setting a time aside to listen to a recording of the session and to practice with past events, and then, as he or she becomes more familiar with the exercise, to begin to use it in daily life in response to difficulties and stressors as they occur.

The following instructions illustrate how concreteness training can be introduced and emphasized as a first-aid strategy to be used by patients in the moment when faced with real-world difficulties:

"You can also use this concreteness exercise as an emotional first aid strategy. Whenever you notice that you are getting stressed, that your mood is slipping, or you are faced with a problem in your daily life, you can use concrete thinking as a first-aid strategy to cope better with the difficulty. Once you have learned and practiced this first aid skill, you can use it whenever you feel the need, at any time throughout the day. We recommend that you practice the emotional first-aid exercise regularly at first, for example, by listening back to the audio recording of this treatment session. After you have practiced this for a while, you should be able to focus on the first aid exercise without the need to listen to the recording.

"Let's practice the emotional first-aid exercise now. For this exercise, focus your attention on the specific details and circumstances of the immediate event as it is happening to you right now rather than having to imagine yourself back into the stressful situation.

"This could be an actual problem, a negative thought, a concern, a worry, or a mood (e.g., feeling sad, anxious, down, bored).

"Is there any difficulty on your mind right now that you can apply the first aid exercise to? [The therapist makes a note of concern and gets some background.] OK, during the exercise we will focus on this concern.

"Please tell me how much this concern [use the patient's term] is bothering you right now from 0, not at all, to 100, as much as possible?

"Tell me how stressed you are feeling right now on a scale from 0, not at all stressed, to 100, as stressed as could be?

"Start the emotional first-aid exercise by focusing on your breathing . . . as best you can focus your attention on your breath . . . [2-second pause]—let the breathing become deep and regular . . . slow . . . steady . . . relaxed . . . noticing how each breath that you take in . . . [2-second pause], allows you to grow more comfortable . . . more relaxed within yourself . . . Breathe in . . . [3-second pause] . . . and . . . out . . . [3-second pause] nice and slow [2-second pause] . . . Calm . . . and relaxed . . . [2-second pause]"

The therapist has the patient focus on sensory details and notice what is specific and distinctive.

"Now, as best you can, focus your attention on experiencing as concretely as possible what is happening in the moment right now . . . [3-second pause]. Notice the specific details of what is happening around you . . . [5-second pause]. Observe where you are. Become aware of your surroundings . . . [3-second pause]. Notice what you can see, notice the specific noises you can hear, scents you can smell, textures you can feel . . . [3-second pause]. Focus on the sensations you feel in your body . . .

[3-second pause]. Notice any feelings, thoughts, or concerns that might be bothering you. Pay close attention to your experience of any feelings, thoughts, or concerns that might be bothering you.

"Focus your attention on the specific details that make your experience right now different from any other moment.

"Tell me briefly, what do you notice about this situation?"

The therapist checks and probes for concrete details (e.g., specific details about surroundings and sensory elements). The therapist gives feedback, examples, encouragement, guidance, rationale, and further prompts if necessary, with a focus on checking that patient is directly connecting with experience.

"What do you notice about this concern [or this thought or this feeling]? What marks this [this concern, this thought, this feeling] as distinct in time . . . place . . . setting . . . circumstances? What makes this unique?

"Now focus your attention on how this situation occurred . . . the sequence of events leading up to this moment, to this live problem and concern . . . As vividly and as concretely as possible re-create the series of steps, of actions and events that led up to [this concern, this thought, this feeling] right now, as if looking out from your own eyes . . . Notice what process, what sequence of events led to this moment, whether over seconds, minutes, hours, days, weeks . . . Notice when the [concern, feeling, thought] started . . . [5-second pause] . . . Briefly tell me how you came to be in this situation?"

The therapist checks and probes for concrete information indicating a sequence and gives feedback, examples, encouragement, guidance, rationale, and further prompts if necessary.

"As you focus on the sequence of events that led up to this moment, spot any clues or warning signs that indicated that this [this concern, this thought, this feeling] was starting. Tell me what signals and cues you can spot."

The therapist checks and probes for concrete information indicating a sequence and gives feedback, examples, encouragement, guidance, rationale, and further prompts if necessary.

"Are there any earlier cues?

"Notice any points where a different decision or action or different circumstances might have changed what happened. Tell me what could have influenced what happened? Now consider briefly how things would change if you moved forward from this difficulty . . . dealt with this problem . . . [2-second pause] . . . Next, focus your attention on the initial steps you can take to move forward . . . how you can make a plan, how you can move forward into helpful action. . . . [2-second pause] . . . Now imagine that you proceed, still looking out from your own eyes, in your own body. . . . Imagine as vividly and concretely as possible what you do next to deal with your situation . . . second by second . . . or month by month . . . breaking the task down into discrete, manageable steps. See the first step in the chain of actions that you can do to deal with this difficult event . . . and then follow the sequence of how one step leads to another . . . imagining it as vividly as possible . . . [5-second pause] . . .

"Briefly tell me, how do you plan to move forward?"

The therapist checks and probes for discrete steps taken, reflecting a sense of sequence and contingency that seem helpful and gives feedback, examples, encouragement, guidance, rationale, and further prompts as necessary.

"Make a mental note of what you have learned and the action you plan to do NEXT.

"Now please tell me how much this concern [use the patient's term] is bothering you right now from 0, not at all, to 100, as much as possible?

"Tell me how stressed you are feeling right now on a scale from 0, not at all stressed, to 100, as stressed as could be?

"What did you notice about looking at this current issue as it happens right now?

"There is another way that you can use the first-aid exercise. You can use it in response to the warning signs you are learning to notice, as a way of preempting problems and nipping them in the bud. For example, if feeling physically tense in your shoulders and neck and feeling your heart rate increase are warning signs that often come just before you start ruminating, then it would be useful to use the emotional first aid whenever you notice this tension. Focus on reducing the tension as the target of the first aid and this might then stop you from ruminating.

"These warning signs for depression vary from person to person. They can be events like conflicts, disappointments, novelty, uncertainties, challenges, risks; they can be physical feelings like tension, butterflies, a 'sinking feeling' in the stomach, tiredness; they can be emotions like anxiety, irritability, frustration; they can be mental experiences like attention becoming narrowed, thinking becoming confused and foggy; they can be situations like feeling under pressure, trying to do too many things at once; they can be thoughts such as doubts and self-criticism. And as you focus on the experience of concrete thinking, make a mental link between your warning signs and the concrete way of thinking. Imagine using the first-aid exercise to shift into the concrete way of thinking in response to the warning signs as an active attempt to cope and improve your situation.

"What do you think are your main early warning signs of depression (of rumination, of inactivity, overgeneralization)? Let's think about how you can use the first-aid exercise when you notice a warning sign. Which of these warning signs—which thought or physical sensation—is the most common or earliest one?

"OK, now make a mental link between this warning sign and doing the first-aid exercise. Imagine that when you next notice the warning sign, you do the first-aid exercise. Imagine that as vividly as you can.

"Make a mental note to yourself—If I notice a warning sign, then I will use the first-aid exercise.

"Focus now on what useful things you could do in response to the warning signs—how you could stop things from getting worse when you notice the warning signs. What are the steps you could take? Focus on that for a few moments."

The therapist checks and probes for discrete steps taken, reflecting a sense of sequence and contingency that seem helpful.

Again, I want to stress the importance of patients being able to practice repeatedly spotting more abstract thinking and then shifting this to more concrete thinking throughout their daily lives (e.g., making thoughts more tied to the particular aspects of the situation, to the what, where, when, and how of the situation). The content of the thought is not important because practice will strengthen the ability to be more concrete and make it easier to do this with more important, more emotional thoughts. Furthermore, regular brief practice will prime and reactivate the more concrete style of thinking, so that even a few minutes of doing it will make this thinking style more accessible.

Guidance for the Therapist: Checking and Prompting during the Concreteness Training Exercise

Throughout the concreteness exercise, the therapist checks that the patient has selected a suitable example for practice and is adopting a concrete style. The therapist guides and prompts toward more specific descriptions if the patient is not being sufficiently concrete. The following are suggestions for how to do this. Additional details can be found earlier in this chapter and in Chapter 3 (Principle 3: Encourage active, concrete, experiential, and specific behavior—the ACES rule).

Choosing Situations for Practice

With respect to the selection of practice examples, the therapist checks that the example chosen is not too upsetting or an event that the patient is highly likely to ruminate about and thus one that it would be difficult to tackle at the start of training. The event selected needs to have distinctive and specific elements that can be identified. If the event does not seem appropriate, the therapist works with the patient to identify another example for practice or changes the temporal focus of the identified example by moving earlier in the chain that led up to the major event, or by focusing on a period of rumination some time later.

The therapist asks the patient to initially set the scene to get a sense of how tractable the event is and whether it is a good training example, and to provide the therapist with details that enable him or her to guide and prompt the exercise in a more informed way.

Focusing on a Specific Point in Time

When setting the scene, I recommend that the timeline for the imagery start at the moment when the problem became evident or is at its most acute. Many difficulties that patients with depression face are often complex and build up over an extended time period or can involve repeated occurrences. It is thus important for the concreteness practice to focus on a specific occasion and on a clear point in the sequence of the difficulty. For the same reason, we need to be clear about the focus of the exercise, and whether it is concentrating on a difficult event (e.g., having an argument with a family member) or the response to the event (e.g., ruminating about it afterwards). Either is appropriate, but the therapist needs to make sure the exercise stays focused on one or the other, not shifting between them. When the difficult event is less amenable to change, then it is often useful to focus on the response to the event.

Prompting for More Sensory Detail

When the patient sets the scene, the therapist seeks enough detail so that he or she can begin to clearly picture it. Useful questions to prompt for more concrete detail include: "What happened? Where did it happen? When did it happen? Who was there? How did it happen? When did it start? When did it stop?" Another approach to shift the patient toward more specific descriptions is to prompt for more contextual, sensory, and perceptual focus in the imagery (e.g., "Notice what you can see in the lounge," "Describe what you can see in front of you"). For social situations, the therapist asks about the patient's and other people's behavior, facial expression, tone of voice, and posture (e.g., "How does he sound?"; "How do you know he was angry?"; "What is it about his behavior/expression that signals that?"; "How are you saying that to him?"). For mental and emotional responses, the therapist prompts for details of physical sensations, exact thoughts, and focus of attention (e.g., "What are you noticing in your body?"; "What thought is going through your mind?"; "What are you paying attention to?").

Prompting for Detail about the External Environment

When helping the patient to notice what is specific and distinctive about a situation, the therapist asks specific questions to draw out information about the external environment (e.g., location, presence of other people) and behavior (including actions, thoughts) that make this situation unique and distinct from any others (e.g., "What was unique about the place, time, behavior, and environment when this happened? What did you think or do differently from other similar situations?"). For example, a patient who points out her headache when she canceled an appointment with a friend may not be seeing the situation as distinctive if she regularly has headaches, but there may be other distinct elements linked to what happened. The more the question itself describes the specific context, the more helpful it will be for generating specific responses. Furthermore, it is useful to highlight potential comparisons within the question and to select the comparison most likely to be meaningful, accessible, and helpful to the patient. If one comparison does not work, try another one. For the patient whose practice example was canceling a meeting with a friend over the phone because she had a headache, questions included, "What makes this time you phoned your friend different from other times you phoned your friend?"; "What makes this event different from times when you have gone ahead and seen your friend?"; "What makes this event different from times when you have had a headache and still gone ahead and seen your friend?" Different questions highlight different aspects of the situation and may generate different alternatives.

Prompting for Details of the Unfolding Sequence

When working through the steps by which events unfold, the therapist needs to ensure there is sufficient detail in the sequence. Patients typically summarize situations in a way that loses temporal detail. It is therefore useful to break down what happened second by second as if in slow motion and use more prompts to identify what thoughts, emotions, and physical sensations the patient was experiencing (e.g., the therapist asks, "What went through your mind at that moment just then? And the second after that, what did you feel, or think, or do?").

Similarly, for the section on next steps, the therapist needs to get a detailed, concrete sense of how things would change, what would be different, what goal the patient would like to work toward. This is usefully operationalized as a behavior, as what the patient would be doing if the problem were addressed rather than as a change in physical or mental state or circumstances (e.g., "What would you be doing differently?"). For a person who was ruminating about the end of a relationship, the desired endpoint could be to resume the relationship, to not think about the relationship, to act in a more confident way, to find a better relationship, and so forth. The therapist would work with the patient to specify the goal in terms of concrete behaviors.

For events in the past that can't be changed, the focus is on learning from the event. The therapist asks questions like: "How can you learn from this event?"; "What can you do differently to prevent or prepare for these problems in the future?"; "How can you change patterns of behavior that maintain this problem?"; "How can you express your feelings about what happened?"; "What would you be doing differently if you let go or moved on from this event?"

The steps taken to solve the problem are most likely to be successful if they are simple behaviors and actions to change the environment or the patient's own response. Across the patients treated with RFCBT, a number of common useful steps keep reoccurring. These include doing one thing at a time; asking someone how they are; expressing feelings appropriately; giving oneself more space; reducing distractions; removing oneself from a stressful situation; recognizing when others are stressed; saying something more positive to oneself; shifting one's focus of attention to more positive things; shifting one's focus of attention outward and onto tasks; getting up and doing something; breaking tasks down into smaller steps.

FA and Thinking Style

Another way to train patients away from abstract thinking is to encourage them to practice FA for themselves (see Chapters 6 and 7; Handout 8, Being More Effective and Handout 9, Being More Effective form). FA forms can be used to help patients consider the discriminative stimuli relevant to a situation (who, where, when, how, and what) and how they influence outcomes.

When describing situations, the patient is prompted to describe the situation in a way that captures the full context, that is, incorporating where, when, how, what, and with whom. For example, "I am a failure" becomes "I failed to go swimming on Tuesday at 2 P.M. when I was feeling tired and my friend phoned to say she couldn't come."

Noting the context relevant to the thought is useful for determining whether the thought and feelings apply to other situations. For example, the thought "I am too tired to do anything. I'll give up on my plan to go out tomorrow" could be contextualized as "I am thinking that I am too tired to go help other people clear the paths at the bird sanctuary tomorrow, while sitting on my own indoors at home at the end of a day where I haven't done anything." This contextualized version has much more detail about what (thoughts and details of activities), where (indoors vs. outdoors), when (today, tomorrow), and with whom (alone, with other people). Reframing things this way can help the patient to see that the tiredness she feels now is not necessarily relevant to how she will be tomorrow, particularly if she enjoys being outside with other people.

Patients can conduct their own FA to recognize more concrete and situational information relevant to the outcomes of their activities. For example, when an attempt at a task is not successful, the patient examines the context in which the failure occurred, what contextual factors (how, when, where, with whom) might have influenced the outcome, and what contextual factors are different between times when he is successful and he is not. For example, following the failure to complete a do-it-yourself job, the patient focused on more concrete information, "I did not do a very good job of hanging a heavy picture this morning, when I was in a hurry and feeling stressed about getting to a meeting, and when I was on my own, and this was the first time I have put up a picture." Introducing more concrete information and making thinking less abstract and less vague tends to make the thought less extreme and facilitates the ability to learn from the situation.

Patients report that being more discriminative makes plans seem more manageable, and it can provide clues as to what to do next. For example, one patient dreaded going to visit her mother and reported it as very stressful, saying "I can't cope with this." She viewed it as a cause of her setbacks. When practicing daily attempts at being more discriminative, she noticed for the first time that she disliked some aspects of going to her mother's house (e.g., sorting out all the chores that needed doing) but enjoyed some other aspects (e.g., sitting and chatting with her mother). Previously she had taken an overly general and abstract view of going to her mother's house as being difficult, rather than discriminating within the situation. By being able to discriminate within the situation, she was able to manage it much better. Further, this increased discrimination provided insight relevant to problem solving (e.g., arranging future visits such that the balance of spending time with mother vs. doing chores was more favorable to her).

In another example, the thought "I feel hungry" can be described within the context in which it occurred (i.e., "I feel hungry at 11 A.M. in my flat, while sitting around not doing much on my own, when I had two pieces of toast for breakfast at 8 A.M."). The contextual details suggest not only that this state may be changeable but that certain factors might be relevant for making a change.

While this is a relatively trivial thought, the same process can be applied to clinically relevant thoughts such as "I feel sad" or "I feel tired," which influence a patient's behavior. By practicing looking at thoughts in this more concrete way, patients may be in a position to shift their view of the stability of this state. For example, a patient could recognize that tiredness may be a factor of the context (e.g., being alone, not doing anything interesting, being indoors) and then recognize that shifting the context could be helpful in reducing the tiredness. These approaches can be further reinforced by talking through examples and practicing more explicit FA using the homework forms (see the FA forms from Chapter 6 and Handouts 6 and 7).

FA can be useful in shifting processing mode when it helps a patient to identify how her own thinking may differ between situations and become aware that different styles of thinking may have distinct effects. When FA reveals distinct styles of thinking, the therapist then guides the patient to more systematically shift into the more helpful form of thinking. This approach has the merit of directly building from the patient's own experience by identifying behavior already in her repertoire and then increasing its frequency.

One patient compared a time when her ruminating about a difficulty was unhelpful with another time when it was more helpful. She identified specific aspects of the context, environment, and her own behavior that influenced the outcomes. The patient first described a recent situation where she had received a bill in the mail and started to feel anxious and tense, with her heart rate increasing and her attention narrowing and closing in. When her sequence of thoughts was tracked moment by moment, the chain of thinking started with a constructive thought ("How am I going to pay my bills?"), but this was quickly followed by more evaluative and abstract thoughts like "I am failure because I am not working" and then a series of ruminative "why"-type questions such as "Why am I useless?"; "Why do people put up with me?"; "What's wrong with me?"; and "What does this mean about me?" This sequence of thinking caused the patient to become more anxious, depressed, tearful, and exhausted, and to retreat to bed. This episode of rumination lasted over 3 hours.

In comparison, the patient reported another time when she felt dismissed by her partner when discussing a decision. This experience also led to her feeling tense and to her heart rate increasing and her attention narrowing. When her chain of thoughts was examined second by second, the first thoughts she had were "I'll probably make the wrong decision," followed by "Why is this so difficult?" These initial thoughts were then followed by a sequence of other questions: "What would someone else do to cope?"; "What is the best way to get a positive result?"; "What can I do differently?"; "How can I handle this?" Asking these questions helped the patient to feel less tense and to make a plan. The period of rumination only lasted 25 minutes, and she was able to get on with her day.

In comparing the two situations, it is apparent that increasing tension and heart rate and narrowing of attention are potential warning signs for rumination. It is also clear that the way she was thinking in the two situations had distinct effects on how she felt and coped. The first example illustrates a common phenomenon in episodes of rumination: an initial attempt to think constructively about a problem ("How am I going to pay my bills?") is highjacked by the tendency to go into more abstract and evaluative "why"-type questions. The second example illustrates naturally and spontaneously occurring concrete "how"-type thinking. When these two situations were compared, the patient was able to see that the latter way of thinking was potentially more helpful than the former, and that it might be useful to increase this in her daily life. These naturally occurring differences in thinking style match the "how" and "why" distinction made earlier and indicate that "how"-type thinking can occur spontaneously in patients.

When this happens, the therapist highlights that the patient is already doing something helpful and then seeks to make its use more systematic and more frequent. For this patient, the therapist followed the six E's or E⁶ precepts (Explore Experience, Experiment with Experience, Exercise and Engage, as described earlier in this chapter) and further consolidated this recognition by trying out a Why–How behavioral experiment in the session. This revealed that the "how" questions were helpful, so these questions were then built into an If–Then plan: If I notice that I am getting tense and my attention is narrowing, I will ask myself helpful questions like "What would someone else do to cope?"; "How can I handle this situation?"

Visualization, Imagery, and Concreteness

Imagery and visualization techniques can be powerful in helping patients to shift from an unhelpful style of rumination to a more helpful concrete style that leads to effective problem resolution. Imagery and visualization exercises have multiple simultaneous benefits for rumination.

First, imagery tends to be concrete, shifting processing away from the abstract thinking characteristic of unhelpful rumination. Second, imagery can help patients to focus on the sequence of actions and the process and mechanics of events. This helps with problem solving and reduces the focus on meanings found in rumination. Third, imagery can help rapidly instill different mind-sets that can shift the style of processing (discussed further in Chapters 10 and 11).

It is important to note, however, that there is no simple one-to-one correspondence between imagery and being concrete. It is possible to be very concrete without imagery, for example by making detailed verbal lists and plans. Moreover, it is possible to have imagery that carries more generic and abstract meanings, such as prototypical images that summarize multiple situations without a specific context. Imagery from an observer perspective (e.g., seeing oneself in the image) is more abstract than imagery from a field perspective (e.g., imagining looking out from your own eyes). For example, a number of anxiety disorders are characterized by generic negative images from an observer perspective (e.g., an individual with social anxiety seeing himself as shaking, sweaty, and with a bright red face).

General Principles for Imagery

For some patients, practicing imagery with straightforward neutral objects may be useful before imagining a personally relevant emotional situation (e.g., imagining an apple in as much detail as possible). Imagery work is most effective when it is done with calm guiding questions, and the patient is relaxed. It is useful to socialize patients into the idea of imagery and help to prepare them for it by having already done some relaxation with them. Patients are asked to evoke and describe the full range of sensory and emotional experience in each situation. Imagery is usually most powerful when it is done in the first person, in a field perspective (i.e., being the actor looking out into the imagined scene, rather than observing oneself in the imagined scene) and in the present tense (e.g., "Imagine yourself in the situation right now. What can you see looking out through your eyes?"). If the patient's description creates an image in your own mind as the therapist, it is probably a suitably vivid image.

Visualizing a Plan

The "visualizing a plan" exercise facilitates better problem solving and a concrete, action-oriented strategy to interrupt imminent rumination about a problem. Patients are asked to concretely imagine and mentally rehearse the steps needed to reach a goal or cope with a difficult situation. Here is an example of relevant instructions:

"It is important to see yourself doing [identified activity] and to hold this picture in your mind. As you imagine this situation, fill in all the details about who, when, where, what was happening. Make the image as vivid and realistic as possible—imagine the shapes and colors you can see, imagine the sounds you can hear, imagine your physical posture, notice any smells, become aware of the feel of your body in the room. Describe to me what you can see. Notice how you feel and as you pay attention to that feeling, let it strengthen and deepen."

This imagery work is based on the finding that it is more effective to imagine the process than the outcome involved in problem solving (Taylor, Pham, Rivkin, & Armor, 1998). Patients are therefore encouraged to vizualize step by step the situation, what is going on, what actions they will attempt, the consequences of the actions, the circumstances surrounding the event, and the feelings they experience. Such visualization can be a useful adjunct to concreteness training.

Visualizing Success, Including Use of a Positive Self-Image

It can be useful to have patients visualize success first and then visualize potential difficulties and how they might overcome them. For example, one patient had spontaneous intrusive images about going to the employment office that made her feel anxious. The therapist worked with her on using imagery to cope.

THERAPIST: This image makes you more anxious and seems to be an early warning sign for rumination. Is that right?

PATIENT: Yes.

THERAPIST: OK, let's use this as an opportunity to practice the contingency plan. The first stage of the plan is to spot the warning sign, in this case, the image. Then what do you do?

PATIENT: Visualize something more positive.

THERAPIST: OK, let's practice that right now. Go on imagining that you are in the same scene, so it is clearly recognizable as the employment office. Imagine how it looks as you go in, right now, looking out through your eyes, as you see the person you deal with—really make it as vivid as you can, see the colors, what the room looks like, see his facial expression, hear the tone of his voice, and run that conversation you were having forward a little bit, see what you are talking about, dealing with, making it as vivid as possible. Spend a few moments building up the image in your mind.

THERAPIST: Have you got a vivid picture in your mind?

PATIENT: Yes.

THERAPIST: Good, and imagine the meeting continuing and see how it unfolds in a positive way. As the conversation moves forward, imagine how it turns out OK—how he is more helpful than you expected. Notice what he is saying and his facial expression and tone of voice as things turn out just as you hoped. Notice how you feel . . . (*pause*)

THERAPIST: What is happening in the situation?

PATIENT: I'm chatting with the guy and things are going pretty well.

THERAPIST: Great. How do you feel now?

PATIENT: A bit calmer, the sensations in my tummy have gone.

THERAPIST: That's interesting. Those feelings in your stomach, could they be another early warning sign of rumination? Maybe we should note that down as well. Let's quickly recap—you have just spent a few minutes imagining the situation in a different way from before. What effect has this had?

PATIENT: I feel calmer and less preoccupied.

THERAPIST: What can we learn from this?

PATIENT: Imagery can have very powerful effects on my feelings.

Visualizing Coping with a Difficulty

When useful coping strategies are identified for patients, repeated imagining of difficult situations that are vivid enough to elicit some emotion, followed by use of the coping strategy (e.g., relaxation, shifting thinking style), strengthens the coping response, consolidates the If–Then contingency plan, and increases the likelihood that it will be used in real-life situations. In the same way, it can be useful to mentally rehearse alternative responses to rumination triggers. This is particularly helpful when the cues to rumination are emotional responses such as feeling tense, down, or irritable; using imagery to induce these feelings in the session, even if only weakly, and then to practice an alternative response, will build an association between this cue and the constructive response incompatible with rumination. In other words, this involves counterconditioning an alternative response to the rumination trigger to learn a new, more adaptive habit (see Chapter 2).

In the example above, the patient who was worried about going to the employment office visualized a meeting that went well. The therapist then helped her rehearse coping with a less positive meeting. The dialogue continues as follows:

THERAPIST: Let's think about going to the next image. Imagine yourself back in the more difficult situation that came up before, but this time imagine yourself coping with it. Let's start by reviewing what you would be doing to cope with this situation. What have you learned that can help you cope with difficult situations? Talk me through the strategies you use.

PATIENT: I can use visualizations, I can try and calm down my breathing, I can try and act and speak in a calm way.

THERAPIST: Excellent, so you have a number of strategies you could use. Now, when you imagine the difficult situation, imagine yourself as best you can using some or all of these strategies. OK?

PATIENT: Uh-huh.

THERAPIST: OK, so re-create the image of yourself in the difficult situation— imagine that you are back in the employment office looking out at the man opposite you, imagine how he is looking. Notice how you are feeling in that situation—that you are feeling a bit anxious and tense. Once you have a clear image, continue to imagine yourself in the situation, and then feel yourself doing the breathing exercise, beginning to calm down. Imagine that you are using a visualization exercise to relax, notice yourself staying focused on positive things. Imagine yourself doing all the coping things, staying calm in the situation. Notice how you might still feel a bit anxious and apprehensive but you go on anyway. Imagine being assertive in a calm way, putting your point of view across. Get as vivid an image as you can of staying in that situation, doing those things we talked about. Hold on to the image of how you are handling this difficult situation, making it as vivid as you can . . . (pause)

THERAPIST: OK, what happened then?

PATIENT: I felt a lot calmer.

THERAPIST: Good, what were you imagining yourself doing to cope?

PATIENT: Just breathing, I do tend to get short of breath when I get upset and then I get shaky and start shouting.

THERAPIST: And what happened in the scene as you imagined slowing down your breathing?

PATIENT: I became a different person. I just thought, I can cope with it. I can think about it in a more positive way.

THERAPIST: So what might be the next step if you are thinking about it in a more positive way—if we think about how to translate thoughts into action? It seemed as if using the image helped cut off the worry. Are there any plans you can make to carry this forward?

Processing Upsetting Events

A visual imagery approach can also be adopted when considering a past event that the patient ruminates about. This approach is useful when patients report repeated rumination about past upsetting events that do not seem to resolve over time. The first step is to check whether the patient is getting in touch with the details and the emotional experience of what happened when she thinks about the past event. It may be that the patient is thinking about upsetting events over and over but is not habituating or fully processing the events emotionally because at the crucial junctures she moves away from the concrete emotional details to more abstract thinking (e.g., asking "Why did this happen?"). To complete successful processing, it may be necessary to get patients to focus on the specific emotionally relevant details of what happened in the situation. Thus, the ACES principle applies as much to the processing of past events as to the response to current problems.

It is fairly common for intrusive memories of past upsetting or difficult events, such as previous trauma, loss, or rejection, to trigger episodes of rumination. These memories typically set off further ruminative thinking about the meaning and implications of the event. Although the initial recall of the memory will tend to involve specific and sensory–perceptual details, particularly for intrusive and involuntary memories, this is often quickly replaced by more abstract and conceptual *thinking about* the event, as the patient tries to makes sense of and understand what happened and why. The effect of such ruminative thinking is that the patient spends very little time with the specific details, emotions, and direct experience of the negative event, making it very hard for her to work through the event, come to terms with it, and habituate to the upset. Instead, the patient is caught up in thinking about the meanings of the event (e.g., "Why did this happen? What does it mean about me?"). Such thinking distances and disconnects the patient from the details of the original event.

Furthermore, when these abstract questions are asked, other similar events and situations often come to mind, so that the patient ends up thinking about a number of different but related difficult events and memories. This makes it even harder to emotionally process and habituate to the upsetting event because the patient is thinking about more than one memory. Thus, a person with a tendency to ruminate can get into a self-perpetuating cycle where upsetting memories can trigger rumination, but the abstract rumination prevents the patient from processing them effectively, so that they keep coming back.

To address such triggers for rumination, the therapist needs to guide the patient to stay with the memory in sufficient detail and for a sufficient length of time that the event is adequately processed, allowing habituation to the upsetting emotion. This parallels the use of imagery exposure to address upsetting and traumatic events in patients with PTSD. This is fully consistent with the ACES principle. It is also consistent with addressing the function of the rumination: one (perhaps unintended) function of abstract rumination is that it avoids the details of the upsetting event and thus is negatively reinforced through reducing acute negative emotion in the short term. In effect, for such upsetting memories, we are engaging in imagery exposure work, which involves carefully and slowly working through the details of a past upset.

The patient is asked to visualize how the problem arose and recall what happened one step at a time: the actions she undertook, the circumstances surrounding the event, and the feelings she experienced during the event. These visualized periods need to be rehearsed repeatedly, as typically done for imaginal exposure work. As the patient recalls and focuses on the memory, we want to ensure that she is fully experiencing what happened by focusing on the concrete and specific details of the event. To ensure habituation to the upsetting event, the patient needs to stay in the moment for each upsetting event and fully experience what happened long enough for the emotional arousal to begin to come down. Because there is often a tendency to shift back into abstract thinking about the memory, as well as a tendency to go through these memories quickly, the therapist may have to keep prompting the patient back to the sensory–perceptual details of the situation (e.g., "What can you see?"; "What did he do next?"). The therapist may also have to prompt the patient to slow things down and to run the memory as if screening a film in slow motion, to ensure there is sufficient time spent on each moment to enable full processing, exposure, and habituation.

One example of processing upsetting events involved a patient who had experienced a painful divorce, where her ex-husband had been difficult and abusive. She reported many memories of events from the final months of her marriage, such as the day when her husband left the family home. These memories triggered bouts of rumination. Her rumination focused on why the divorce happened, what it meant about her, and what she had done wrong. When the therapist explored these memories and her rumination in further detail, it became clear that although these intrusive memories were frequent, she was only spending a few moments on the details of each memory before going into more general rumination *about what* had happened and what it meant. After identifying this, she collaboratively agreed with her therapist to experiment with trying something different, namely, spending time exploring one of those memories, the day her husband left, focusing on the details of where she was, what she felt, what he did and said, and so forth. The therapist planned for a longer session (2 hours) to increase the chance that her feelings would begin to decrease as exposure to the situation continued. The therapist also recorded the session so that the patient could repeat the exposure daily as homework.

After a week of practice listening to the recording, the patient came back and reported that she was feeling a lot sadder. However, when the therapist looked at her depression scores, the symptoms had significantly abated. Moreover, her levels of rumination had been significantly reduced. It appeared that spending detailed time on the memories of the divorce had put her in touch with the normal response of feeling sad following a significant personal loss, while reducing her rumination had begun to ameliorate the depressive symptoms. Over subsequent sessions, other specific events were worked through. She also got in touch with feelings of anger toward her ex-husband for how badly he had treated her. The rumination may have prevented her from working through her primary emotional response to the divorce, such as sadness and anger, instead getting her stuck in secondary responses like self-blame. If the rumination hadn't been stopped, it may not have been possible to help her emotionally process the upsetting event and come to terms with the past.

CHAPTER 10

Shifting Processing Style

Absorption

As described in Chapter 9, patients in RFCBT use directed imagery to vividly create a more helpful thinking style (e.g., concreteness), in order to directly counter rumination. One useful set of memories are of times when the patient is completely absorbed in an activity. These may be "flow" or "peak" experiences of being creative, being immersed in sensory experience, or involved in highly focused physical activities like rock climbing or skiing. During such periods of absorption, the patient is unlikely to be ruminating. Moreover, an absorbed mind-set tends to involve a concrete, process-focused, action-oriented style, and it is associated with a direct connection with experience and increased engagement with activities.

The focus on increasing absorption to reduce rumination is based on several principles. First, rumination is characterized by high levels of self-consciousness, self-criticism, negative evaluations, and conceptual–evaluative thinking. Often, rumination can be experienced as having a mental "running commentary" that compares and judges the individual, his or her mood, and performance. Becoming fully absorbed in a task is therefore a good counter to rumination because when someone is fully immersed in what he is doing, he no longer has this running commentary and is no longer aware of himself.

Second, rumination is often characterized by an outcome focus where the individual evaluates how well she is doing (e.g., see Dykman, 1998, for a discussion of validation orientation), and the motivation is to check performance and avoid mistakes. This orientation can be contrasted with a process-focused way of thinking, where individuals are interested in how things are happening and are motivated by learning and discovering (a growth-seeking orientation, Dykman, 1998).

For example, when writing a research paper, you could be focused on outcome—on what you need to do to get it published—or you could be focused on process and be interested in exploring the ideas involved in writing the paper. The outcome-focused approach can be useful in defining what you need to do to get the paper published and in checking how your work meets those criteria. The outcome-focused mode is an important and essential mode. However, if it were the only mode you used when writing the paper, it would probably be very hard work, feel like a chore, and would be associated with thoughts about what was going to happen if it was not accepted. The process-focused mode would be more creative, more motivated, and more fun. Ideal working practice probably involves healthy switching between the two modes.

The outcome focus is associated with a conceptual–evaluative style of processing (asking why, making comparisons), typical of that found in rumination. In contrast, process focus is associated with a concrete style of thinking, which should help people to break out of rumination. Research indicates that the growth-seeking orientation produces greater resilience in the face of difficulties and an ability to learn from and overcome mistakes and errors, leading to better performance relative to the validation-seeking outcome-focused approach (Dykman, 1998). Encouraging absorption in activities is a powerful way to induce the process-focused approach and to shift into a more growth-seeking orientation.

Third, abstract rumination can distance individuals from the world around them, from their environment, and from possible reward. When someone is stuck in rumination, she is caught "in her head" rather than "in the world." This is hypothesized to make her less sensitive to what is going on in the world around her, to potentially miss important cues and signs, and to make it hard to learn from events (Watkins, 2013). This can feed into difficulties with other people. It can also contribute to a reduced ability to experience pleasure and reward, as the person is not fully in contact with possible reinforcing activities (Killingsworth & Gilbert, 2010).

This is further exacerbated by abstract thinking, where the individual is thinking about what he is doing and evaluating it, rather than directly experiencing it. In this way, it is hypothesized that rumination can interfere with the ability to experience pleasure and reward even when doing previously positive activities. This will particularly be the case if there is a running commentary on the behavior or activity.

For example, someone with depression who used to enjoy playing a musical instrument might be trying to increase this activity to improve his mood, perhaps within activity scheduling during cognitive therapy, but even as he does this homework, he is having ongoing evaluative thoughts like "Why this is so difficult?"; "Why can't I do this as well as before?" Experiencing such thoughts while doing the activity would take the shine off it and block any possible benefit. I therefore hypothesize that rumination may contribute to anhedonia and reduced motivation in depression. This is consistent with my clinical experience, where patients have come back from completing activity-scheduling assignments and reported that "I did the plan but I felt worse." A recent large-scale experience-sampling study confirmed this hypothesis with negative mind wandering associated with reduced pleasure from normally pleasurable activities (Killingsworth & Gilbert, 2010).

On closer examination, we often find that in these circumstances, the patient is ruminating during the activity and this impairs her ability to gain benefit. Shifting into an absorbed mind-set and getting immersed in the process of doing an activity, rather than thinking about it, is therefore designed to circumvent this rumination and help patients connect with positive experience and benefit from increasing their activities. The handout on connecting with experience (Handout 10, Engaging with Life through Concreteness) provides further reading on this topic for patients.

The RFCBT approach to increasing absorption is twofold. First, the therapist works with the patient to identify memories of being absorbed and coaches the patient in experiential imagery exercises designed to recapture this experience and reengage the same mind-set that facilitates absorption. Second, plans are made to increase activities in daily life that are likely to be absorbing and that will shift the patient out of the abstract–evaluative processing characteristic of unhelpful rumination. These absorbing activities are chosen based on reviewing past memories of absorbing activities and informed by FA of when the patient is more and less likely to be absorbed.

The goal of absorption experiences is for the patient to be able to re-create the experience of being caught up in a task, in a state of "flow" or "in the zone," in order to use it to interrupt rumination. This is done by helping the patient to identify a relevant memory of being absorbed, then talking the memory through and prompting the patient to vividly reimagine her state of mind during this memory by imagining being back in that situation. To make this induction of the absorbed state of mind as powerful as possible, the therapist focuses on creating a holistic experiential shift that incorporates memories and images of thoughts, feelings, posture, sensory experience, bodily sensations, attitude, motivation, facial expression, and action feelings.

Key Elements in Shifting Style

There are several key steps in helping patients to recapture the experience of being absorbed. Our experience is that this takes a certain amount of preparation and socialization into the idea of using imagery. It often works better when patients have already used some relaxation or imagery, which makes this approach more familiar.

First, the therapist works with the patient to find vivid memories and imagery of being in the process-focused absorbed state. These are then explored and reviewed in detail to establish the context and sequence of what happened. This information helps the therapist to later prompt the patient into reexperiencing the memory.

Second, the therapist works with the patient to re-create the mental state of being fully absorbed by guiding the patient to imagine herself back into the remembered situation, with prompts based on the reviewed memory and instructions to adopt a present-tense field perspective. These prompts need to develop the full holistic experience by prompting for sensory experience (e.g., "As vividly as you can, see what you are looking at. Describe what you can see"); motivation and attitude (e.g., "Focus on your motivation for doing this activity"); posture (e.g., "As you become more absorbed, notice your posture of relaxation. Notice and recapture how you are holding your body"); physical sensations (e.g., "Notice the sensations in your body"); emotional feelings (e.g., "Experience and hold on to your feelings, letting them deepen"); facial expressions (e.g., "Notice the expression on your face as you become more absorbed"); urges to action (e.g., "What do you feel like doing right now?"); and attention (e.g., "What do you notice? Where are you focusing your attention? What is capturing your attention?").

Recapturing the experience of being absorbed can be used in several ways. First, the therapist can use the experience to kick-start the concrete, process-focused mind-set associated with being absorbed. It can be used to illustrate an alternative to rumination, for example, within a behavioral experiment, or to get patients in a more helpful frame of mind before attempting activities. Therapists can use the induction of the absorbed memory as a coping strategy within a patient's If–Then contingency plan to shift away from the ruminative mode. When the patient is faced with a problem, engaging with a memory of being absorbed can facilitate a more constructive mind-set in which to address the real-world situation. Moreover, exploring times when the patient was deeply immersed in an activity can be used within FA to work out what facilitates the patient becoming absorbed, identify useful activities, and make future plans.

In adopting a FA approach, the therapist identifies times when the patient has had the experience of being absorbed. Useful questions to identify these memories include:

"Can you think of a time when you were absorbed in the process of doing something?"
"What happens when you are involved in the process of doing something?"

"Describe a time when you were caught up in doing something—tell me about where it was, what you were doing, what you were paying attention to, how you were thinking, what was going on in your body, what your facial expression was, how you held your body."

Many people are concrete and process focused when they are being creative, whether thinking up new ideas or being artistic. Therefore it is useful to ask when the patient has felt creative, original, and open to new ideas. Similarly, the concrete, process-focused mode may have come when an individual was deeply focused on the details of a task, solving a problem, or using skills like working with one's hands. People can also become absorbed when performing a physical action like those in sports (e.g., swinging a golf club or casting a fishing rod). This is the same kind of experience sometimes referred to as being in "the zone." Overlearned and well-practiced routines, when carried out skillfully, may also contribute to the same mode. Importantly, there is no specific type of activity that is more or less likely to be absorbing. Which activities are more absorbing will be individual and idiosyncratic to each patient.

These questions then lead into attempts to recapture the process orientation by asking the patient to imagine a memory of being absorbed. For example, the therapist says:

"Reflecting on past experience, can you think of times when you were immersed in an activity? As best you can, relive and reexperience that situation. See what you were looking at during that time, re-create how you were thinking, notice what you were attending to. As best you can, recapture and hold on to that feeling of being absorbed in the process of [specify activity reviewed] . . . Focus on what you can see in this situation. Notice what you are paying attention to. Tell me what you can see in this situation. Tell me what you are doing in this situation."

The patient's descriptions of sensory experience and activity are then used by the therapist to further reinforce the experience. Patients often describe particular aspects of sensory experience (e.g., light, colors, shapes, textures, sensations) when they describe these situations. By refocusing and prompting attention to these elements, the therapist guides the patient further into the processing mode and engages it more strongly.

For example, one patient recalled painting the picture of a landscape 20 years ago; she was totally focused on the form and colors of the paint and felt that she was capturing the essence of the scene. In this case, the imagery would focus on the sensory and perceptual details relevant to this experience, for example:

"Imagine the picture in front of you. Notice the details of the colors, see how the paint changes to convey changes in light. See the view across the hills as clearly as you can in front of you. Watch your hand and fingers as you paint the next detail—see the exact movements of the brush on the canvas. Notice how you are deciding what to paint next. Observe what you are paying attention to—the focus of your concentration. Describe what you can see. Feel how you choose each movement. Focus on your feelings of concentration and absorption in the picture. As you continue to paint the picture, feel that feeling of being caught up in the painting get stronger and stronger. Feel more and more absorbed in what you are doing as the sensations become more and more vivid. Notice your feelings as you stand looking at the painting you are working on."

The recollection of creating this painting produced very strong feelings in this patient, shifting her away from an evaluative mode to a here-and-now experiential absorbed mode. The memory also shifted her back to a context when she felt more on top of things and made her thinking concrete and focused on how to do things. All of these changes had the effect of reducing rumination, making her feel lighter, freer, and less anxious, and increasing her motivation to get on with some artwork. This was an important step for her as previously she had avoided doing any artwork because she always felt she had other things she should do, even though the artwork seemed to be relaxing and beneficial for her. The therapist then encouraged her to use imagery of this memory and of other similar memories as part of an If–Then plan whenever she noticed her warning signs for rumination. Recognizing that she found painting and drawing absorbing, further behavioral plans were also made to increase these activities.

The second step in helping patients recapture the experience of being absorbed is asking patients to compare their experience when recalling an absorbing memory versus an alternative memory of doing the same or a similar activity but when less absorbed and finding it hard to concentrate. An example in which the patient ruminates while performing the activity provides a good comparison condition for the FA. A behavioral experiment comparing these two memory inductions tests if the patient experiences differences between the two processing modes (i.e., absorbed versus nonabsorbed). This exercise parallels the Why–How behavioral experiment described in Chapter 9. Patients often report that when they access the process-focused absorbed memories they feel more open-minded, more comfortable, more relaxed, more assertive, their mind quiets down, and they feel less self-critical. By comparing the two modes experientially, the therapist is able to label and explain the difference between focusing on outcome and focusing on process, and between being absorbed versus being disconnected from experience when ruminating. Following such an experiment, the therapist points out that the two modes are out of balance for the patient and that therapy will try to redress the balance. The therapist also summarizes the patient's experience of the two modes (i.e., the absorbed mode was more helpful).

When the experiential exercise is effective in the therapy session, the next step is to use the absorbed memories and imagery to kick-start the process mode, encouraging patients to rehearse imagining those situations daily, as well as before any situation where it would be good to get into an absorbed mode. Furthermore, by looking at when the absorbed mode occurs more often, the therapist works at changing aspects of the environment or the patient's attention and behavior to encourage this mode. The imagery to induce an absorbed mind-set is an important strategy to include in effective contingency plans for rumination.

Because being absorbed usually involves learning, growing, exploring, or discovering, it is useful to ask patients directly to adopt perspectives that support those values, for example:

"Try and approach things in the spirit of discovery."
"How would I approach this situation in an exploratory way?"
"What is an exploratory way of doing this?"

Flow

The literature on "flow" (Csikszentmihalyi, 2002) provides a useful scientific and theoretical background to inform the absorption intervention. Flow is described as a deep and effortless involvement in an activity that occurs when individuals are fully engaged and immersed in what they are doing. It is typically associated with improved mood and better performance. The literature on flow has identified a number of characteristics that can increase the likelihood of entering a state of "flow" and that also help us to tell whether a patient is genuinely in a state of absorption or not. These pointers can help the therapist to judge whether a selected memory is likely to be one that will facilitate absorption (Csikszentmihalyi, 2002).

A Merging of Action and Awareness

For an absorbed or "flow" state, there is a merging of action and awareness. An individual simultaneously acts, notices the effects of her actions, and adjusts the response accordingly. Perception and action become closely entwined. For example, a rock climber will be focused on feeling for the next handhold or grip, and her perceptions and actions will be fused. This fusion leads to fast, efficient performance without second-guessing. When there is a merging of action and awareness, the subjective experience is of being and doing rather than thinking. In an absorbed flow state, there is no internal running commentary. If you ask someone who is in flow what he is thinking, it may be difficult for him to answer because instead of having verbal thoughts, he is more likely to be working directly within experience. This is what we look out for when inducing this state. It also suggests that activities that have a strong sensory–perceptual or proprioceptive body-based element are more likely to lead to flow than conceptual, abstract activities.

Challenges Are Balanced with Skills

Flow is more likely to occur when there is a balance between challenge and skills. It is easier to get absorbed in a task if it is neither too easy nor too difficult. Tasks that are too easy will be boring, done without needing focused attention. Tasks that are too difficult will be frustrating. A task is more likely to promote absorption when it is challenging and stretches the individual but is within her reach and capabilities. A good example is playing tennis with an opponent who is perhaps a little better than you but whom you can beat. This balance between difficulty and skill is important when planning absorption exercises and activities. Another way of looking at this is that the patient needs to sense that he can control the activity.

Focused Attention on the Task

Flow is characterized by focused attention on the task at hand. When checking whether someone is absorbed in a memory, the therapist checks where the patient is focusing attention; this provides a good clue as to whether the induction attempt was successful. When the patient is absorbed, attention is focused on the appropriate details to accomplish the task. This is often attention to sensory and perceptual details in the world, but it can also be a focus on internal sensations, depending upon the activity. Attention is usually controlled and focused rather than jumping around among different targets and topics. Volatile and movable attention is typical of a distracted, less absorbed state. The focused attention in a state of flow can be narrow—honing in like a spotlight on the key aspects of a task, or expansive and broad, enabling the individual to be aware of all that is going on around him, but it is usually stable, steady, and not jittery.

Prompting the individual to focus attention on the appropriate task elements can facilitate an absorbed flow state. For example, to increase the likelihood of engendering an absorbed state, shift the patient's attention away from the self, especially from judgments about the self, and toward the outside world and the sensory–perceptual details of what the patient is doing (e.g., the sound of music being played; the feel of the racket being swung, and the angle of the ball). Similarly, encourage patients to hold their attention steady and focused, rather than constantly moving around. For example, the induction includes the following prompts: "Your attention is focused on the task at hand; the more you attend directly to what you are doing, the more absorbed and connected you will become."

A Focus on the Immediate Present

Absorbed flow states are characterized by the individual attending to the immediate "here and now" present moment. This is clearly related to the narrow attentional focus. We want patients to be in the here and now when imagining a past absorbing experience or trying an engaging activity, not focused on what happened in the past or might happen in the future. When recalling a past absorbing experience, the goal is for the patient to have the experience of being back in the situation as if it is happening now. The therapist prompts to facilitate the induction of this narrow temporal focus state and checks to see if it has been induced. If the patient is looking back on it as a past memory, she might then compare it with the current situation, leading to unhelpful contrasts and discrepancies (e.g., "Why can't I do that anymore?"). Instructions to patients emphasize this narrow temporal focus (e.g., "Your attention is focused on the immediate, present moment, on what is happening in the moment right now, rather than on the past and the future").

The Activity Has Goals and Rules and Offers Immediate Feedback

Absorbed flow states involve clear goals and rules, and immediate feedback. This is a critical setting condition when selecting potentially absorbing exercises or activities. To become absorbed in an activity, it needs to be structured so that the effects of the patient's actions can immediately be perceived and assessed against the goals or rules of the activity. These goals and rules don't need to be explicit or formal as in sports and games. Rather they reflect the implicit properties of the tasks. For example, when playing an instrument such as a guitar, you immediately hear the notes played and know whether the sound made is pleasing or not. Thus, there is an aesthetic rule as to what sounds are pleasant, even if this is not explicit or formal. Likewise, when painting, you have a sense of when a brushstroke captures the effect you are striving for, that is, the goal or rule being applied. This close combination of goals, rules, and immediate feedback is essential in order to have the merging of action and awareness and the connection between environment and activity central to entering flow. This can be explained to patients as follows:

"The activity you choose should have clear goals, rules, and immediate feedback. It is easier to get absorbed when you know what you are trying to do and for every action you take there is an immediate and direct response—for example, when playing a musical instrument, you immediately hear what note was played; when painting you can directly see the effect of the brush on the canvas."

A Lack of Self-Consciousness

States of absorption and flow are characterized by a loss of self-consciousness—the individual is no longer aware of herself, is not self-focused, and does not have an internal running commentary about herself. This is a key signifier that absorption has been attained. It also indicates why absorption is a state that acts counter to rumination. A person can be aware of herself in terms of sensory experience and bodily sensations, but not in terms of evaluating the self. When a patient reports not being self-conscious during the absorption exercise, this is a good indicator that the exercise was successful.

A Changed Perception of Time

Another characteristic of flow states is a changed perception of time. When absorbed in an activity, people often report that the subjective experience of time speeds up or slows down. We all have had the experience of being immersed in what we are doing where hours have passed without our awareness. People also sometimes report feeling like time has slowed down. People playing sports report being in a zone where they see the ball as if in slow motion. These changes in subjective temporal perception presumably reflect the amount of attention paid to the task relative to an internal clock. Asking patients about their perception of time is another good way to check if they were absorbed in an activity. Too much focus on time and deadlines can impede absorption. When individuals are in a hurry and feeling under time pressure, they often find it harder to become absorbed in what they are doing. Clock watching and sensitivity to the passage of time seem to interfere with becoming fully absorbed in a task.

Connection with the Environment

Flow states involve a connection with the environment in a way that directly guides behavior (overlapping with immediate feedback principle above). The absorbed person is not conceptually analyzing the situation and determining what to do but rather directly responding to his sensory–perceptual experience. Absorption is more likely when attention is paid to the relevant aspects of the environment that can guide the target activity, for example, when rock climbing, the relevant aspect of the environment would be potential footholds and handholds in the rock. Guiding the patient's focus of attention can help to induce a state of absorption and assessing attention can indicate whether absorption has been induced.

Environmental factors may also help or hinder the state of absorption. When the environment is conducive to the activity at hand, absorption will be easier, for example, sitting down to write in a quiet study. In contrast, writing in the middle of a noisy and busy household is less conducive to absorption. Unwanted distractions or unnecessary stimulation do not guide activity. Internal states are also an aspect of the environment with the potential to impair absorption, for example, ongoing concerns and associated thoughts about other issues.

The Nature of the Activity

The nature of the activities chosen influences the likelihood of entering a flow state. Activities that are intrinsically rewarding and valued as an end in their own right (i.e., autotelic) are better for becoming absorbed than extrinsically rewarding activities done only as a means to an end. Of course, it is important to recognize that there will be large idiosyncratic differences in which tasks and activities patients find intrinsically rewarding. This is where the FA is important, because the function of an activity rather than its form is critical: depending on its function and context, the same activity could be intrinsically rewarding in one circumstance but not another, whereas two different activities could have the same function of being intrinsically rewarding. For example, reading a therapy monograph could be absorbing when picked up voluntarily with curiosity about learning something new (intrinsic reward), but could be less absorbing if given as homework on a tight deadline to pass a course for formal accreditation (extrinsic reward). Often patients in a state of flow may be doing the activity out of curiosity, to see what happens or to learn and improve.

It is important to consider the function of an activity before using it either as the focus of a mental absorption exercise or in activity scheduling. For example, one of my patients reported a memory of knitting as a potential example of when she was absorbed. On the face of it, this seems a plausible example for absorption, as knitting can involve direct sensory focus on the here and now and can be intrinsically rewarding. However, when we talked through the memory to check it before going to the imagery exercise proper, we found that during the knitting, the patient had been focused on the endpoint of the knitting—to make a sweater for her grandson—rather than on the process of the activity itself. This suggested that knitting might not be a good choice for an absorbing activity.

Here is an example of how to illustrate this point to a patient:

"The activity needs to be rewarding in itself. What you are doing is valued because the process of doing it is interesting, rather than because of what you might achieve by doing it. For example, playing a sport might feel good as you are doing it because of the feeling in your body, whether you win or lose."

Related to this, the motivation for the activity is important. When the goals are discovery, learning, growth, curiosity, and playfulness, flow states are more likely than if the goals are to complete an activity or to master a situation. When the motivation is to build self-potential, there is more chance of absorption. Function triumphs over form: the same activity can be performed with different motivations and goals at different times and this influences absorption. How an individual approaches a task will influence the likelihood of becoming absorbed.

Activities are also more likely to be absorbing when they in some way reflect the individual's values and what is important and meaningful to the person. For example, walking in the countryside and paying attention to nature is likely to be absorbing for someone who appreciates the natural world. Learning to play a musical instrument is likely to be absorbing for someone who values learning. Common personal values include increasing connection with others and with nature, honesty, kindness, warmth, growth, learning, playfulness, experiencing life fully, sensation seeking, and curiosity. Activities that embody these values are more likely to be absorbing for people who share them. When selecting absorption exercises, it is therefore important to check if suggested memories reflect important personal values for the patient. Further, the flow literature would suggest that a patient is more likely to be absorbed in an activity when he is encouraged to focus on those aspects of a task that reflect his values (e.g., when talking to a friend, emphasizing how this relates to his values of being connected to others, or when practicing a skill, focusing on what he can learn and how he can grow). Likewise, when an activity is found to be absorbing, this suggests that it reflects important personal values for the individual, which can inform further planning.

Presenting the Rationale for Absorption Exercises

Here is an example of a script illustrating how to introduce the absorption exercises. It covers how they might be helpful, and what they might involve. The same points are also made in Handout 10, Engaging with Life through Concreteness.

"Depression often makes it hard for people to fully connect with experience, to fully engage with life. You can be doing something you previously enjoyed but not feel anything, or feel disconnected. You could be talking to a friend or playing with your children but not feel anything. You're there but you're not there; you are not fully attending to or connecting with the experience.

"Spend a few moments reflecting on those times when you are not fully there. These might be times when you feel a bit numb, spaced out, distanced, or when you feel like you are going through the motions. Can you identify times like this?

"Not being connected to experience can contribute to depression in two main ways. First, you don't get the benefit of doing something enjoyable. You can do something that would normally be rewarding, but it does not make you feel better. Thus, whatever you do, your mood will not improve. Second, if you are not connecting with experience, you are not able to notice what is going on around you, to notice changes, or learn from success and failure. You are likely to keep repeating the same mistakes again and again, since there is no chance of realizing what you could do differently.

"Both rumination and overgeneralization contribute to not being able to connect directly with experience. When people ruminate, their minds are full of thoughts going round and round about their problems, and they are not really paying attention to what they are doing. Likewise, when people jump to conclusions from an event and think about what it might mean about their futures and themselves (overgeneralizing), they are moving away from the direct experience of what is happening and into abstract thoughts about the experience. Thus, too much abstract thinking can stop you from connecting with experience and prevent you from getting the benefits of directly connecting with the world around you.

"We can also lose connection with direct experience because we are trying to avoid thinking about upsetting or emotional events, or trying to avoid unpleasant feelings, new challenges, or risks. By trying to avoid threats or possible failure, we often reduce our activities. This results in having fewer positive experiences as well. Avoidance can increase until there are very few activities where you have any chance of feeling alive or fulfilled, further fueling the depressed mood. Avoidance can close life down. To reduce depression, you need to open up your options and try exciting and rewarding activities.

"The way to reconnect with experience is to pay attention to what you are doing and to the world around you. Focus your attention on an activity that you find interesting and in which you can become completely absorbed and immersed. You can do this through a mental exercise that re-creates the experience of being absorbed in an activity. You can also reconnect with experience by deliberately increasing the activities that you find interesting and absorbing. We often find that when depressed, people drop the activities that excite and absorb them, while carrying on with the chores and duties they feel they should do. You can end up doing all the dull activities that you find tiring and draining but not doing any of the interesting and fun activities that make you feel better and give you more energy. It is important to get the balance right between chores and positive activities because the former drain your batteries while the latter recharge your batteries. If you are doing too many chores and not doing enough fun, engaging activities, you are going to wear yourself out.

"The kinds of experiences that we are looking for are those where you feel completely absorbed, immersed, or caught up in the process and details of what you are doing; where you lose all sense of self and time and experience a sense of being completely focused in the present moment. Such absorbing experiences are sometimes described as flow experiences or peak experiences. People who play sports refer to being in the zone. Whether such experiences are created through mental exercises or through actually taking part in activities, they are a strong antidote to rumination, overgeneralization, and inactivity, and act as a powerful antidepressant.

"Different people find different activities absorbing. Absorbing activities can include doing something creative, musical, or artistic, focusing on the natural world, participating in dance, sports, or challenging physical activities, or taking part in activities that involve intellectual stimulation and learning. Specific examples include sensation-seeking, high-adrenaline activities like rock climbing, scuba diving, horseback riding, surfing, or sky diving, where you are completely focused on the experience of what you are doing, such as focusing on where next to put your hands when rock climbing. Or absorbing activities could be creative activities like painting where you are focused on the patterns of light and dark, on color and texture, and where to put the brush next.

"There is no right or wrong way to become absorbed. Try and think of times when you have been completely absorbed in an activity. You can use these memories for mental exercises where you will imagine one absorbing situation as vividly and concretely as you can. You will imagine that you are there right now, looking out onto the scene through your own eyes, experiencing the sensations of being in your own body, using all of your senses to become fully aware of your experience in the moment. You can use these exercises to get into a frame of mind more directly connected to experience and as a means to fully experience what you are doing. Practice the absorption exercise to get yourself into the right frame of mind before starting an activity. It can increase your chance of getting started and increase your enjoyment of what you are doing."

Absorption Exercise to Inform FA

The examples that patients provide for the absorption exercise give useful information. The therapist should check with the patient on how many of the absorbing activities she has stopped doing or is doing less frequently. Also ask the patient which of the activities that she would like to do more often. This can then lead into activity scheduling to build up absorbing activities as a means to improve mood and as an antirumination strategy.

Conducting a FA helps to identify the behavioral and environmental factors that enhance or impede absorption. Compare the times when the patient has been absorbed in an activity with times the same activity has not been absorbing. The factors that influence absorption will probably reflect the characteristics noted above in the discussion of flow. They will, however, vary from individual to individual. They may include how the patient behaves (e.g., state of mind, state of tension, focus of attention, goals) and aspects of the environment (preceding events, amount of distraction, amount of time and space available). Identifying these influences will facilitate absorption. Preparation before an activity can facilitate the patient becoming absorbed and increase the likelihood that she will get the full benefit of doing the activity.

As for cognitive interventions such as thought challenging, the successful desired state of mind will not be successfully induced in full every time. However, it should be possible to shift patients into a process-focused and absorbed approach to events, which in turn will increase the likelihood of the patient experiencing a state of flow. This approach is probabilistic: although it is not always possible to directly induce flow, the aim is to increase the likelihood of the patient engaging in it by putting in place the right conditions so that over time there is accumulated benefit from more frequent absorption experiences.

Problems with Absorption

A common concern that has been raised when I have taught RFCBT workshops is that it will be difficult for patients with depression or other emotional disorders to identify past memories of being absorbed. Based on my experience in treatment trials and clinics, this is often less difficult than anticipated: the majority of patients are able to identify one or more memories of being absorbed. The literature on flow suggests that such experiences are universal and that nearly all people have them.

Patients are asked about times when they were immersed in a task with a focus on behavior, rather than on feeling good or happy. This seems to bypass the negative schemas and mood-congruent biases that make it harder for depressed patients to recall positive experiences. Patients who have clear and distinct periods of being depressed versus periods of remission can typically detect memories of being absorbed. Patients with long-standing histories of depression, including those with a dysthymic presentation, who cannot report any sense of a self without depression, may find it more difficult.

When faced with difficulty in obtaining a suitable memory of absorption, the solution (as is so often the case!) is to follow the ACES principle. Before moving to absorbing experiences, it is helpful to further practice the use of imagery and relaxation to make the recall of experiences more vivid and more accessible. The therapist prompts with more specific questions highlighting activities or periods in the patient's life that previous questioning has suggested may involve more beneficial processing. Moreover, it can be helpful for the therapist to operationalize the "absorbing" experience in more detail with respect to the flow principles and to use these as specific prompts to identify and strengthen a potential memory. For example, the therapist asks whether the patient has had experiences when he has lost self-consciousness or his perception of time has changed.

A more serious issue concerns whether the imagining of an absorbed memory is helpful or not. When recalling a past positive situation, a patient can be immersed in the experience of that memory, recapturing some of the emotions and mental state associated with it in an adaptive way and thereby benefiting. In contrast, she could instead be evaluating her current state and comparing it to the memory, with the potential to feel much worse. Recalling a time when things were going well without being "in the experience" can lead to negative contrasts and comparisons like "Why can't I do this anymore?"; "Why are things so difficult now?"; "I am worse now than I was then," and so on. It is therefore critical to optimize the chances that absorption exercises will result in immersion rather than comparison. The focus on all aspects of the holistic experience is central to this, as is repeated therapist prompting toward a flow state, as outlined in detail above. For this reason, I recommend that therapists review a possible memory in some detail with the patient before attempting the imagery exercise, in order to confirm it is a suitable memory for absorption and to garner details to further prompt the patient into the sensory–perceptual experience. Similarly, therapists need to check carefully against the flow criteria to see if the exercise was successful or not.

On the basis of the six E's principle (Explore Experience, Experiment with Experience, Exercise and Engage; see Chapter 9), I do not encourage a patient to use the absorption exercise outside of the session until it is clear that she is immersed in the experience and not comparing the memory against her current state. If the behavioral experiment in the session resulted in a comparative experience, we then look at the nature of the comparative thoughts coming up and what triggered them (ABC analysis) to inform ways of bypassing this in a future attempt. We would also seek another memory of being absorbed that may be more effective.

Another potential problem with absorption exercises is that the activity chosen may not serve an adaptive function, for example, it may be a form of distraction or avoidance. This is why it is important to keep in mind the function of the planned behavior and tie it back to FA. The goal of absorption activities is to connect the patient with an alternative mind-set that is at odds with rumination, which facilitates effective processing of situations and problem solving, and enables close and direct engagement with the world, particularly with its potential rewards and contingencies. Thus, the function of absorption is to bring an individual closer to the world and to his or her direct experience. It is not to provide temporary relief through daydreaming, distraction, or avoiding thinking about real difficulties.

As intended in RFCBT, absorption exercises and activities involve approach into the world and build resources for the patient, whether these resources are practical (e.g., getting better at writing, painting) or emotional (e.g., feeling calmer and more energized to tackle a problem). Because any behavior can constitute either constructive engagement or avoidance, it is not possible to specify in advance which behaviors should be permitted or proscribed; a FA of the behavior is required. Behaviors (and memories) that reflect the flow principles are more likely to be constructive and less likely to be linked to avoidance and distraction. For example, when an activity is done to avoid an unpleasant and unwanted state, its motivation is extrinsic, not intrinsic. Nonetheless, consideration of function is important when planning absorption work with patients.

Some patients with depression engage in cognitive activities to take their minds off their problems (e.g., puzzles, crosswords). It is possible for such activities to be absorbing and engender flow when the right combination of processes and dimensions are aligned (e.g., the person enjoys playing with words and does the puzzle for intrinsic pleasure and to enhance vocabulary), but the therapist needs to explore and check this first. Look at the antecedents and consequences of recent times when the patient engaged in crossword puzzles as well as his experience during the completion of the puzzle. This will clarify the function of the behavior.

We also want to look at activities that tend to build resources, skills, and competence over time: activities that leave patients in the same state they were in when they started are less likely to be helpful. For the same reason, more active relative to passive pursuits are encouraged for absorbing activities. The patient needs to be an active and effortful agent in the activity rather than simply a passive recipient. Activities where the patient interacts with the world and others and creates something are encouraged. Watching TV or reading a book is not likely to encourage absorption. Of course, there are no hard-and-fast rules here, and a close examination of the function for individuals is important. Under some circumstances, reading a book can be an active and effortful pursuit where the reader is generating images and ideas from the words on the page and carefully parsing the meanings and allusions in the text. In this context, reading could be absorbing in a constructive sense. However, getting caught up in turning the pages of a genre thriller may simply be distraction. Similar analyses could be made for listening to music or watching TV.

An increasingly common example raised with me by other therapists is the playing of computer games. Computer and video games are designed to be engaging and immersing and are engineered in a way that meets a number of flow criteria, such as balancing challenge and opportunity (as a player progresses through levels of difficulty), requiring direct focus on the immediate task, providing immediate feedback, and having clear goals and rules. However, games may not meet the criteria of intrinsic value and personal growth. Again, FA is necessary to determine whether or not a game is helpful for each individual patient. For one patient (or in one circumstance), gaming may be a form of distraction and avoidance, whereas for another it may enable development of personal skills and resources.

Remember that the absorption exercise is used to elicit a processing mind-set of high concreteness and engagement, which can then be applied to the patient's current real-world situation. Generating an absorbed mind-set is not the final goal of the process. The goal is to mentally prepare patients with this mind-set to tackle their current situation. For example, a mental absorption exercise can be incorporated into an If–Then plan as follows: the patient identifies a trigger to rumination (such as increasing tension in the shoulders) when anticipating a difficult conversation. She would then focus on an absorbing memory to interrupting the onset of rumination and engender a more outward, open, energized, and concrete processing mode in order to engage in this conversation in a more productive way.

An Example of a Dialogue Introducing Absorption and Identifying an Absorbing Memory

The following dialogue continues the therapy of Emily, who was introduced in Chapter 7. Having successfully introduced environmental changes and the practice of concrete thinking to Emily, the therapist now considers absorption as an intervention.

THERAPIST: Up to now you have practiced stepping out of rumination by looking at how you can do things, by asking yourself helpful "how" questions rather than "why" questions. Another way to step out of rumination is by focusing on an opposite experience, by concentrating on times when you have been doing something that you are really focused on, really absorbed in for minutes and hours. In these experiences, you are completely focused, absorbed, caught up in what you are doing, completely at one with it, not bothered by thoughts, not having any running commentary on what you are doing. When you are immersed in what you are doing like that, it is not possible to be ruminating. Can you think of any recent examples of activities when you have been doing that, where you have had that experience of being absorbed?

EMILY: Yes, yesterday, playing the piano yesterday.

THERAPIST: Great. Describe to me in more detail what you were doing and where you were.

EMILY: I was sitting in our front room, at the small piano we have, and I decided to try and take a shot at playing the piano again. I started to think about an old piece of music I knew and where to play the keys to get the right notes. Then I was thinking about the interplay of the different notes and sounds and playing around with tunes on the piano and imagining how I could make different combinations of sounds.

THERAPIST: It may be useful to re-create and imagine as vividly as you can being in that situation, to see that situation as if you are there right now, looking out from your eyes, as you focus on the piano. Notice where you are, what colors and shapes you can see. Get a strong picture of the scene directly in front of you. What's immediately in front of you? What can you see?

EMILY: The black and white keys of the piano, and beyond that the shelf behind the piano with the books and flower pot on it.

THERAPIST: What are you noticing and paying attention to?

EMILY: I am trying to find a structural harmony but also playing with the notes, how they are arranged together to make a pleasant sound.

THERAPIST: Notice any sensations in your body or muscles. Notice any feelings and emotions that you are experiencing as you become totally focused and absorbed in playing the piano. Notice where you are putting your attention.

EMILY: I am putting my attention on the movement of my fingers across the keys and the patterns of sound, the tune I can hear.

THERAPIST: Imagine a few seconds' worth of being in this situation, focusing on what's in front of you, noticing what pattern you can see and hear, focusing on the sounds you can hear, and the feel of your hands on the piano keys. As this becomes more vivid, reexperience what is going through your mind. What are you aware of?

EMILY: I am focusing on the coherence and harmony of the melody as I look down at the keyboard and hear the variations on the tune I am messing about with. I keep seeing interesting and unexpected juxtapositions that spark new thoughts about the tune.

THERAPIST: How are you feeling?

EMILY: Absorbed, interested, exploring, and useful.

THERAPIST: Anything else?

EMILY: A feeling I can do this, this is interesting, lots of things could come out of this.

THERAPIST: What is your mood like?

EMILY: Positive, more confident, imaginative in a good way.

THERAPIST: OK, let's take a step out of this imagined situation and back into the therapy room here. Did it change how you are feeling right here, right now?

EMILY: Yes, I feel more capable, I have a kind of renewed vigor for arts and sciences.

THERAPIST: How was that situation you just reexperienced different from the times when you are ruminating and dwelling on difficulties?

EMILY: I was physically doing something, it was not about me, it was about design and theories, more creative.

THERAPIST: What was the most important thing as you were focused on playing with the sounds and tune on the piano?

EMILY: Not so much to get it right as to see what came out of it. I wanted to keep doing it, and I was curious as to what I might see.

THERAPIST: That sounds like it might be an interesting difference from when you are ruminating and brooding about problems: Here your focus was not so much about getting things right and being concerned with the outcome, as it is during rumination, but more about exploring, looking at the process and playing with ideas. Does that sound about right?

EMILY: Yes.

THERAPIST: Does this experience happen much?

EMILY: Not that often now. I can think of other situations like that further back in the past. For example, more day-to-day things in which I can get absorbed, like gardening. The focus was opposite from what I am doing in rumination—I am using different bits of my mind, I am focusing outward rather than inward.

THERAPIST: Anything different in what you were doing when more absorbed?

EMILY: I am focused on the sensory details of what I am doing rather than how I am feeling.

THERAPIST: Do you think it might be possible to practice reliving and recapturing this more confident, exploring, creative way of thinking when you notice an early warning sign for rumination, such as your mind fogging up? What do you think would happen?

EMILY: It is about getting my mind back into that zone and out of the rut that leads into rumination.

THERAPIST: (*after summarizing the session*) What came out of what we have been trying out today?

EMILY: I have moved on, it was most interesting. It was about using my brain more. It definitely lifted my mood just now.

Inside the Therapist's Mind: Decision Points and Reflections with Emily

The dialogue above provides a flavor of how the therapist works with Emily to induce an absorbed state and how she benefits from this state of mind. This example indicates how a memory is found and how the therapist prompts imaginal reexperiencing of the memory. You can see how directing the focus of attention is an important part of the process of becoming absorbed. The responses from Emily suggest an open, creative, sensory–perceptual type of thinking, which is typical of a more absorbed experience. It is a good sign when patients provide detailed descriptions of what they can see and hear and touch, as well as talking about more creative responses.

As the absorbed state is facilitated, the therapist asks further questions to identify potential elements and dimensions that might facilitate and influence the induction of an absorbed state of mind. Identifying these factors is useful both to further prompt and deepen the imagery exercise but also as useful pointers to build into behavioral plans to increase the likelihood of absorption in planned activities. In this example, important aspects include a focus on the external sensory world rather than on the self, a focus on the process of what is being done rather than the potential outcome, and adopting a curious, wanting-to-learn, explorative motivation and approach to the activity. This suggests that for Emily, plans to increase absorption in other situations would benefit from highlighting process and being motivated by learning and curiosity.

When the therapist discusses the differences between the times Emily is absorbed versus not absorbed, one potential next step is to run this as a behavioral experiment in the session, comparing imagining the situation from these different perspectives. A similar comparison could be between an episode of being absorbed versus one of rumination to determine what is different between them. Each of these approaches would help to further consolidate the idea that being absorbed is useful and identify what helps to increase absorption.

Next, the therapist needs to ensure repeated practice of the absorption exercise and link it to an If–Then plan as an antirumination strategy. This idea is introduced at the end of the dialogue, but the therapist needs to develop this further, perhaps with another practice and by collaboratively exploring whether Emily can use the absorption exercise for homework, perhaps by listening to the relevant section of the audio-recorded session.

The therapist follows up this exercise by exploring ways to increase absorbing activities in Emily's daily life as a means to increase positive affect and reduce rumination. For Emily, it could be useful to increase an activity like playing music or gardening through activity scheduling plans.

CHAPTER 11

Shifting Processing Style

Compassion

In the previous chapter, we looked at absorption as an alternative form of processing that directly counters rumination. Another useful type of experience is that of compassion to the self or to others. Compassion is here defined as an emotional and cognitive response to the suffering of oneself and others that involves feelings of kindness and care and that motivates a desire to help, support, and nurture. It thus overlaps with sympathy and empathy but is more involved, incorporating active desire and efforts to alleviate suffering and to project care and concern. It typically manifests in terms of being kind, warm, tolerant, caring, nurturing, nonjudgmental, and supportive to oneself or to others. Such experiences of being compassionate are at odds with the depressive rumination style, which tends to involve critical, evaluative, and judgmental thinking about the self and others. Hence, shifting into a compassionate mode can be an effective means to shift away from ruminative thinking. Research in depression and anxiety has highlighted how these disorders are often characterized by a lack of self-soothing, and instead by repeated attacks on the self and prolonged self-criticism in forms such as rumination (see Gilbert, 2009, for detailed discussion).

Why Compassion in RFCBT?

I identified the development of compassion as an important element of RFCBT in the light of functional analyses of patients. Two functions that regularly surfaced for rumination were to motivate oneself by putting pressure on the self ("spurring oneself on") and to avoid becoming a feared or unwanted self (see Chapter 2 for further details). Thus, a patient might constantly point out the mistakes she was making in an attempt to push herself to perform better. Alternatively, a patient who was afraid of being a selfish person might repeatedly berate himself about how insensitive he was. In both these cases, the rumination may be reinforced because it has an avoidant function despite making the patient feel bad. As discussed in Chapters 6 and 7, the aim is to find an equivalent strategy that is incompatible with rumination while also serving its beneficial functions without the negative consequences. The ability to be compassionate to self or to others seemed a useful strategy to address rumination's motivational functions.

Compassionate self-talk is another way to motivate oneself. Being validating and encouraging does not have the downside of self-criticism and pressuring oneself. In most cases, while ruminating about one's mistakes, and exhorting oneself to do better may be effective in the short term for acute problems, it can prove to be demoralizing and dispiriting in the longer term. Validating and encouraging oneself, being forgiving of one's limitations, is likely to be more beneficial in the long run. For example, one patient said that if she was not checking up on herself, she would get lazy, unmotivated, and complacent. We therefore looked to use compassion as an alternative to motivate her that does not have the negative effects of rumination.

For an alternative to the function of avoiding a feared self, therapists require a behavior focused on approach rather than avoidance. Rather than trying to avoid a particular outcome, therapists want patients to work toward a more constructive outcome. For example, rather than ruminating to avoid being a selfish person, the patient can develop strategies to work toward being a more thoughtful and caring person. Learning ways to adopt a more compassionate style of processing is consistent with this shift into approach goals. It fits with many of the positive values to which a patient may aspire to move toward (e.g., kindness, warmth, thoughtfulness). Compassion exercises thus fit neatly into the functional-analytical framework of RFCBT as a means to address the reinforcing functions that may underlie rumination. Again, as with all strategies in RFCBT, the use of compassion is dependent on FA of the patient's difficulties.

The approach adopted in RFCBT to induce the experience of compassion is similar to that used for absorption, as described in Chapter 10. The patient identifies and explores specific memories of experiencing compassion. This state of mind is then induced through imagery, using the reexperiencing of that state as a means to shift processing. The techniques and guidance for inducing absorption are thus all relevant for generating compassion. In other words, building on the patient's own experience, compassion is imagined and rehearsed with cues and prompts from the therapist to strengthen the experience, with repeated practice when the specific memory of compassion is found to be useful. This approach organically follows from the emphasis on FA and self-empowerment within RFCBT.

This approach to training compassion contrasts with the compassionate mind training approach of Paul Gilbert (see, e.g., Gilbert, 2009, 2010, for details), which developed in parallel to the current RFCBT work. Gilbert's work has been central to highlighting the importance of compassion in therapy and to the development of therapeutic models. Moreover, it builds from a well-established theoretical basis, with emerging evidence of the efficacy of enhancing compassion for mental health. While both approaches emphasize the use of vivid and holistic imagery to induce a self-compassionate state, the RFCBT approach has focused on imagining past experiences of compassion, reflecting its BA and FA background, whereas the compassionate mind training approach utilizes a wide range of imagery, including imagining avatars and symbolic representations of compassion that then interact with the patient (Gilbert, 2009). RFCBT is not prescriptive about which approach to use: both imagery building on past personal experience and more open-ended compassionate imagery (Gilbert, 2009) appear to be effective and can be used within the RFCBT framework. I recommend that those interested in compassion explore the work of Gilbert, who is the world leader on compassion-focused treatment. His work is extensive, thorough, and deeply informed by considerable clinical contact and acumen.

When to Choose Compassion as an Intervention

Consistent with the general principles of RFCBT, the use of compassion exercises and activities is secondary to FA of the patient. A focus on compassion may emerge as a consequence of examining the functions of the patient's rumination and then be chosen as a strategy to replace rumination with a more constructive alternative. Compassionate responses may also emerge in comparisons of effective versus ineffective attempts to address problems. Work on compassion may seek to build on this preexisting repertoire to make its use more systematic and frequent. Thus, compassionate exercises are not necessarily done with every patient but are selected for those patients where it reflects the formulation arising from FA. This analysis informs whether the focus of the compassion work is on compassion to self, compassion to others, or both.

For example, a patient's FA indicates that irritability with others is a warning sign for rumination, and that this rumination may function to address that patient's fear of being selfish and inconsiderate. For this patient, compassion to others is a sensible strategy to use as an alternative to rumination. If the same patient is also often down on herself and unnecessarily blaming herself, practicing self-compassion is also indicated. We need to carefully evaluate the function and consequences of introducing compassion as a strategy. As for other strategies, we aim to build constructive approach behaviors rather than unhelpful avoidant behaviors. For example, practicing compassion to others is intended to be of value to the patient in providing a more adaptive and approach-focused means to address negative responses to others in a way that makes the patient feel calmer and more positive. Compassion to others is not intended to make the patient less assertive or to put other people's needs before her own.

Introducing Compassion to Patients

I often use experiments similar to those described in earlier chapters to introduce the potential value of developing a compassionate mind-set. For example, we might compare a situation where the patient was being down on himself with another situation where he was being compassionate to another person experiencing a similar difficulty. This is used to illustrate the potential benefits of being supportive and to highlight how the patient may not be compassionate to himself.

For example, the therapist says:

> "Let's look at how you might talk to yourself when things aren't going well. Think about something difficult you have had to deal with. Identify a time when you had a bad outcome and you were down on yourself about it: when things did not turn out as well as you hoped or when something went wrong. Maybe you applied for a job and went to interview but then did not get the job. Recall that situation as vividly as you can. Spend a few moments recalling that event in your mind as if you are there now."

The therapist then explores what the patient was saying to himself and how he was speaking to himself (e.g., "What was your inner voice saying? What was the tone of the voice like? What kinds of things were you saying? How were you saying them to yourself [tone, volume, speed]?").

The therapist then introduces a comparison situation where the patient had been compassionate (or where someone else had been compassionate to the patient). For example, the therapist might say:

> "OK, let's now try and do something a bit different. Think of someone you care about and want to help, like a close family member or a best friend. Think about the difficulty you just imagined earlier, but now imagine that your close friend or family member is facing it at the moment. Imagine that he or she comes to speak to you about it. What would you say to help

your friend? Try to make a list of things that you would say to your friend or family member. How would you say it? What do you notice about your voice (tone, volume, pace, content)?"

These two situations would then be compared to identify the differences between them in terms of what is said and how it is said, and to raise the possibility that it might be helpful to find ways to be supportive to the self as well as to others. Highlight the difference between the negative judgmental and evaluative thinking characteristic of rumination and being encouraging and supportive. Here is an example of how this can be introduced.

"Most of us have an 'inner voice' that we use when we talk to ourselves. Often when we are depressed or stressed, this voice can be extremely critical and unpleasant, and it is frequently present in rumination, for example, saying things like 'Why can't you get things right?' 'You're pathetic,' and so on.

"While it might seem that the critical voice is 'spurring us on' to be a better person, it is doing this in a harsh, upsetting way. This can make you feel less motivated and make it harder to get on with things. At other times we might experience a more gentle and kind inner voice that feels supportive, helpful, and is encouraging us to better things.

"We know that the way in which we talk to other people influences how they react and feel. You wouldn't be surprised if your friend was upset, hurt, and deflated if you shouted at her and told her how ugly and useless she was. After what you said, she might be less likely to try new things and might just want to curl up and hide. So is it surprising that how we speak to ourselves changes how we feel and what we then do?

"To reduce rumination, anxiety, and depression, it is extremely helpful to be kind to yourself. Rumination can often include very mean, critical thoughts that blame you or point out all of your faults. Changing your frame of mind and being kinder in the way you talk to yourself can get you unstuck from that cycle of negative thoughts and emotions, and can get you feeling ready to take action to solve the problem."

It is important to acknowledge that developing skills in compassion, and especially self-compassion, can be difficult, challenging, and threatening for people with histories of depression, particularly those with chronic histories and past histories of abuse and/or neglect. This has been my experience within the development and delivery of RFCBT treatment. The challenge of engaging people with depression and long-standing mental health difficulties in self-compassion has also been extensively reported by Paul Gilbert. Being kind to oneself can be very threatening and scary for some patients, in part because it is a very different approach to tackling their difficulties.

It can fly in the face of years of avoidance, as well as repeated external and internal messages that they do not deserve kindness. Moreover, being kind to the self feels risky: patients may have little experience of self-soothing, coupled with a fear that being nice to themselves may simply rebound and lead to worse difficulties. Many patients feel that they do not deserve to support or encourage themselves and are afraid of what might happen if they let up on themselves. It is important to recognize the potential difficulties in becoming self-compassionate in advance and to build this into the treatment to optimize the chance of success.

Be up front with patients about the difficulties and note that while developing skills in compassion can be very helpful, it can feel odd, strange, and uncomfortable at first. Further, existing habits of blaming the self or avoiding being nice to oneself will resist this new approach. It is essential to work together to identify a hierarchy of difficulty with respect to practicing compassion and to then work through this hierarchy in a systematic way, gradually working up through the levels of difficulty. In this respect, it is helpful to think of practicing compassion as a form of exposure. For many patients, the ultimate goal is developing improved skills in self-compassion; however, it may make more sense to start with practice at being compassionate to others and then build up to compassion to the self.

Key Steps and Principles for Encouraging a Compassionate Mind-Set

As with encouraging absorption, facilitating a compassionate mind-set takes preparation and socialization into the idea of using memories and imagery. It often works better when patients have already practiced other imagery and relaxation approaches. For this reason, I often use the compassion work later rather than earlier in therapy.

Therapists should start with situations where it is easier for the patient to be compassionate (e.g., to someone the patient cares about who was experiencing a difficult situation, such as a parent or child), and then move to a situation that was a little harder (e.g., a person the patient cares about who was being difficult, or someone the patient does not know), to still more difficult situations (e.g., a time when it was difficult to be caring to another close person), and so on, until the patient is successfully practicing compassion to himself. As with exposure treatment, therapists do not proceed to the next level in the hierarchy until there is successful habituation and processing in the current level of the hierarchy; therapists want to see that any negative feelings toward self or other have been reduced by a good degree before moving on. The patient needs to be provided with a positive experience of staying with compassion and learning that it is not as threatening as feared. For the same reasons, therapists need to allow sufficient time to work through each example and for the benefits of compassion to become manifest. In practice, this means that it is prudent to book longer sessions (1½–2 hours) for the introduction of compassion to ensure that a satisfactory point can be reached before the session finishes. Therapists want to avoid ending a session when a patient's anxiety has been aroused but before he has begun to become more comfortable.

When faced with difficulties in engaging with compassion, a useful first step is to break down the situation and to determine if a smaller alternative step in the hierarchy can be tried, coupled with further use of successful prompts into the compassionate mind-set. In the same vein, it is helpful to adapt the exercise so it focuses on overcoming barriers experientially, rather than on discussing and talking about the difficulty (Principle 3: Encourage active, concrete, experiential, and specific behavior—the ACES rule). For example, when working on practicing self-compassion, the therapist can gainfully explore what perspective or representation of the patient may help her to engage in compassion as a first step. For example, one step to minimize the distance between compassion to others and compassion to self is to consider situations in which the patient easily and strongly felt compassion for others and when she experienced a similar situation herself. Another approach is for the patient to imagine being compassionate to herself as a child. This can bypass some of the resistance to being kind to the self.

An important dimension is the perspective adopted during attempts at self-compassion. We have observed that attempts at self-compassion are often less successful when the patient imagines being compassionate to himself but adopts an observer perspective, in which he sees himself physically in the scene. The observer perspective can trigger more abstract–evaluative thinking, moving the patient away from compassionate experience. Furthermore, it can be tied to concerns about self-image and body image, which can act to further trigger negative thinking. Attempts at self-compassion tend to be more effective when they are experienced from a field perspective and are fully embodied (i.e., the patient imagines looking out through his eyes and experiencing the internal sensations of compassion spreading through his body).

The therapist encourages the patient to re-create the mental state of being compassionate by guiding the patient to imagine himself back into the experience of feeling compassionate, instructing the patient to adopt a present-tense, field perspective and using prompts based on the reviewed memory. These prompts need to develop the full holistic experience and will include prompts for sensory experience, motivation, and attitude (e.g., "Focus on your wanting to help another person"), posture, physical sensations (e.g., "Focus on feelings of calmness, warmth"), emotional feelings (e.g., "Experience and hold on to your feelings, letting them deepen"), facial expressions (e.g., "Notice the expression on your face as you feel compassion—how your face softens"), urges to action (e.g., "Focus on feelings of wanting to help, to hug or hold the person"), and attention.

As with the absorption exercise, the therapist ensures that the patient is fully immersed in the experience of compassion and not entering a conceptual or evaluative state in which she is *thinking about* the time she was compassionate. Abstract and analytical thinking will drop the patient out of the direct experience and can often lead to negative evaluations, such as "Why can't I be compassionate more often?" The therapist checks on the effect of the experiential exercise and uses prompts and imagery to strengthen the induction of a compassionate mind-set. For example, when a patient describes an aspect of her experience of being compassionate in physical, emotional, or symbolic terms, such as feeling kindness inside, the therapist encourages the patient to focus and concentrate on this aspect of the experience to strengthen the experience. Focusing on feelings or elements of the experience that work reinforces the overall experience.

When a patient finds this more difficult, the therapist needs to provide more scaffolding, prompts, and reminders, guiding him back into the experience by referring to previously successful descriptions. The therapist looks for shifts in and out of experiential processing and into abstract–evaluative processing and then tries to redirect attention back to engaging in the experiential exercise. The ACES principle applies here: when abstract–evaluative processing is observed, rather than discussing what is happening, it is recommended that the therapist look for ways to reengage the patient in direct and concrete experience.

Consistent with the RFCBT focus on changing habits, we want the patient to stay with the compassionate experience and to work through it in detail and on repeated occasions, until being compassionate to self or others becomes a habitual response. It needs to be practiced on multiple occasions in the therapy session and audio-recorded so it can be practiced repeatedly outside the treatment session. There should be repeated pairing of rumination triggers and warning signs (e.g., feeling irritated) with the alternative response of being compassionate to self or others. Being compassionate and self-soothing then becomes an automatic response to these cues (Principle 5: Link behaviors to triggers and warning signs).

A central aspect of developing compassion in RFCBT is the importance of validating the patient's experience. The therapist needs to model self-validation to the patient and look to facilitate validating self-statements, in which the patient's feelings and opinions are acknowledged, heard, respected, and valued. This follows the principles of normalizing the patient's experience and empowering the patient, which run throughout RFCBT (Principle 8: Focus on nonspecific factors). As a first stage in compassion training, validating the patient's own experience is a potent means to reduce distress and a useful skill for the patient to learn to apply for herself. The therapist models this approach and guides it in patients. When a patient reports a distressing emotion, it is helpful for the therapist to reflect that back and to value the patient's own experience. This is, of course, a central tenet within the principles of RFCBT and within the application of FA.

Several different types of statements can be helpful for the therapist in shaping patients toward validation and compassion, and to provide a structure for patients to develop more self-compassionate statements. I introduce these statements as pointers to help patients to become kinder and more supportive. The therapist goes through the different categories of compassionate things that the patient can say to himself to structure this for someone less experienced at being compassionate.

The following are five categories, which provide useful instructions and steps as to what the patient can say to himself, along with further explanation and examples that therapists can give for patients to use:

1. *Normalize the situation.* Remind yourself of the fact that everyone makes mistakes. No one is perfect.
2. *Focus on any progress made.* Point out all the hard work you have already done, the steps you've already completed, the progress you've already made, focus on positives rather than negatives, focus on the answers you got right rather than wrong. Look at what you can learn from this situation.
3. *Highlight success and strengths.* Remind yourself of other times that you have succeeded. Think about these times in detail.
4. *Put the situation into perspective.* Think about how this was a difficult situation, and it is not surprising it did not go well. Remind yourself that a bad mood will pass, and other opportunities will come along. Focus on the process rather than the outcome, for example, what you might be learning even if you have not mastered a situation, that it is important to keep trying, and that with effort, the difficulty will be overcome.
5. *Encourage yourself to go on to the next step.* Tell yourself that you can do it, that's it is just one step at a time, that you are strong. Break down the problem into smaller steps and focus on getting the next step done.

When patients find it hard to be self-compassionate, it often helps to explicitly run through these exemplar statements and work with them to develop their own self-statements in each category for particular situations. In this way, the therapist builds patients up into compassion step by step.

The nonverbal qualities of internal speech are also critical. The tone, pitch, and quality of the "voice" used have a big impact on the consequences of self-talk. Encouraging statements are more likely to be effective when they involve a calm, warm, gentle, confident, firm, persistent tone of voice that is not too loud or quiet and does not have any irony or sarcasm. In contrast, ruminative self-critical thoughts often have a critical, sarcastic, overbearing tone and can be cold or acidic. Such negative rumination can be an internalized version of a critical other, such as a parent. When patients practice shifting what they say to themselves, it is essential to look at how they say these different things. Different forms of internal dialogue and their distinct effects can be revealed during FA of helpful self-talk (compassionate) versus unhelpful self-talk (critical). The lessons from these functional analyses then feed into developing more self-compassion.

Acting in a Compassionate Way

In addition to practicing mental exercises, therapists want to encourage patient actions and behaviors that are compassionate. Paralleling the work on building up absorbing activities, the aim is for the patient to act in a more compassionate way toward herself. The therapist encourages the patient to ask herself the following two questions and then to make plans in response to these questions:

"What would I do more of if I were caring more for myself?"
"What would I do less of if I were caring more for myself?"

Changing the pattern of activities to be consistent with self-compassion will consolidate its benefits for the patient. Moreover, as a patient looks after and cares for himself more, he will find that he has more self-respect, which will build up his confidence. It will also reduce his chances of getting into stressful situations and increase his resilience to stress.

Common examples of activities to increase when acting in a self-compassionate way include spending more time with positive people; good self-care such as sleeping well, eating well, exercising more, resting and relaxing after stress; rewarding oneself more; trying new activities; respecting oneself more; putting one's self and one's needs first; and increasing chances for success through good planning and preparation.

Common examples of activities that people reduce when acting in a self-compassionate way include: doing less and having a less pressured schedule; avoiding people who take advantage; avoiding harmful situations; drinking less alcohol and not using drugs; not leaving things to the last minute; not rushing things; not pushing oneself too hard. Once activities to increase and decrease are identified, the therapist works with the patient to develop detailed and concrete plans that break the changes into smaller, more manageable steps.

An Example of Facilitating Compassion

The following dialogue reflects a session in which compassion was first discussed and then practiced with Emily, who was introduced in earlier chapters. The actual dialogue is generic, reflecting a composite of our experiences with a number of different patients. Emily responded well to concreteness training and absorption training but was still experiencing negative rumination. Her rumination was hypothesized to serve the function of motivating herself and preventing herself from developing her feared traits of being selfish, insensitive, and arrogant. In this context, it was judged that learning to be more compassionate would be a good alternative strategy.

Emily was one of the first patients in RFCBT treatment, and we were still developing the compassion technique. This dialogue, therefore, has strengths but also some weaknesses and limitations that we have subsequently addressed in the therapy. The dialogue is interspersed with reflections about what the therapist was doing, lessons learned, and ways to improve what was done.

THERAPIST: We have started to talk about tolerance and compassion and about how this might be helpful for you. We have spotted lots of thoughts that you have about being a bad person. Rather than dwelling on these thoughts as a way to avoid being a selfish person, we talked about doing something positive to make you a better person and to help you to feel better. As a first step toward this, I previously asked you to try and come up with these feelings of compassion and tolerance for other people, and you talked in detail about the example of providing advice at the health center. I want to focus on a memory when you caught those feelings at their strongest. Can you think of a particular incident when you remember having strong feelings of compassion?

EMILY: I can remember talking with a young mother who was having difficulties making ends meet. Saying "I am so sorry you are having these difficulties, I will try and help." I was trying to reach out and understand where she was coming from.

THERAPIST: OK, let's focus on this situation in a bit more detail. Notice where you are and what you can see and hear in this situation. Describe the scene to me.

EMILY: I am at my office sitting down talking to this teenage mother.

THERAPIST: What does she look like?

EMILY: She is quite young and thin, and clearly very anxious. She tends to talk really fast and finds it hard to sit still.

THERAPIST: What is happening? What are you and she doing?

EMILY: She is telling me all about her problems with her on-and-off boyfriend, with caring for her baby, and with paying the rent, and is getting tearful. I am trying to find ways to help.

THERAPIST: It sounds like you have a very vivid picture of this scene. Is that right?

EMILY: Yes.

THERAPIST: How much compassion and kindness are you feeling toward her?

EMILY: I felt very compassionate toward her.

THERAPIST: This sounds like a good memory to focus on. What would be interesting to try for a few moments would be to re-create that experience in your mind. Would that be all right with you?

EMILY: Yes.

THERAPIST: So it is as if you are back in that situation right now looking out through your eyes. Really focus on those feelings so you can try and re-create that feeling of compassion and that attitude of caring in yourself . . . And let that feeling get as strong as possible—making it as vivid as possible. Make that experience as vivid as you can. As best you can, recapture that experience. (*Pause.*) Let it grow and deepen. (*Pause.*) What are you noticing? How are you feeling emotionally inside?

EMILY: A feeling of softness, caring, a wish to make it better.

THERAPIST: Good. Can you concentrate on that feeling of softness and caring? See if you can get more and more caught up in it . . . becoming more and more absorbed in that feeling, becoming caught up in it, feeling it strengthen and spread throughout you. (*5-second pause*) How does that feel?

EMILY: It's sad but it is good.

THERAPIST: What are you noticing? What is your experience?

EMILY: A feeling of love and wanting to help. Just maybe hug the person or hold her hand.

THERAPIST: Good, focus on the feeling of softness and concern, as it continues to deepen and stay with that feeling of wanting to hug and hold her. What else are you noticing as the feeling of compassion grows? What are you noticing in your facial expression or body posture?

EMILY: I notice my face softening, I feel more relaxed inside. I feel that maybe I won't be able to help enough. There is hope for the other person and the hope that I can help them make it.

THERAPIST: How strong is that feeling of care and concern for her?

EMILY: Very strong.

THERAPIST: How does it feel to have that feeling?

EMILY: Good.

THERAPIST: As you focus on that feeling of compassion, was there anything that helped to bring it to life? What helped to bring that feeling of compassion to life as you are sitting there with this young mother? What are you paying attention to? What are you saying to yourself?

EMILY: I am focusing on her face, not what her background or status might be, thinking just we are all the same, we all have feelings, we all get hurt, we all cry, we all get afraid.

THERAPIST: So, there is quite a lot going on there; there are physical changes, change in expression . . .

EMILY: Feeling a bit weepy.

THERAPIST: Yes, that's right, feeling sad but good, having thoughts like trying to understand what it is like, wanting to help, images of hugging or holding hands . . .

EMILY: Just being kind.

THERAPIST: Being kind, thoughts like we are all the same, we all have different feelings. So if we stop for a second, and if you go back into this compassion feeling, try to pull it back up again. Bring it up as strongly as you can. Refocus on that experience of feeling kind for a moment and let it deepen and strengthen as you focus on the feelings of softness, of wanting to hug and hold her, of focusing on her face, on knowing we are all the same . . . (5-second pause)

EMILY: (Looks calmer and more relaxed, nodding.)

THERAPIST: Are you able to get it?

EMILY: Yeah.

THERAPIST: OK, notice those changes in posture and facial expression—face softening, the emotion coming up—it's sad, but it's good, the attitude that we all have feelings, trying to understand, wanting to help, the feeling inside of wanting to hold and wanting to hug her, as the feeling of compassion and warmth becomes stronger and stronger. Focus on these feelings. Pull it up as strongly as you can. What are the best words to describe how it feels?

EMILY: Very powerful, overwhelming feeling of wanting to support. A strong feeling of kindness and warmth toward her.

THERAPIST: How does this make you feel inside?

EMILY: It feels good.

Inside the Therapist's Mind 1: Decision Points and Reflections with Compassion

The dialogue above illustrates several important principles and common issues that occur when using the mental exercise to engender a compassionate mind-set. First, it shows how to identify a memory of feeling compassionate and to begin to explore it in detail to get a sense of whether it is an appropriate memory, one that the patient can vividly imagine. This memory is chosen because it was relatively easy and at the bottom (easiest end) of the compassion hierarchy. This description is relatively brief here both for conciseness and because Emily was good at imagery work, so the therapist was confident that a detailed memory was imagined. With other patients, more background work might be done to build a vivid picture of the event, asking about what happened and where, when, how, and with whom it happened, and seeking out detailed descriptions of the sensory–perceptual experience. Emily is then guided to imagine herself back into this situation, with the therapist prompting her to pay attention to the full holistic range of the experience (feelings, sensations, attention, attitudes, facial expression, action urges, etc.) and using suggestive prompts to encourage the compassionate mind-set. These details of the elements that contribute to the experience are noted by the therapist because focusing on them later may be helpful for activating the compassionate mode in more difficult situations.

You may have noticed that there was a brief moment when Emily moved out of an experiential mode of processing into a more abstract, evaluative, and comparative mode typical of her rumination. It was when she said, "maybe I won't be able to help enough." This signals moving from an emotional, experiential way of processing into an intellectual, judgmental mode. If this persisted, it would disrupt any induction of a compassionate way of being. Rather than challenging or discussing this difficulty, the therapist maintains a focus on the experience of compassion and returns Emily to the detail of the experience, consistent with the ACES principle, asking her to bring up those feelings of compassion again. As the session continues, Emily is encouraged to repeatedly practice shifting out of the default abstract–evaluative mode into the nonjudgmental experiential compassion mode.

Having successfully induced compassion for one other person, the therapist wants Emily to further practice this skill to other cues and for more difficult situations. The next step is to move up in the compassion hierarchy and practice compassion for a more difficult other. This is consistent with the six E's principle (see Chapter 9): once an exercise is found to be effective, it is further practiced and extended. Relevant to the dialogue below is that one of Emily's cues for rumination is feeling irritable.

THERAPIST: I'd like you to keep hold of that kindness feeling and hold on to those cues—your face softening, sensations of softness inside, wanting to help and to hold, keeping that feeling of compassion. Can you hold on to that feeling to apply to someone else? Let's move from applying compassion to the young mother to someone else. Thinking of what we talked about before, let's think of someone who would be a good person to practice being compassionate to but with whom this is not too difficult a step.

EMILY: My mother.

THERAPIST: Does that . . .

EMILY: I could be much more compassionate to my mother. I can be much more understanding to her.

THERAPIST: Is that a good step to take? I wonder if it is too big a step?

EMILY: Yes, maybe start somewhere else, say, my best friend because I have seen her when she has been difficult.

THERAPIST: All right. Would it be easy to be compassionate to your best friend?

EMILY: Yes.

THERAPIST: Is there a time when it would have been a bit more difficult with your best friend? When your best friend has gotten on your nerves or irritated you a bit?

EMILY: Yes.

THERAPIST: Have you got a clear memory of that happening?

EMILY: Yeah, there was a time recently when she was more irritable with me. That would be a good time I could have been more understanding.

THERAPIST: When was this?

EMILY: It was a couple of weeks ago. She was having stress at work and was a bit short-tempered and when we got together for a drink, I was a bit late, and she was quite sharp with me, and I got a bit annoyed back.

THERAPIST: Can you get a vivid memory of that time when you met your friend and felt a bit irritable?

EMILY: Yes.

THERAPIST: How does that feel right now as you get into that memory?

EMILY: Slightly annoying but not terribly annoying.

THERAPIST: OK, do you get some of that feeling of being irritated?

EMILY: Yeah.

THERAPIST: How strong would you say that feeling is out of 10?

EMILY: About 5.

THERAPIST: OK. How are you noticing that irritation with your friend right now?

EMILY: I am feeling a bit hot and tense.

THERAPIST: Starting at that point where you are feeling a bit irritated with your friend, I want you to bring up those feelings of compassion and focus on them, using what you have just done when you felt compassion for the young mother, using your friend as the person you are focusing those feelings on. As best you can, re-create those feelings of compassion, focusing on the feeling of softness, the attitude we are the same, wanting to understand and help her. Spend a few moments trying to do that as best you can . . . (10-second pause)

EMILY: Yes, OK.

THERAPIST: Good, just let those feelings deepen and strengthen and focus on them as best you can. Notice them as much as you can. What are you noticing as you focus on those feelings? What's happening?

EMILY: Umm, just a feeling of, you know, calmness and forgiving, we all make mistakes, we can all be insensitive at times.

THERAPIST: And the feelings of irritation and annoyance, what happens to those?

EMILY: (Shakes her head.) They seem less important.

THERAPIST: What would you say they are as you continue to focus on those compassion feelings? How strong are they now?

EMILY: Probably 2 to 3.

THERAPIST: OK, and if you hold on to these feelings of compassion, and stick with them for a bit longer, trying to build up those feelings as strong as they were. Focusing on how you are feeling inside, concentrate on those feelings of warmth, softness, and kindness. Focus on your face softening, as you become more and more absorbed in the feeling of compassion, encouraging those changes in your posture and facial expression. As you focus on her face, and focus on those thoughts that we are all the same and we all have feelings, let the feeling of kindness and warmth strengthen and deepen. Re-create those feelings of kindness.

EMILY: OK, I get a stronger feeling—it is not important what was annoying.

THERAPIST: How do you feel? What has happened to the feelings of irritation?

EMILY: They have gone away.

THERAPIST: So what is that 1 or 0?

EMILY: 1.

THERAPIST: And how do you feel having done that, as you hold on to those feelings?

EMILY: Better, more worthwhile, I suppose. Glad that I have been able to do it. Happy that I can be nice and understanding.

Inside the Therapist's Mind 2: Decision Points and Reflections with Compassion

In the dialogue above, the mental exercise of becoming more compassionate to others is practiced again, this time in a slightly harder situation in which a close friend is being annoying, reflecting the next step up the hierarchy. Furthermore, the exercise reflects the six E principles (specifically Exercise and Engage) by having the patient practice becoming more compassionate in response to a warning sign for rumination. Previous sessions had identified that feeling irritable toward others is often a cue for Emily's rumination. The therapist thus asked her to recall a time she felt irritated to elicit some of these feelings (i.e., a mood challenge) so that in the practice, being compassionate is directly paired with feeling irritated, and compassion, rather than rumination, is used to reduce the irritation. This affords the patient practice similar to real-world circumstances where it may be most useful, and increases the generalizability of this strategy outside of the session. Repeated pairings of irritation and compassion will make it more likely for compassion to become an automatic response to future periods of irritability, replacing the rumination habit (Principle 5: Link behaviors to triggers and warning signs; Principle 6: Emphasize the importance of repetition and practice).

It is important to note that at the beginning of this dialogue, Emily suggests her mother as the next person to practice being compassionate with, but the therapist queries this and looks for an alternative example. The therapist knows that Emily has a difficult relationship with her mother and has already established that being compassionate to her would be less straightforward and higher up the hierarchy.

This section of the treatment session demonstrates the use of prompts to direct the compassion experience and heighten the effect. The therapist continually encourages Emily to stay with the experience to further its impact. The final sentences indicate how powerful this compassion approach was at removing the feelings of irritation and acting as a functional alternative to rumination. The exercise also helped her to feel calmer, more forgiving, and more worthwhile. This suggests that the use of the compassion exercise was addressing the desired function formulated from the FA. The exercise can also be viewed as a behavioral experiment that implicitly challenged Emily's negative view of herself. She believed that she was not capable of being kind and considerate to others, but this exercise convincingly indicated that she was easily able to feel compassion. The next section repeats the exercise to further practice generating compassion to others in difficult situations, moving further up the difficulty hierarchy.

THERAPIST: So hold on to those feelings of kindness and compassion, and don't let them go away, keeping the focus on those feelings of being nice and understanding. Let's move on to practicing with another person and another situation. So who would be a step up from your best friend?

EMILY: I suppose my mother.

THERAPIST: So is there a situation you can remember where you were getting irritated with your mother?

EMILY: (*very quickly*) Yes.

THERAPIST: It sounds like one is coming up quite easily there.

EMILY: Yes.

THERAPIST: OK, what is the situation that is coming to mind?

EMILY: Umm . . . it was a few weeks ago, I went to see my parents and my mother was being very difficult. We were talking about my future plans and she was being very dismissive. She was also being really picky with my dad. She kept going on about how we were being selfish and not supporting her. She was just blaming everybody, picking on people, and going on about things. (*Sounds more and more annoyed, voice tense, louder, speaks faster, sits up in her chair.*)

THERAPIST: So as you reimagine that situation, what feelings are coming up?

EMILY: Angry (*said very definitely*). I can feel that anger.

THERAPIST: How are you noticing that anger? Any physical effects? What are you noticing?

EMILY: I get tense and I feel hotter, more alert.

THERAPIST: And how do you feel right now? How strong would you say that feeling of anger is?

EMILY: Quite strong, I'd say about 8. (*annoyed tone*)

THERAPIST: So keeping that situation in mind, imagine that you are in that place right now, staying with those feelings of irritation. Again try and pull up those feelings of compassion. Try and focus on those cues and elements that we talked about before—focusing on the feelings of kindness and softness, the attitude that we are all the same, the physical sensations of loosening and softening, the posture and facial expression, building from those previous situations and transferring across to this situation. As best you can, get hold of feelings of compassion, concern, and softness, bringing up those feelings as strong as you can. And, as you notice those feelings, just let them grow and become more and more absorbing, just spend a few moments trying to make that as vivid and as powerful as possible.

EMILY: OK (*looking a bit calmer, sounding less irritated*).

THERAPIST: How is that going?

EMILY: Good.

THERAPIST: What are you noticing?

EMILY: I am feeling calmer again.

THERAPIST: How are you feeling toward your mother?

EMILY: Feeling more tolerant.

THERAPIST: What are you noticing as you become more tolerant?

EMILY: Just that she has reasons for being that way. Not so angry about it, taking more of an empathetic view.

THERAPIST: What is happening to that feeling of anger?

EMILY: It is less.

THERAPIST: What has it gone down to?

EMILY: A 2 or 3.

THERAPIST: What's holding it up still? Any particular things you are holding on to that are keeping the anger going?

EMILY: Yes, I am not focusing on one thing at a time. I have thoughts of other things that she has done that annoy me.

THERAPIST: OK, as best you can, stay with that original situation and focus on those feelings of compassion. Focus on whatever you can, whatever cues help you to pull it up as strongly as possible. Spend a few more minutes so that you can really dive into that feeling, and let those feelings come up and spread throughout you, deepen and enrich, and apply those feelings of warmth, kindness, and softness to those other thoughts that are coming up . . . taking that feeling of compassion that you experienced earlier and focusing on those feelings as you become more and more absorbed in the feeling of compassion . . . (*10-second pause*)

EMILY: OK, it's good, it seems like, it feels like it spreads out from my center, from my heart.

THERAPIST: OK, and if you focus on that, go with that, let it take its course. If that seems to help, focus on that, concentrate on that feeling spreading out from your heart.

EMILY: I suppose the irritation has been replaced by concern for her well-being. I guess she is difficult because she wants everything to be just right and finds it hard to come to terms with her own health issues.

THERAPIST: So how are you feeling now?

EMILY: Better, better about her.

THERAPIST: What feelings are you experiencing? What are you concentrating on now?

EMILY: I feel bad for not being more tolerant before.

THERAPIST: The anger has gone away and been replaced with guilt?

EMILY: Mostly. It's only about a 1.

Inside the Therapist's Mind 3: Decision Points and Reflections with Compassion

This dialogue illustrates the value of identifying a memory that genuinely activates an emotional response and a warning sign for rumination (in this case irritation), and practicing an alternative strategy to that response. It is clear that the emotion was still very real and alive for Emily, making this an excellent opportunity to practice doing something different to an active feeling of irritation. This section also illustrates the value of staying with the experience and prompting it with more concrete and specific cues to enrich the imagery. This enabled Emily to overcome a block and experience stronger feelings of compassion. Using a patient's language can increase the impact of the exercise: metaphorical and symbolic phrases like "it seems to spread out from the heart" capture a sense of deep engagement with the experience. Similarly, pay close attention to a patient's nonverbal signals and body language, as this provides clues as to whether she is experiencing compassion (with associated softening and relaxation), becoming more irritated, or finding it a struggle.

At the end of this dialogue, there is another shift back from experiential thinking to conceptual–evaluative thinking, and this provides a decision point for the therapist as to what to do next. In the actual session, the therapist chose to move from practicing compassion for others to practicing compassion for self. The introduction of the feelings of guilt seemed to provide an excellent opportunity to do this. With more experience, I now suggest that this is not likely to be the best course of action. As noted earlier, self-compassion is often scary, difficult, and challenging for patients to attempt. I now recommend building up to it more gradually. This may involve having several weeks' practice at being compassionate to others to consolidate this skill before moving on to compassion for self. Alternatively, if starting with self-compassion, the therapist works out a detailed hierarchy of difficulty and practices the use of compassionate self-statements before moving into the imagery exercise. All of the tips noted earlier, such as identifying a hierarchy of difficulty, ensuring the patient is fully embodied in the experience, and having an effective set of prompts and cues, are necessary to develop a self-compassionate mind-set.

The dialogue continues below as the therapist focuses on developing self-compassion. It illustrates some of the potential difficulties and ways past these problems. Even for this early session, when the therapist is persistent and creative at employing the ACES principle, some headway is made in giving the patient an experience of self-compassion.

THERAPIST: We could practice being compassionate to lots of people. I wonder if you could try to apply those feelings of compassion to what is coming up now, to those feelings of guilt coming up. Would you be willing to try?

EMILY: All right.

THERAPIST: OK. Now take all those feelings of kindness and warmth, attitudes like we are all the same that you have applied to others . . . getting that sense of compassion as strong as you can, that feeling spreading out from your heart . . . and keeping that feeling, as best you can, apply that feeling to yourself and to those thoughts about feeling guilty. Let it spread with yourself as the focus . . . let it spread, focusing inward, and again as you do that let the feelings becoming stronger and deeper. Noticing your facial expression softening, relaxing your posture . . . Feeling like you want to hug yourself, letting that feeling of softness spread throughout yourself making those feelings of kindness stronger and deeper. And if it wavers, pull in those feelings from the previous practice. Spend a few moments letting those feelings of kindness to yourself deepen and strengthen.

EMILY: (frowning, looking tense) It doesn't work. It just seems different. It can work on a certain level, like we all make mistakes, that kind of thing. Trying to apply it to myself, it just feels like I am not worthy of it.

THERAPIST: Did this thought come up with any of the other people?

EMILY: No, not with any of the others.

THERAPIST: Let's go back then and re-create the feelings of compassion when you were applying it to another person such as your best friend, where you were able to experience the feeling of kindness very powerfully. Bring that feeling back up again. Let's re-create that feeling again. Go back to the images you had before when recalling this feeling. Getting that feeling as strong and as deep as you can.

EMILY: OK, I can get that completely.

THERAPIST: What is happening as you are doing that?

EMILY: I don't feel so tense, it is almost like my arms are more open, not closed up. Just more relaxed, more full of warmth and energy.

THERAPIST: And as you focus on those sensations, what happens to the feeling of compassion?

EMILY: The feeling of wanting to help gets stronger.

THERAPIST: OK, so keep focusing on what you are noticing, getting the feeling of kindness and softness as strong as you can. Is there anything else you are noticing or doing as you notice that feeling of compassion get stronger?

EMILY: I suppose, just a sense of wanting to hold and to comfort.

THERAPIST: How do you experience that? Is it an image or a feeling in the body almost?

EMILY: A feeling in the body, but also an image.

THERAPIST: What is the image?

EMILY: I see an image of someone in tears, of someone who is distressed, and an image of myself wanting to hold, comfort them. That is very strong.

THERAPIST: Can you focus on that feeling inside your body and try and notice that as much as you can? What are you noticing as you do that?

EMILY: The feeling is in the heart and across my chest. (*Gestures across her chest.*)

THERAPIST: OK, good, stay with those feelings and focus on them and let them become stronger and more powerful. Keep those feelings and hold on to them. You mentioned this example from the other day when you were sitting at home, feeling upset and ruminating about your difficulties, can you visualize yourself in that situation?

EMILY: (*Nods.*) Yes.

THERAPIST: What do you see?

EMILY: Someone who is unhappy.

THERAPIST: What are you experiencing as you get that image of yourself?

EMILY: Contempt.

THERAPIST: How are you feeling right now?

EMILY: Not so good, because in order to have a visual image of myself, I need to see myself and I don't like what I see.

THERAPIST: So that feeling of contempt, how strong is that?

EMILY: Quite strong, I see myself as useless, for not being able to cope and for letting myself get taken advantage of.

THERAPIST: How strong are those feelings?

EMILY: About 9 out of 10.

THERAPIST: So you are seeing yourself in that situation. Now stepping aside, imagine it is someone else, not you, another person in that situation, in all other aspects the situation is exactly the same, so what they are thinking, what they are feeling is the same although it is a different person, what they are experiencing and the events that happened before are the same as they were for you in that situation. Can you now take that feeling of compassion and tolerance and forgiveness, and wanting to hold and wanting to comfort, and apply it to that person? Imagine applying the feeling of softness and compassion to that imaginary person.

EMILY: Yes, it is easier to do that.

THERAPIST: As best you can, do that. Apply those feelings—it could be almost anyone who has had the same experiences and has the same thoughts and feelings as you do. Someone who has had those experiences and you can see them. They are going over those things in their mind, making themselves feel bad, and criticizing and doubting themselves. Imagine sending those feelings of support and compassion to that person, re-creating those feelings in your body and your heart, your face softening, getting that feeling as strong as you possibly can, applying it to that person, getting that sense of wanting to hold or to hug that person, embracing them with those feelings of softness and warmth. Are you able to get that?

EMILY: Yes.

THERAPIST: Keep focusing on the feelings, getting them as strong as you can.

EMILY: When I think of me, it stops.

THERAPIST: OK, let's just keep it as not you for the moment and stay with the feeling, sinking deeper and deeper into the feeling. Notice those feelings of softness, kindness, caring getting stronger and stronger. What do you notice?

EMILY: I feel more tolerant toward the person.

THERAPIST: What effect does it have on you as you become more tolerant?

EMILY: I suppose I feel calmer, I want to help.

THERAPIST: And those feelings, those really strong sensations—of softness spreading through your heart and chest and through your body, are you getting those? The feeling of wanting to hold and comfort?

EMILY: It is harder to get.

THERAPIST: OK, spend a bit of time staying with those feelings, applying them to that person you can imagine, who is in the exact same situation as you, and experiencing the same distress as you.

EMILY: OK.

THERAPIST: And let those feelings get as strong as possible, so you can feel them absolutely coursing through you, through your body, really powerful, overwhelming, really strong, as you direct those feelings toward that person.

EMILY: OK.

THERAPIST: And as you focus on those feelings, what happens?

EMILY: It's the same. It's positive. It's kind of all-embracing.

THERAPIST: Keep that all-embracing feeling, let it grow and develop. If we switch back and that person in this difficult situation is you, what happens?

EMILY: (*Shakes head.*) It doesn't seem right.

THERAPIST: OK, putting that thought to one side for a moment, keep focusing on those all-embracing feelings of warmth, softness, kindness, wanting to heal—those feelings spreading out from the heart—doing what you have done all the way through today, focusing on that feeling in your own body of wanting to hold and comfort, and those physical sensations inside of kindness and softness, of comforting, hold on to those feelings and let those feeling stay, as you focus on that image of the other person in your situation.

EMILY: OK. (*sounding tentative*).

THERAPIST: Keep re-creating all those feelings of wanting to hold and help, and understanding, why that person is feeling the way they are, and being more tolerant, feeling those feelings spread out from the heart . . . judgment and irritability being replaced with concern, and focusing on the person's face, getting those feelings of wanting to hold and comfort, really let them grow and stay.

EMILY: OK.

THERAPIST: What is happening as you are doing that?

EMILY: Umm. It's a bit better. I can visualize this person as me up to a point and feel these feelings for them, I know it is me, but when I physically see myself, it is more difficult.

THERAPIST: So you can have the feelings when it is you without seeing yourself directly? Is that still having some effect on you right now? Are you experiencing some sympathy toward yourself? Do you know it is yourself you are sending it too? What effect does that have?

EMILY: It is hard to describe. It's nice. It's nice to feel that.

THERAPIST: When you say it feels nice, what are you noticing? Focus on that feeling of nice, of compassion, make that as strong as you can.

EMILY: Kind of a feeling of maybe I am actually all right. To a certain extent, I deserve compassion as much as the next person.

THERAPIST: Just stay with those feelings and stay with them, explore those feelings of tolerance and being all right. (*5-second pause*) And if you focus on the physical things you noticed before, like your posture opening up, can you re-create that? (*pause*) And focus on those feelings you were having of face softening, let your face soften, and those sensations of kindness, softness spreading out from your heart to your arms and face, holding on to those, focusing on those, as you keep becoming more and more absorbed in the feeling of compassion and tolerance, applying it to yourself, becoming immersed in that feeling, spreading it to your whole body, your feelings, and your thoughts, holding it in your body right now. (*5-second pause*)

EMILY: Yes (*looks more relaxed, less tense*).

THERAPIST: Opening up those feelings to yourself, embracing yourself internally, holding and comforting yourself.

EMILY: OK.

THERAPIST: What is happening as you do that, as you spread those feelings of compassion out to yourself and immerse yourself in those feelings? As you get those feelings as strong as you can?

EMILY: I feel less uncomfortable with myself.

THERAPIST: Concentrate on that feeling—on feeling softer and more tolerant of yourself, let that spread, work its way through you, so that you become softer throughout, relax into that feeling throughout your body. (*pause*)

EMILY: (*Nods.*)

THERAPIST: What is happening as you do that?

EMILY: I suppose just the feelings I had for other people coming to myself, a sense of it physically changing, it feels odd, me doing it.

THERAPIST: Are you feeling those feelings of kindness you were sending out to other people?

EMILY: A bit. Not as strong.

THERAPIST: How does it feel having those feelings?

EMILY: Nice, comforting, but sad, because I have not had them before.

THERAPIST: OK, so it is nice and comforting but sad because this is new, a new step for you. And if you think about the situation you were imagining, when you were dwelling on all those things, what is happening to the feelings you were having about that?

EMILY: That I need to let go of them because they are damaging.

THERAPIST: And that feeling of contempt that you had for yourself in that situation, what's happened to that as you have been focusing on the feelings of softness and compassion?

EMILY: It is less to the person inside but not to the physical me. It is a bit better. I feel kinder to myself.

THERAPIST: What effect does that have?

EMILY: The world is a less frightening, less threatening place.

THERAPIST: And thinking of that situation that we were talking about, where you had all that contempt toward yourself, what happened to that?

EMILY: It turned into concern and care.

THERAPIST: Is this a different feeling from what you were feeling toward the other people we practiced with? Is it the same feeling of compassion?

EMILY: I have been trying to do that really hard, it is the same feeling but not as strong. I feel they deserve it more than I do. I am going to have to work on that.

THERAPIST: Having given yourself just a little bit of that kindness, how is that different from what you were doing before?

EMILY: It is completely different. It is a glimpse of thinking of myself as someone I like, instead of someone I don't like. Or seeing myself as someone that has got faults, has made mistakes, but who is forgivable.

THERAPIST: And when you start thinking like that, what effect does that have?

EMILY: It is soothing. I feel like it might be possible to open up to the future like I can carry it all around. I feel calmer.

THERAPIST: So how would you say you were feeling right now, having done this exercise?

EMILY: OK, it seems a good thing to use, yes I can try, a feeling of wanting to try and be nicer to myself.

THERAPIST: We have seen that it can have quite powerful effects, both when you apply it to other people and to yourself. How could you try to hold on to those feelings and build on them?

EMILY: I think it will work if I can apply it to myself.

THERAPIST: And when you turn these feelings of compassion directly onto yourself, what happens then?

EMILY: A sense of things being OK, that I am OK—in a small way.

THERAPIST: In a small way, well, that's a good start. We have worked through quite a lot of difficult stuff today. What are you taking away from what we have done today?

EMILY: A sense of wanting to try harder at looking after other people and looking after myself.

THERAPIST: So there is a sense that you haven't been looking after yourself? It seemed that that was the bit that was hardest.

EMILY: Yes.

THERAPIST: And what do you think you can learn from what we have just been doing?

EMILY: Everybody needs to be kinder to themselves.

THERAPIST: And when you are being kind to yourself, what happens?

EMILY: It gets easier.

THERAPIST: And did that feel pretty weird?

EMILY: It did feel pretty weird. It felt odd that I was bothering to do that for myself. That I was out there supporting myself.

THERAPIST: And, if you were going to start somewhere, with being more compassionate in general, where would be the best place to start?

EMILY: I don't know whether to start with physical feelings or emotions. So I can start with feelings, when I get irritated, start by asking is it reasonable to be irritated, have I got reason to be irritated?

THERAPIST: I guess what we are talking about here is taking what you have practiced here today—being more compassionate—and using that as an alternative to one of your triggers for rumination, for example, getting irritable. And it sounds like when you are being compassionate one of the things you are doing is saying more reasonable things to yourself, that mental side is coming up, the attitude of we all are human, etcetera. But the sensations, the physical feelings were important too. What will make it easier to get there?

EMILY: Practice.

THERAPIST: And how do you feel about doing that?

EMILY: I feel OK about it and I know this is the right thing to do in this context, but I know that I am going to go away and try and do it and think this is selfish.

THERAPIST: And if you apply the being compassionate to . . .

EMILY: To that thought,

THERAPIST: To that thought, what happens?

EMILY: Yes, it might seem selfish, but it is a process you need to go through.

THERAPIST: And what would make something not selfish?

EMILY: If I was doing it for someone else. If I was doing it to help other people. But I suppose you can look at it as if I make myself a better person, or a happier person, then I am in a better position to help others, to make others happy, because I have my own experience to draw on.

THERAPIST: That's an interesting idea. What do you make of that?

EMILY: That's probably a good way to go. Because it is not so me, me, me.

THERAPIST: Are you kind of saying that if you are feeling more compassionate to yourself then it is going to be a lot easier to be compassionate to other people, whereas if you are beating yourself up all the time, it will be harder?

EMILY: Yes.

THERAPIST: Does that sound like being selfish to you?

EMILY: No, that is why I think this could be a useful way to look at it.

THERAPIST: So if you hold on to that idea, it may be easier to do. And when you practice being compassionate, it may be a good idea to practice both sides of it, to apply compassion to someone else, then to apply it to yourself. Starting off with applying to someone else and then applying it yourself. So you are not being selfish because you are practicing both. How does that sound?

EMILY: Good, cool.

THERAPIST: And in terms of practicing it, what do we think? How often?

EMILY: I think linking it with checking myself when I get upset and start going over and over things.

THERAPIST: I agree it sounds like it would be good to do at those points. But you might need to strengthen it up a bit before then. You might need to practice it a few times perhaps by listening back to the tape of this session.

EMILY: OK, perhaps I can add that to my visualization before I start the day, to practice it every day, and then try to use it throughout the day when I spot a warning sign.

THERAPIST: That sounds like an excellent plan.

Inside the Therapist's Mind 4: Decision Points and Reflections with Compassion

The extended dialogue above makes clear how difficult it can be for patients to shift into being compassionate to the self and the kinds of hurdles that can come up. Attempts at self-compassion can be blocked by difficulties staying in an experiential nonevaluative mode of processing. Emily shifts back into the comparative–evaluative mode tied into taking an observer perspective and seeing herself, and concerns about not being worthwhile enough, not feeling deserving, and feeling selfish, weird, or uncomfortable for being kind to the self.

Lessons that my colleagues and I learned from our first attempts at engendering self-compassion, as illustrated in this example, include the importance of not rushing into this practice but setting it up slowly, in small steps, and preparing a hierarchy in advance. One mistake of this session was moving straight from practicing compassion for others into practicing self-compassion. Now I recommend that therapists practice the former more and consolidate this before moving on to the latter. A more explicit hierarchy of the difficulty in being self-compassionate is explored with the patient before trying the exercise in detail.

It also becomes clear that inducing self-compassion works better when the patient is able to adopt a field perspective where the experience of compassion is embodied within the patient and experienced as an immersive internal state, rather than imposed on the outside of the person. Within this dialogue, there are points where this is prompted and it seems to be helpful, but in other places, the language refers to having an image of oneself, which may prompt Emily into the observer perspective and which seems much less helpful. When Emily saw images of herself, this activated her self-comparison and self-judgment, cutting out any feelings of compassion. The therapist could have spotted this earlier, worked toward the embodied experience, and been more systematic in encouraging this. Our later experience suggests that this strengthens the creation of the compassionate mind-set.

Strengths within this session included the following: persistence staying with the compassion experience; repeated detailed prompts into multiple aspects of the full holistic experience; creative attempts to bypass blocks to fully engaging in the compassion by shifting to alternative images; linking the compassion experience to warning signs and cues (If–Then plans); repeated checking and feedback on the experience; not finishing the exercise until Emily had made some progress and had a positive experience; reinforcing the positive experience and tying this into ongoing practice plans. For example, when Emily first tried to be self-compassionate and it failed to work, we see a clear example of being able to think about compassion intellectually but not being able to connect with it experientially or emotionally. This emphasizes the value of helping the patient to stay with the experience but also the difficulty of engaging with this experience. The therapist at this point chose to return to the feelings of compassion for another person (her best friend) to pull these feelings up strongly and return to a more positive state, as a potential jumping-off point back into practicing self-compassion again. The therapist then looked for a way to gradually build Emily toward self-compassion in easier steps that did not immediately activate self-evaluation. He asked her to imagine another person experiencing exactly the same situation that she experienced and bringing compassion to this faceless avatar, before then moving this to herself directly.

The blocking role of self-image was highlighted by the experience of seeing herself. However, with persistence, a small but meaningful first experience of self-compassion was achieved. Other, potentially better ways to build up self-compassion are to develop the internal embodied experience of compassion, which avoids the observed self, and to imagine the self as a younger person. This is also where developing completely new images that represent compassion, as advocated within compassionate mind training (Gilbert, 2009), could be useful.

Incremental small changes and repeated practice are critical to building up self-compassion. A session lasting nearly 2 hours was necessary to reach a positive endpoint. I do not recommend trying this with a shorter session, at least for the initial sessions. Although only a small glimpse of compassion was achieved, this is significant when patients have very limited experience of self-soothing. This breakthrough is then reinforced and consolidated with repeated practice, for example, with the patient listening to an audio recording of the therapy session to re-create the experience every day until the next session. It is also helpful to give more feedback to Emily about how hard she has worked and to reinforce how even a small step here is big progress. The therapist can also inculcate the idea that all difficulties are potentially grist to the mill, wherein compassion can be applied to any hurdle as it arises.

Values

A focus on the patient's personal values can be important for both absorption and compassion. By values I mean the direction that the patient wants to pursue in life. Values are distinguished from goals in that goals have concrete endpoints that can be achieved. Getting married, passing a test, or getting a job are each distinct goals. Values can never be definitively achieved; one can only align one's actions with values and either be heading in a direction consistent or inconsistent with values. For example, to be honest or to have closer relationships are values.

Attempts at absorption and compassion are more likely to be successful when they are aligned with the patient's deep-seated values, for example, when an attempt to become immersed involves the patient's concern for the natural world, or when increasing compassion addresses the patient's desire to be a more considerate person. Connecting exercises and plans with the patient's values is a means to motivate and consolidate an exercise's benefit. Moreover, what the patient finds absorbing will provide clues as to his or her personal values. Patients will find it hard to become engaged in activities that do not capture what is important to them.

When we ask patients about their personal values, common themes emerge. Typical values include closeness to others, closeness to nature, personal growth, kindness, honesty, learning, being considerate, being responsible, humor, freedom, caring for the environment. Personal values often seem to reflect moral and social qualities. This is an interesting contrast to much of the content of depressive rumination, which is focused on evaluative and comparative thinking about achievement, competence, material success, and status, which are somewhat at odds with the personal values described above. It appears as if rumination is often about internalized and introjected values from others, relating to coming across well, "keeping up with the Joneses," not letting others down, not being a disappointment, and other culturally supported values. It can be helpful to get patients to identify their own values and to consider how their actions and situation relate to these values, as this often cuts out unnecessary rumination. For example, a patient who was ruminating about how poorly she is doing in terms of her financial situation and the difficulties in her low-paid work, which made her feel like a failure, identified being close to others as her most important value. When she examined herself against this value, she was doing much better—she had close and good relationships with her partner and her children. Reorienting her to her values removed all of this rumination.

It can be helpful to focus on the values that are important to the patient when attempting to change behaviors. These values can improve motivation, increase the likelihood of changes being implemented, and maximize the benefit of any approach behavior. We don't just want people to go into "positive" situations or to increase arbitrarily chosen activities generally deemed to be reinforcing. To get the maximum benefit, we want patients to focus on the intrinsic value within the task and approach those elements of the situation that are of most value to them.

I have found the following questions useful in asking patients about their values:

"What is important to you?"
"What values give your life meaning?"
"What values make activities seem worthwhile?"
"What gives your life purpose?"
"What do you dream about happening?"

The therapist also asks patients what they are paying attention to when they feel most absorbed and interested in a task, or when the task seems positive and significant. These questions give a clue as to what the person values. Useful questions include:

"Can you think of a time when you were absorbed in the process of
    doing something?"
"What were you paying attention to then?"
"Which aspects of the process were meaningful to you?"

Once the therapist and patient have collaboratively ascertained the values
that are most important to him, it is beneficial to ask the patient to imagine
carrying out a plan and focusing on the aspects of the plan he values. Imagining the feeling of value that would come from the activity helps motivate
the patient to put the plan into action.

The therapist asks questions like:

"What qualities and values that are dear to you can you bring to bear
    on this present moment from which you can derive satisfaction?"
"What process that you value can you focus on in this situation?"
"How would you be acting if you were going in the direction of these
    intrinsic values?" "What would you be attending to if you were act-
    ing in line with your intrinsic values?"

These latter questions about acting in the direction of your values can be
particularly useful for keeping patients on track in the long run and for orienting the patient toward more helpful activities.

For example, one patient tended to focus so much on how badly things
were done when he went to rehearse in a play that he did not gain in positive
mood from this activity. We recognized that something he valued was learning new things, so we planned for him to try and focus on what new things
he could be learning at the next rehearsal. This shift in perspective caused
him to find the rehearsal more enjoyable and absorbing.

This approach is powerful at maximizing BA. It can also help to cut
down on rumination, since rumination can be triggered when people feel
that they aren't doing as well as they should. Sometimes when people make
these evaluations, they are ignoring their values, and if they shift their thinking to include their values, they see that they are doing OK. "How are you
progressing in living your values?" can be a useful question. Encouraging patients to work toward their values is likely to reduce their ongoing
depression and rumination. It helps to orient patients to what they want
to achieve, while taking off some of the pressure that comes from having a
concrete goal. It is not really possible to fail at a value—one is either moving
closer or further away from it.

PART III

APPLICATION AND
EXTENSION OF RFCBT

CHAPTER 12

A Case of RFCBT
from Beginning to End

This chapter pulls together all the elements described previously, using the example of Stephen (a generic case) and outlining his background assessment, formulation, and session-by-session activities. I have split the description of the session-by-session activities into two sections: the initial assessment, rationale, and FA (sessions 1 and 2), followed by the remaining sessions, which involve more active interventions, the introduction of contingency If–Then plans, behavioral experiments, visualizations, and increased approach behaviors (sessions 3–10). This split does not reflect any distinction within therapy, as the use of FA and interventions are continuous throughout the therapy. Rather, it is used to enable the reader to reflect on potential formulations and therapy plans before reviewing the formulation of the therapist and the actual treatment delivered.

The background, presenting history, and developmental history, plus the detailed examples based on recent episodes of rumination, were all gathered in a detailed assessment during the first few sessions of the therapy.

Initial Assessment: Sessions 1 and 2

Stephen, a 30-year-old man who works in the media, sought therapy for a long-lasting episode of depression. His therapist reviewed his current symptoms, background, and recent history using the introductory questions in Chapter 4. Stephen lives alone in his own apartment. He reported a history of recurrent depression, with at least three previous episodes of depression during his late teens and early 20s, including a serious suicide attempt involving an overdose of painkillers. The most recent episode started 2 years ago, following a stressful time at work and then a period of sick leave. He is hoping to return to work part-time. When asked about his current symptoms, Stephen reported extremely high levels of rumination and preoccupation (score on the Response Styles Questionnaire [RSQ] = 83), high levels of depression (Beck Depression Inventory [BDI] score of 18), anxiety, and poor concentration. He reported feeling overwhelmed by rumination about his difficulties and his life, spending much of his time dwelling on his failures and problems. His main concerns were worries about not earning enough money and not being successful in his profession. When asked by his therapist about his goals for therapy, Stephen reported that he wanted to be more confident, to worry less, and to feel better in his own skin.

The therapist checked with Stephen to see whether rumination was a major problem for him. After reviewing its effects and observing that it exacerbated his anxiety, depression, low self-esteem, and poor concentration, Stephen and his therapist collaboratively agreed that rumination would be a good target for therapy. Having established rumination as a primary focus of the therapy, the therapist sought further information about the background to Stephen's rumination and asked about recent examples of rumination (see questions in Chapters 4 and 6).

The therapist started by asking about Stephen's general experience of rumination: when and where it tended to happen, what Stephen tended to dwell on, and the antecedents and consequences of his rumination. Stephen reported that he ruminated nearly every day for several hours, and that he often ruminated when he was not busy, when he was lying in bed in the morning and at night, and that it made it difficult for him to fall asleep. Common situations where he would start to ruminate included when he faced conflict with another person and had to assert himself or when he felt insecure and made negative judgments about himself, for example, when he saw people who looked more successful than him. His rumination was often about how he was responding to other people and how he was coming across to others (e.g., "Am I overreacting?"; "Should I complain?"; "Am I being unreasonable?"; "What does he think of me?"; "What does this mean about me?"; "Am I being oversensitive?"), and included dwelling on his problems and feelings (e.g., "Why can't I be more capable?"; "Why do I always have to feel like this?"; "Why can't it be easier?"). The consequences of his rumination were often to feel worse, more depressed, and less confident.

The therapist then asked about Stephen's history of rumination, and when he remembered it first starting. Stephen reported ruminating since an early age, from "as early as he can remember." He reported having a number of early upsetting memories that intruded into his mind. These revolved around concerns that he would get into trouble with his parents, who were strict and had very high standards, for example, worrying about how his father would respond when he saw Stephen's grades in school and whether he would be punished for not getting good enough grades.

The therapist also asked about Stephen's experience of his parents, how they treated him, and whether he might have learned his rumination from either his mother or father. Stephen reported that his mother had suffered from anxiety and that she was always worrying about what others would think. Stephen described his father as a very angry, aggressive, stern, and critical man, who had very high standards and often flew into a rage when things weren't done as he wanted or expected. He described his father as being very easily angered, with his temper on a hair trigger, and that when he was angry, he would shout and scream and be verbally abusive in a very hurtful and contemptuous way, with this sometimes spilling over to lashing out physically. If Stephen managed to hide away and be inconspicuous as a child, then he did not upset his father and avoided his anger. As a child, Stephen never knew when his father was going to attack or criticize him or his mother.

Based on this initial assessment, the therapist discussed with Stephen a personalized rationale for why he might ruminate and how the therapy might be helpful (see Chapter 5). The therapist noted how it was normal to ruminate about difficult situations to try and make sense of them and to avoid trouble, and how this could be learned so that it become a frequent habit in particular circumstances. He suggested to Stephen that it made sense that Stephen learned rumination as a habit when he had both a mother who modeled worrying to him, and an unpredictable and aggressive father. The therapist discussed with Stephen how he would have spent a lot of time thinking about what might set off his father as a coping strategy to try and avoid getting into trouble. They collaboratively agreed that this was probably an effective strategy in this difficult situation. The therapist raised the possibility that this response might have become overlearned so that Stephen was now second-guessing and overanalyzing other people's responses in other situations, where it may not be helpful. The therapist introduced the idea that the therapy might help Stephen by coaching him to replace the ruminative habit with more helpful habits. This would involve spotting the warning signs for his rumination and finding alternative strategies to practice. The therapist checked whether this made sense to Stephen and whether he was willing to try this approach. Stephen indicated that he wanted to tackle rumination and was hopeful that this therapy could be helpful.

The therapist then explored a specific recent episode of rumination in detail with Stephen, looking at what happened moment by moment, with the rationale that this would help them spot warning signs and think about alternative strategies. Stephen reported that a few days before, he had started to feel tense when he felt that a friend had taken advantage of him. He had lent his friend some money when he was doing better financially, and his friend had just called him up to say he wasn't going to pay it back on schedule. The first sign that Stephen noticed was feeling tension in his shoulders and arms. This was followed by a chain of thoughts like "When I am going to get it back?"; "How long is it going to take?"; "Should I complain to him?"; "Why does he treat me like this?"; "Why isn't he being fair about this?" As this rumination continued, he became angry, feeling tense, irritated, worked up, and hot. There was then a series of thoughts about being angry, including "What if I lost control?"; "Complaining could make things worse and escalate into an argument or a confrontation"; and "I might lose my temper." In response to these thoughts, Stephen tried to be reasonable and had a series of thoughts like "It could be worse. I am being unfair" and "I am overreacting." This attempt at being reasonable escalated into self-critical rumination. Stephen began to feel sad and self-critical. As his rumination continued, these feelings and thoughts escalated and became more extreme: "I am weak"; "I am a coward"; "I am a wimp." He described feeling more and more depressed as this bout of rumination continued. His thoughts became more negative as the rumination continued, focusing on his feelings of impotence. As the rumination continued, Stephen reported feeling hopeless, powerless, and tired. This bout of rumination lasted for several distressing hours until Stephen decided it was reasonable to be assertive. At this point, he phoned his friend and asked for some of his loan to be paid back. After a detailed conversation, his friend agreed to pay back some of the money over the next week.

The therapist summarized this detailed example back to Stephen, highlighting that it indicated how rumination was unhelpful for Stephen and contributed to his feeling down on himself. The therapist also raised the possibility that the positive response of his friend indicated that the several hours of rumination may have been unnecessary, and that it might be helpful for Stephen to find ways to step out of the rumination and get to this active problem solving more quickly. He also checked whether this pattern of response was typical of how Stephen ruminated, and whether this happened often when he felt irritable. Stephen confirmed that this was how he usually responded. The therapist pointed out how this example suggested that getting tense and irritable could be warning signs for Stephen's rumination habit. He also used it to illustrate how Stephen did sometimes take effective action—in this case, talking to his friend—and that therapy would look at ways to make this happen more frequently and more systematically, building on learning from Stephen's own experience.

For his homework in these initial sessions, Stephen was given the handouts on rumination and self-monitoring (Handout 1, Key Facts about Rumination; Handout 4, Self-Monitoring) to read, asked to listen to audio recordings of the therapy session before the next session, and encouraged to complete the rumination self-monitoring forms (Handout 5, Tracking

Rumination and Avoidance; Handout 6, Rumination Episode Recording Form).

In the second session, Stephen brought in another example of rumination that had occurred that week (see Stephen's filled-in Rumination Episode Recording Form, Figure 12.1). The therapist reviewed this example in detail to see how it unfolded moment by moment. Stephen was putting off talking to his manager about arranging to go back to work part-time because he had concerns about being seen as an awkward person and about how his manager would react. In anticipation, Stephen started by planning how he is going to do this, for example, when to call his manager and what he would say. However, these thoughts were quickly followed by abstract thoughts and questions about the meaning and implications of the call, such as "How will I be come across?"; "Is this reasonable or not?"; "Will he think I am trying to see how much I can get away with?" These questions were then followed by an image popping into his mind of his manager being annoyed at him, which led to a series of "why"-type questions such as "Why is this so difficult?"; "Why can't get this sorted?"; "Why can't I be more capable?,"

Date	Time	What happened just before the rumination started?	How did you feel before?	Duration	What were you thinking about?	What were the consequences of rumination— for mood and actions?	What stopped the rumination? What did you try to stop it? Was it useful?
Tuesday	10 A.M.	At home, thinking about phoning manager to discuss coming back to work part-time.	Anxious, tense in shoulders	3 hours	Concerns about not being seen as an awkward person, started making plans, had thoughts about how I would be perceived, "Is this reasonable or not?"	Feel down on self, less motivated, give up.	It went on for hours.

FIGURE 12.1. Rumination Episodes Recording Form completed by Stephen.

followed by negative comparisons to other people. Stephen imagined others as forceful and capable but saw himself as falling short. As this bout of rumination went on, he became less and less motivated and gave up. The therapist reviewed this episode with Stephen and explored how he had started with an attempt at problem solving but that his thoughts were then hijacked by abstract thinking about meanings and consequences, focused on his own insecurity. This example was used to reinforce the idea that tension could be a warning sign for Stephen's rumination, that his rumination was often concerned with what others would think of him and how they would respond to him, and that there was scope to stay with problem solving rather than getting stuck in rumination.

Stephen completed a rumination episode recording form every week for several weeks. This was reviewed and discussed with the therapist each session, with the nature of his rumination examined. Collaboratively, it was identified that much of his rumination was about analyzing the meaning of situations or checking up on actions (thinking "Why?"; "What does it mean?"), rather than focusing on solving problems (thinking "How?").

The rest of this chapter summarizes the actual treatment that Stephen received. Compare what you planned with the RFCBT he received.

Self-Test: FA and Formulation of Rumination for Stephen

Use the information above to create an initial formulation for Stephen, taking into account that your goals are to identify antecedents and consequences of rumination, identify potential moderators, and hypothesize possible functions for the rumination.

Useful questions to reflect on include:

- What comes before the rumination?
- Does this suggest possible changes in environment or patient behavior to reduce cueing of rumination?
- What follows the rumination? What are its effects?
- How might the rumination have developed?
- How might this knowledge contribute to the rationale given to the patient?
- What does this suggest about possible functions of the rumination?
- How can I further test this hypothesis?
- What other information do I need? What do I need to check in more detail when discussing specific examples?

See the second box on page 279 for the formulation produced by Stephen's therapist.

Self-Test: Treatment Planning Options for Stephen

Based on the information above, think through what treatment components your intervention for Stephen might include.

The following questions are useful to reflect on as a therapist to guide your formulation and treatment planning:

- What are possible external environmental moderators that influence the frequency, duration, or usefulness of his rumination?
- What are possible behavioral or mental state moderators within Stephen that influence the frequency, duration, or usefulness of his rumination?
- What might be informative and therapeutically useful behavioral experiments to do in session?
- What next steps might be possibilities for interventions?
- What monitoring might be useful for Stephen?
- What changes in environment and routines might interrupt the cues to rumination?
- What might be good alternative behaviors for him to practice within an If–Then plan?

See the box on page 280 for the treatment planning options produced by Stephen's therapist.

FA and Formulation of Rumination for Stephen

Antecedents and triggers: First thing in morning when he wakes up; when he is not busy or has nothing scheduled; feeling insecure; any situation leading to negative comparisons with others, for example, seeing people who are more successful, needing to assert himself with others (e.g., with his friend), feeling irritated or angry.

Consequences: Feeling overwhelmed and powerless, tense; avoids acting assertively (e.g., complaining); it becomes harder to act; more depressed and tired; less angry; less motivated.

Themes: Concerns about upsetting people; concerns about being an unreasonable person; concern about becoming too angry; comparing himself with others.

Hypothesized functions: Containing anger; avoiding being angry with others; avoiding expressing feelings; checking on whether his own behavior is appropriate; avoiding a negative response from others; trying to work out the "logic" of the world to avoid punishment; trying to "sort things out" in his head.

Other avoidant behavior: Tries to block and suppress upsetting concerns and emotions; tries to be as invisible as possible (a strategy from childhood).

Therapist's Treatment Planning Options for Stephen

What are possible external environmental moderators that influence the frequency, duration, or usefulness of his rumination? Stephen's rumination appears to be worse when he has to be assertive, when he is faced with situations that engender negative comparisons, when he is exposed to irritations, and when he is not busy. Many of these situations depend on other people, and so may not be amenable to environmental modification.

What are possible behavioral or mental state moderators within Stephen that influence the frequency, duration, or usefulness of his rumination? The shift from focusing on active problem solving to asking "why?," making comparisons, and thinking through implications appear to be important moderators of the duration and usefulness of his rumination. The extent of his anger and irritability appears to moderate the frequency and duration of his rumination.

What might be informative and therapeutically useful behavioral experiments to do in session? It could be useful to conduct the Why–How experiment to compare different thinking styles. It could be useful to compare approach versus avoidant responses to dealing with anger and irritation (e.g., assertiveness vs. putting himself down). Comparing times when Stephen has been compassionate instead of critical toward himself might be useful to identify alternative ways to respond when faced with situations that induce negative self-comparisons.

What next steps might be possibilities for interventions? Possible interventions include teaching Stephen relaxation as an alternative means to contain anger; encouraging assertiveness to reduce the situations that produce irritability; concreteness training to reduce abstract "why" thinking and improve problem solving; compassion to provide a counter to negative self-comparisons.

What monitoring might be useful for Stephen? It would be helpful for Stephen to spot any additional warning signs for rumination to test the hypothesis that irritability is a trigger for rumination.

What changes in environment and routines might interrupt the cues to rumination? Finding ways to build in more activities so that he is busier may interrupt cues to rumination.

What might be good alternative behaviors for him to practice within an If–Then plan? Relaxation, assertiveness, concreteness, and compassion are all potential alternative strategies to rumination.

Summary of Stephen's Treatment: Sessions 3–10

Session 3: FA to Explore the Role of Rumination and Altering of Environmental Contingencies

Based on the assessments conducted in the first two sessions, the therapist hypothesized that one major function of the rumination was to reduce anger and to avoid negative responses from other people. Stephen and the therapist collaboratively agreed that much of the rumination was about trying to contain anger, as identified in one of the examples discussed in sessions 1 and 2. It was agreed that it was important to keep monitoring the rumination and to look out for the early warning signs for rumination, because spotting these signs was the first step in changing the habit. The therapist worked with Stephen to identify potential triggers to rumination in the environment, such as not feeling very skillful, or not being busy. The therapist looked for possible environmental contingencies that triggered rumination, which would be relatively straightforward to change. Stephen and his therapist worked collaboratively to find effective ways to address the times he was not busy and his sense of not being skilled. Stephen had previously done some voluntary work for a charity, using his IT and web-development skills and had found this quite fulfilling. As a problem-solving measure, plans were made for him to try some charity work in order to reduce his empty time, while he was also building back his time at work. This approach successfully increased his activity and improved his sense of mastery. It increased his confidence about returning to work. Monitoring of his rumination and symptoms each week indicated that this intervention had a positive effect.

Session 4: Shifting Thinking Style and Introducing If–Then Plans

Recognizing from their work in sessions 1 and 2 and from Stephen's monitoring forms that Stephen often shifted into abstract thinking rather than staying with problem solving, the therapist further explored differences in thinking style. Recognizing how attempts at problem solving were hijacked by these abstract concerns pointed up the value of using more helpful questions to keep problem solving on track. The Why–How behavioral experiment was used to discover the effects of shifting an abstract thinking style to a concrete style (see Chapter 9). It became apparent to Stephen that the concrete "how" style of thinking was more adaptive and effective, giving him a greater sense of control and improving problem solving. Stephen was encouraged to practice asking the useful "how" questions when faced with the warning signs for his rumination, such as getting tense. The therapist also explored the function of the "why"-type questions, examining what Stephen got out of asking these questions. It appeared that he was asking these questions to try to ascertain whether he was making reasonable or unreasonable demands of other people. The therapist introduced the idea of If–Then plans, and an If–Then plan was made for Stephen's homework: If I notice that I am getting tense, then I will ask myself questions like "How can I solve this problem?"

Session 5: Consolidating If–Then Contingency Plans and Increasing Concreteness

Building on the Why–How experiment, the next step was twofold: first, to introduce more action-focused questions to keep problem solving on track, and second to further challenge the idea that the "why"-type questions were helpful as a means to work out how to respond to other people. The therapist started by discussing with Stephen the relative pros and cons of "trying to sort things out in his head" versus "sorting it out in the world by action." The need for a balance of thought and action was reviewed: it may be useful to think things through, but thinking is not helpful if it only leads to more thinking; to be more helpful, thinking needs to lead to action. Furthermore, the therapist raised the possibility that trying things out in the real world may be more effective and enable more learning than just thinking things over again and again.

As a further behavioral experiment to test out these ideas, the therapist and Stephen made a plan for Stephen to be more direct and assertive to see what would happen. This shifted him away from trying to work things out in his head, with its avoidant function, and toward deliberately approaching problems in the real world. For example, Stephen had spent several hours being upset by his friend not honoring his loan, ruminating about it, thinking "Is it bad enough to complain yet?" and putting himself down for being oversensitive. After several hours of distress and self-critical rumination, he eventually approached his friend and got some money back. The behavioral experiment was to compare waiting and thinking things through with what would happen if he directly asserted himself within 15 minutes of another issue coming up with his friend. Together the therapist and Stephen made predictions about all the different things that could happen and rated their likelihood. In the end, Stephen discovered that rapid action with his friend was more helpful and without any of the downside of ruminating about things over and over again.

In tandem with the behavioral experiment, the therapist further reinforced the use of action-plan "how" questions on how best to reach goals. When faced with a problem, Stephen was coached to use the following questions: "Is this a useful thought? Is this emotionally useful? Is it helpful for me? What can I practically do? What do I want from this situation? How can I make things move forward toward my goal?" In particular, Stephen repeatedly practiced replacing "why"-type questions with "how"-type questions that were adapted versions of his "why"-type questions, (e.g., "Why can't it be more straightforward?" was replaced with "How can I make it more straightforward? How can I make it easier?"). Stephen practiced using these questions in response to his warning signs for rumination, such as irritability or making negative comparisons between himself and others.

Stephen was also encouraged to focus on those thoughts and behaviors that encourage action sooner rather than later. The therapist encouraged an experimental approach to gathering information, and encouraged Stephen to look at the advantages of direct feedback for himself and others. For example, the therapist and Stephen explored whether directly responding to others and actively trying things out could make his judgments more accurate. Stephen was asked, "How will you learn to get better at this without feedback?" To consolidate the benefits of the behavioral experiment, the therapist encouraged Stephen to (1) deliberately look for further opportunities to practice being more assertive and (2) set up opportunities to test things out directly in the real world as an alternative strategy to rumination. Specific examples coming up over the next weeks were identified and plans made to practice assertiveness (e.g., making a request of his manager and recording the outcome).

Sessions 6 and 7: Finding Functional Alternatives to Rumination

Stephen's concerns about his behavior being unreasonable were central to what triggered his rumination and avoidance. His rumination apparently served the function of checking whether his behavior was reasonable or not. Based on this formulation, a logical next step was to find effective alternatives to address this concern. This involved finding ways to challenge the idea that Stephen's behavior was unreasonable, and to normalize it in comparison to others. The therapist set up experiments to test the idea that being annoyed is OK and that other people are more used to encountering annoyance in others than Stephen believes. The therapist introduced some alternative questions for Stephen to try in social situations: "Is it really important what this other person thinks?"; "What is the worst that could happen?"

Through review of his experience and experiments, it became clear that a major fear for Stephen was that he was like father, that his temper was uncontrollable, and that if he got angry, he would lose control and act in a nasty and aggressive way. His rumination dampened these feelings of anger and was hypothesized to function to avoid his becoming this feared self (i.e., angry and uncontrollable). Because this was such an aversive state for Stephen, the rumination was negatively reinforced even though it made him feel down. Thus, the therapist reasoned that a functional alternative to controlling his anger was called for based on the FA.

With this in mind, Stephen was taught progressive muscle relaxation using breathing and imagery exercises in session 6. Using the normal format for applied relaxation, he practiced using the relaxation twice a day and in response to rumination triggers (i.e., as part of an If–Then plan). As well as providing an alternative to rumination as a means of dealing with anger, the relaxation provided the added benefit of reducing tension. The relaxation exercises involved generating specific images of relaxing places, such as a calm spot out in the countryside. Practicing relaxation was the homework for the following week.

In session 7, the therapist reviewed Stephen's progress at learning relaxation and practiced relaxation again. Stephen was beginning to learn to relax when he noticed he was tense or irritable, and this was reducing his rumination. To further improve how Stephen managed his anger, the therapist also encouraged Stephen to become more assertive—to express his opinion clearly, firmly, and calmly to others. The intention was to develop another useful alternative way to manage anger and irritation, and to help Stephen to constructively address the potential causes of his irritation. The therapist reviewed with Stephen examples of when he had been assertive before and it had been helpful (e.g., the earlier behavioral experiment with his friend). The therapist also emphasized the value of being assertive as a way to address difficulties through approach rather than through avoidance. The therapist modeled how to be assertive in different situations, and then Stephen practiced being assertive, using a series of role plays with the therapist. Over these sessions, repeated practice at relaxation followed by assertiveness in response to feeling angry proved to be a helpful strategy for Stephen, further reducing his rumination, as monitored in Handouts 5 and 6. Stephen continued to practice relaxation and assertiveness through the rest of therapy, with the therapist monitoring progress each session. To support this practice, he kept a monitoring chart, in which he recorded every time that he experienced a warning sign for rumination (e.g., tense or irritable) and checked off every time he responded with relaxation or assertiveness.

By using this alternative strategy, Stephen was able to learn that he was not like his father and that he was able to control his temper. In fact, through attempting this approach, Stephen and the therapist established that his experience of his father's temper led him to be quiet and considerate of others to avoid getting into trouble. As a child, this was a useful strategy because it stopped him from receiving his father's verbal abuse. However, the strategy was overlearned and continued into his adulthood and into other situations where it was no longer appropriate. Stephen was encouraged to label this response as a learned pattern and to think about how it was or was not relevant to his current circumstances. The repeated practice at using relaxation in response to irritability began to produce a new, helpful habit to replace rumination.

Session 8: Working with Values

Another theme of Stephen's rumination concerned repeated social–evaluative comparisons regarding his career and material success. The therapist assessed how much these concerns reflected Stephen's values. For example, the following questions were asked: "What are your intrinsic values? What is most important to you? How relevant are these values to the comparisons that you are making?" Stephen's important self-concordant values concerned moral and spiritual issues rather than material concerns. He valued empathy, understanding, imagination, and having fun. Material trappings were not relevant to these values. Stephen was encouraged to use his own values, not other people's values, when making comparisons. It was also useful to reiterate the value of returning to specific, concrete plans rather than using abstract evaluations (e.g., "How useful is it to make these comparisons? What is a better thing to do?"). Stephen was encouraged to check on the motivation for these actions: "Am I doing this because it is useful or because I want to appear nice?" He found this useful in consolidating the changes he had already made, such as increasing his time back at work, practicing relaxation, and assertiveness.

Sessions 9 and 10: Relapse Prevention and Preparation for the End of Therapy

The final two sessions were spent recapping the previous work done in therapy, making consolidation plans, and reviewing anything that was particularly helpful. Stephen and his therapist reviewed all of his warning signs for rumination and his If–Then plans, and the formulation for his rumination. This was used to identify which strategies had been most useful and to encourage Stephen to continue using them. The warning signs were reiterated and clear plans made for what he would do in response to them in the future. The warning signs were also used to generate potential risky situations that could come up in the next 6 months to 2 years—for which Stephen generated specific contingency plans (e.g., possible conflicts or confrontations that could come up, and how he would handle them). These relapse prevention plans were written down in detail. In addition, Stephen and his therapist reviewed how he could continue to consolidate the skills learned, and how he could continue to practice alternative strategies to ensure that his helpful habits were maintained. This included making specific plans for repeated practice (e.g., to practice relaxation every day for the first month, and then 3 times a week for the next month), and reinforcing the cues in response to which he would practice alternative strategies.

Outcome

At baseline, Stephen's score on the BDI was 18, reflecting a moderate level of depressive symptoms (range = 0–63). His score on the RSQ was 83, reflecting a very high level of depressive rumination (range = 22–88). In his initial weeks completing Handout 5, Tracking Rumination and Avoidance, his weekly frequency of rumination was 35%, average duration 2–3 hours, intensity 80%, and level of interference 80%, all indicating high levels of rumination.

After 10 hour-long sessions, Stephen's score on the BDI was down to 5, which reflects a minimal level of depressive symptoms (i.e., no longer depressed). His RSQ was down to 46, reflecting that self-reported depressive rumination was significantly reduced and now in the normal range for rumination. On Handout 5, Tracking Rumination and Avoidance, Stephen's weekly frequency of rumination was 5–10%, average duration a half-hour, intensity 40%, and level of interference 25%, again indicating a level of rumination that was no longer pathological.

CHAPTER 13

Adaptations of RFCBT*

The RFCBT described up to now pertains to an individualized face-to-face intervention used to treat acute depression and anxiety. However, RFCBT has been adapted into other formats to increase its dissemination and accessibility: a group format (group RFCBT) and an Internet-delivered format (Internet RFCBT). The group variant has been used in standard clinical settings and within research trials, both as an acute treatment for current depression in various health service settings and as an intervention within a prevention trial for people at high risk for depression because they have elevated worry and rumination. The Internet variant has been used predominantly within a research context, also as an intervention to prevent depression in people at high risk for the disorder. In this prevention trial, Topper et al. (2016) found that both group RFCBT and Internet RFCBT outperformed a no-treatment control in reducing rumination and prodromal symptoms of depression and anxiety and preventing the onset of cases of major depression and GAD over the following year (see Chapter 1 for further details and the rationale for this study).

At this point, the group form of RFCBT is better developed than the Internet form in terms of wider clinical dissemination and general use. My colleagues and I have convergent evidence from both clinical trials and use in everyday clinical services that the group variant of RFCBT is a practical way to extend the use of RFCBT. The principles and techniques of group RFCBT are very similar to those of individual face-to-face RFCBT.

In contrast, the use of Internet RFCBT is still in the research phase and limited to our research group. The delivery of Internet RFCBT requires access to a specially programmed Internet package and the acquisition

---

*This chapter is in part based on work conducted with Maurice Topper and Thomas Ehring, both of whom commented on a draft of this chapter that I wrote.

of specific therapeutic skills used in providing online feedback, and thus this format is not yet widely available to clinicians. This chapter therefore focuses mainly on providing details about the group variant of RFCBT in order to present material that clinicians can easily adapt for use with their own patients. In contrast, information on Internet RFCBT is presented only briefly to provide awareness of this treatment option, which has considerable future potential but is still undergoing development.

Group Therapy

My colleagues and I have adapted RFCBT for use in groups consisting of between 6 and 12 patients and with one or two group therapists. Group RFCBT covers the same material as individual RFCBT, although the method of delivery is adapted to include more structure, psychoeducation, and group discussion. Group RFCBT has been used in the National Health Service (NHS) depression clinic at the Mood Disorders Centre, University of Exeter, United Kingdom; within a clinical service in Western Australia; within a prevention intervention trial conducted in the Netherlands (Topper et al., 2016); and in a randomized trial comparing group RFCBT to group CBT for adult patients with major depression in Denmark. This trial found RFCBT significantly outperformed CBT (Hvenegaard, Watkins, Gondan, Grafton, & Moeller, 2015).

Across five consecutive groups totaling about 60 patients within our local U.K. NHS clinic, we found a reduction in depression of 10–15 points on the BDI after 10 sessions, each lasting 90 minutes. As described in more detail in Chapter 1, the prevention trial, using group RFCBT, successfully reduced rumination, depression, and anxiety relative to a no-treatment control.

The program for group RFCBT follows the sequence outlined in Table 13.1. We have typically delivered group RFCBT over 6 to 10 sessions, each lasting 60–120 minutes, and occurring weekly or fortnightly. In this chapter, I outline group RFCBT delivered over 6 sessions lasting 90 minutes each because this is the form we have used most extensively and for which we have the strongest evidence (Topper et al., 2016), because it is the most cost-effective and efficient for treatment delivery and because it provides a full account of all elements of group RFCBT. However, variants of group RFCBT have been run with up to 10 sessions, following exactly the same content and order of the 6-session RFCBT. In these extended variants, some content has been presented over two shorter sessions rather than in one longer session to enable more practice and repetition of key skills and strategies (sessions 4, 5, and 6 are split into two sessions each, with two sessions devoted to FA; two sessions for experiential exercises such as absorption and compassion; an additional session to work on increasing approach behaviors; and an additional session at the end of therapy for further revision of skills learned and relapse prevention). The number of sessions will depend on the particular constraints of service delivery, although it may be helpful to have more sessions for patients with current depression, where more practice is indicated for the full benefit of therapy to be realized. Table 13.1 shows the content of each session.

The content of the group sessions includes the key elements of RFCBT as described in previous chapters, albeit presented in a more structured and didactic way. Participants are asked to complete symptom measures (e.g., the Beck Depression Inventory-II or Patient Health Questionnaire-9 for depression) for all sessions, and rumination rating scales (see Chapter 5) and

TABLE 13.1. Outline of Content of Group RFCBT for Targeting Rumination

Session 1

Introduction, handling stress, introduce idea of worry/rumination, examples of worry and rumination generated within the group, introduce rumination as a habit, generate consequences and functions of rumination, introduce self-monitoring. Handouts 1 and 4 to read; Handouts 5 and 6 to complete.

Session 2

Noticing warning signs, stepping out of habit—introduce If–Then plans, idea of changing circumstances to prevent triggering of habit, increasing activity and approach behaviors. Handouts 2 and 3 to read.

Session 3

Introduce different styles of thinking, experiential alternatives to rumination (e.g., concrete thinking, Why–How experiential exercise), link into If–Then plan, practice using different processing skills with warning signs (e.g., when in sad or angry mood).

Session 4

Functional analysis; identifying and planning alternatives to rumination that serve the same function; useful rules of thumb to discriminate helpful versus unhelpful rumination (unanswerable questions, 30-minute rule, does it lead to action?), introduce idea of absorption, increasing absorbing activities. Handouts 8 and 9.

Session 5

Introduce self-compassion, compassion experiential exercise, acting in a more caring way toward self, increasing compassionate activities.

Session 6

Interpersonal effectiveness, comparing effective versus ineffective strategies, resilience; review skills, plan for ongoing activity, relapse prevention plans, review experience of group.

recording forms (Handout 5, Tracking Rumination and Avoidance; Handout 6, Rumination Episode Recording Form) for at least the first few weeks. In the first session patients learn how to complete the recording forms, and later sessions use examples from the forms for functional analyses and practice of strategies. At the beginning of the therapy, patients are informed that new strategies will be introduced and that each week a new strategy will be practiced. At the beginning of each new session, there is a review of the previous week, and the therapists check on how homework progressed. At the end of each session, there is a summary of what was covered, and homework is assigned.

I recommend that each group has two therapists, as this enables one therapist to be talking and responding to the group while the other therapist is observing. Having two therapists provides more scope to catch up with each of the individual patients within the group. The larger the group, the more useful it is to have two therapists. Nonetheless, it is possible to conduct RFCBT with a group of 10 patients and only one therapist.

A more detailed description of the six-session group program for RFCBT follows.

Session 1

Introductions and an Icebreaker

The therapists welcome the group and then get the participants actively engaged by asking them to form pairs. The participants are then asked to introduce themselves to each other and share a hope (what the patient hopes to achieve) and a fear (any concerns the patient may have) about the group therapy. The larger group then reforms, and each member of a pair introduces the other member to the whole group along with the person's hope and fear. This serves as an icebreaker, as well as informing the therapists about participants' motivations and concerns for the group. The therapists also contribute a hope and a fear to set the tone for the group. Useful hopes to share include that the group will help participants, participants will find the group safe, participants will feel able to accept help from others, and that participants will be supported in new ways of acting. Useful fears to share include that participants will only help others and forget to help themselves and that participants may feel overwhelmed by the new things to learn (but with the hope that these things will soon become familiar and helpful).

Ground Rules

The therapists lead a group discussion of ground rules for the conduct of the group. Key principles for group therapists to emphasize include confidentiality and respect within the group, for example, not speaking over others; respecting others' opinions; and not tolerating unkindness or abuse. Therapists ask participants to commit to attending sessions for themselves and for the benefit of group as a whole. Punctuality is emphasized. Arriving on time allows the group to start and finish on time. Participants are asked to let the therapists know if they are unable to attend a session. Therapists also emphasize the value of approaching the sessions with a spirit of curiosity, of patients being open to trying new things, to give things a try and see what they learn, and of being compassionate to themselves and to others. Establishing these principles up front helps them to permeate the therapy. These principles, of course, support the absorption and compassion exercises.

Overview of RFCBT: Rumination as an Unhelpful Habit

The idea that rumination, avoidance, and other unhelpful coping behaviors are habits is introduced and discussed in the first session and further elaborated in later sessions. The therapists introduce the idea of helpful and unhelpful ways of responding to stress and introduce rumination and avoidance as unhelpful strategies for coping with difficulties. The therapists start by discussing rumination, in a way that is similar to how it is introduced in individual RFCBT (see Chapter 5). The therapists ask for recent examples of worry and rumination from the participants within the group and look for the consequences of rumination. Handout 1, Key Facts about Rumination, is given out and worked through. With each example, the therapist draws out the typical warning signs and cues for rumination and then asks patients to discuss the effects and the consequences of their rumination. The therapist looks for the following consequences to be generated by the group: worsens mood, interferes with problem solving, saps motivation, causes fatigue, prevents attention to changing external realities, disconnects one from the world and from positive experiences; causes insomnia; interferes with learning new things; impairs relationships with others. Therapists single these out from the discussion and summarize them, indicating how rumination is typically unhelpful. If the group cannot spontaneously generate these examples, then the therapist asks more directly about specific consequences.

Therapists ask for examples of prior habits that have developed and were changed to illustrate that habits take time to learn, require repeated pairing with a particular cue and are followed by a positive outcome, and are typically resistant to change. The general approach and rationale of RFCBT are reviewed as detailed in Chapter 5: patients are informed that the group sessions will coach them in new strategies to replace the rumination habit and that the group sessions will work to help them spot the habit and practice a range of different alternative strategies. Each session, one or two new strategies will be introduced and practiced. Different strategies will work for different people, and thus it is worth trying out each of the different strategies, and then concentrating on the ones that work best for each patient.

Introducing Self-Monitoring

The therapists introduce record keeping and monitoring form completion in order to learn patterns of behavior in the first session. Self-monitoring is emphasized as a means to become more aware of habits and to spot the cues for habits as a first step to changing them. Patients are given the handout on self-monitoring (see Handout 4) and this is talked through. The therapists explain that writing down activities and how you feel allows patients to spot links and patterns in mood, situations, and activity. This record keeping helps patients to spot examples of rumination and of its warning signs, and to identify when they feel better or worse, and what factors might be influencing their mood.

Guided by the therapist, the group brainstorms an example and fills in a section of the Rumination Episode Recording Form (Handout 6). This is written out on a blackboard, whiteboard, or flip chart. Participants then practice filling in a chart for yesterday and today, with the therapist checking on this by going around the group. Homework is to complete the form every day for the next week.

Throughout the sessions, we recommend that therapists prepare examples to illustrate each session's key ideas and then draw out relevant examples from the patients' recent experiences. It is a good idea to collect patients' forms at the beginning of each session and scan through them. Examples can then be drawn from them to illustrate strategies.

We have found that a particularly useful homework exercise in terms of monitoring and recording is to ask each patient to identify a time when he felt good and a time when he felt bad each day. For each situation, the patient is encouraged to note the context, his emotional response, what happened just before (antecedent), whether he ruminated (and if so about what), what he did, and the consequences of what happened next. This can then be used to illustrate the effects of actions and context on mood and to make plans to build positive activities.

Session 2

Spotting Warning Signs

Session 2 is used mainly to review the recording forms and to identify the warning signs for rumination from the completed Rumination Episode

Recording Forms as a starting point for If–Then plans. In a group discussion, the therapists try to brainstorm warning signs for rumination and stress with the group participants.

If–Then Plans

Therapists explain that once warning signs are identified, the plan is to replace rumination with new alternative responses. Once patients are familiarized with the idea of looking for warning signs, the idea of If–Then contingency plans is then introduced. The session includes some exercises in developing If–Then plans on the basis of examples generated within the group (i.e., identifying "if" parts of the plan—including warning signs such as feeling tense, being self-critical, and asking "Why?"—and identifying the "then" part of the plan for steps to take in response to warning signs, such as slowing down, setting priorities, and doing things step by step). Simple activities that I have typically found to be useful are introduced to group participants, such as building up activities, getting into helpful routines, and doing one thing at a time.

Changing Circumstances to Prevent Triggering of Habits

The therapists also note that one way to stop unhelpful habits is to remove potential cues to the rumination habit, if those cues reflect easy-to-change aspects of the individual's circumstances or routines. The therapists highlight any examples of modifiable environmental triggers for rumination that were generated by the group participants and discuss simple changes that could be made. Triggers to be looked for include particular routines around getting up, going to bed, or coming home from work; particular places that cue rumination; being in a rush and under pressure; reminders, such as photos, that trigger rumination; listening to sad music or watching sad films; having nothing to do; untidiness or messiness around the house. Each of these is potentially modifiable with a simple plan that could be part of the homework for the relevant patient (e.g., changing routines around getting up or going to bed; building in more activities to reduce unfilled time; listening to different music; scheduling activities so that the patient is in less of a rush; removing upsetting reminders; cleaning up the house).

Reducing Avoidance and Increasing Approach

The idea of modifying environment and routines leads naturally into the therapists briefly introducing the importance of reducing avoidance and building up positive activities. The idea of opposite action is introduced here as a potential "then" part of an If–Then plan—rather than the current typically avoidant response to a situation, participants are encouraged to find an approach behavior instead that acts in the opposite direction (e.g., when feeling sad, to do something active and positive, rather than withdrawing; when feeling anxious, to do something relaxing).

Session 3

Different Thinking Styles—Concreteness

Session 3 starts by reviewing the monitoring forms, identifying any new warning signs, and checking on the progress of the If–Then plans made in the previous session. Feedback from these plans across the group is used to reinforce the use of the plans by participants, to trouble-shoot any problems, and to highlight successes. Successful If–Then plans are shared with the group because a plan that worked for one patient may be helpful for another patient. The therapists then consolidate the use of alternative strategies in response to the warning signs for rumination by introducing the alternative of shifting one's thinking style. The comparison between concrete and abstract thinking is illustrated through the Why–How experiment. The imagery script used should relate to a common event many people are likely to have experienced (e.g., waiting for someone in a café and the person does not show up, or the car failing to start when you are on the way to a very important meeting). The therapists use prompts to make it as real as possible and to engage the participants in the experiential exercise (see Chapter 9). The group is asked to imagine this event, first asking "why" questions and then asking "how" questions. The therapists then seek feedback from the group on how the two conditions affect mood and thinking. Although there is typically variability among group members in how the different processing styles are experienced, a preference for concrete relative to abstract thinking usually emerges. The different effects of How versus Why thinking are summarized by the therapists. When the concrete thinking is found to be helpful, participants are encouraged to incorporate it into If–Then plans and to practice it over the following weeks. The therapists emphasize the importance of practice using concrete thinking in response to patients' daily warning signs, especially when patients are in a sad or angry mood and using the alternative strategy is most needed. If possible, it is useful for patients to practice using the strategy when experiencing a negative mood (e.g., the therapists can ask participants to think of a time when they felt stressed before they practice using "how" questions).

The next week's homework is to build an explicit If–Then plan using "how" questions in response to warning signs. This homework is set up by asking participants to note down likely triggers and situations in which rumination will occur for them over the next week, and to then prepare useful "how" questions to ask themselves as part of their plan. In the next group session, it is important to check on whether there are times when rumination is helpful or not helpful, and whether "how" questions have been helpful in replacing "why" questions. Another useful homework exercise is to ask patients to look out for instances of rumination (noting triggers and consequences) and to practice concrete "how" thinking as an alternative at these times.

Session 4

Functional Analysis

After reviewing homework and refining plans from the previous week, Session 4 builds on the earlier sessions that plan alternatives to rumination by including further FA of rumination. There is a group discussion about the importance of understanding the purpose of rumination. The therapists ask, "When is rumination bad?"; "When is it helpful?"; and "What are the reasons why we do it?" The therapists seek to generate possible reasons and functions from the group, looking for the following functions: making predictions of things that could go wrong; thinking deeply; trying to understand difficulties and problems, with the belief that this can help to solve problems; to push oneself, motivate oneself, and drive oneself on; to keep one's feared self in check (e.g., having to understand a situation better to prevent oneself from acting in a rude way and possibly offending someone else; to keep from becoming insensitive or selfish); mind reading and second-guessing to avoid getting into trouble with others; to control and change emotions; putting off doing unwanted things; doing things "in the head" rather than "in the real world" as a means to avoid taking the risk of things going wrong. Ideally, the group will generate many of these possible functions, but if not, the therapists guide and point out these common functions. Patients are then asked to identify which of these functions tend to be the ones that occur for them. This helps to develop more individualized plans for each patient within the group, in which alternative strategies (increasing activity, concrete thinking, opposite action, absorption, compassion, assertiveness, etc.) are chosen to match the functions of rumination.

Having identified potential functions, the therapists then examine the effectiveness of rumination and what would be a good alternative. Useful questions to pose to the group include "What would happen if you *did understand the problem*? [or substituting another named function]." Alternative responses to reach these outcomes are also asked about (e.g., "What else can you do to reduce feelings of sadness/anger?"). It is useful to explicitly talk about "unanswerable questions," where it is difficult to resolve a situation through logical analysis, for example, when trying to understand one's own feelings or other people's behavior. The therapists distinguish between trying to work things out in one's head and actually trying to work them out in the real world and look for examples where learning is best achieved through intuition and by trial and error.

Next the therapists and participants discuss how we know when we are in a situation where rumination is not helpful, to help patients to discriminate between when rumination is effective and when it is not. It is useful to suggest that rumination tends to be less useful in situations that are multifaceted and dynamic (i.e., constantly changing, with the current state directly influenced by the previous state) and that have long histories. In contrast, analytical thinking about problems may be more helpful in a closed system, where there are definite solutions and a limited set of answers (e.g., doing a math assignment, cooking, putting together a piece of Ikea furniture, resolving a computer problem). Reflecting the core precepts of RFCBT, the key question for rumination is "Is it helpful or unhelpful?"

Within the group therapy, the therapists provide clear heuristics to help participants discriminate helpful from unhelpful avoidance and rumination. For example, avoiding an acute, external situation can be helpful, whereas avoiding internal states or chronic problems is usually not helpful. Similarly, there are three useful rules of thumb to help individuals determine whether rumination is likely to be helpful or not. First, is it asking an unanswerable question? Rumination about abstract, existential, complex, or philosophical issues, as exemplified by asking "Why me?" or "What does this mean?," are unlikely to have a definitive simple answer, and thus such rumination can be readily identified as unlikely to be helpful.

Second, does it lead to an action, plan, or decision or to more thinking? Repetitive thinking can be helpful when it is more concrete and leads to detailed, contextualized plans (i.e., when it is in the service of problem solving). However, repeated thinking that is more abstract will tend to lead to more thoughts and more questions, expand into other situations and topics, and thus continue to persist and be elaborated. Therefore, checking whether the thinking is leading toward an action, a plan, or some kind of decision is a good way to discriminate helpful versus unhelpful thinking early on.

Third, how long has the bout of rumination lasted? Most adaptive thinking, such as problem solving, will make some progress toward a solution, even if it is only a step rather than the full solution, within a fairly brief time period. This period of time will vary with the problem and the circumstances, but most individuals, if asked to compare times when dwelling on a problem was helpful versus not helpful, can distinguish that helpful thinking occurred within a particular time period. A good starting point is around 30 minutes. Often continued thinking that goes over that time period without any further progress with respect to personal concerns is unlikely to make significant gains, and becomes increasingly subject to diminishing returns. It is useful to ask patients to consider whether there will be significant gains in the solutions achieved for the additional time spent thinking something over.

FA is introduced later in group RFCBT than in individual RFCBT because in individual RFCBT the FA can be thorough and detailed and guides all therapeutic decisions, whereas it is not possible to conduct individualized FA in such detail in the group format. Rather, in the group RFCBT, participants are given the rationale of changing habits and then practice a menu of different options to change the habits. Because FA cannot be done in as much detail, it is introduced later and conducted in a simpler and more pared-down way.

Absorption

The therapists also teach absorption as a potential alternative to rumination. The rationale is to increase connection with the world and is similar to that provided in individual RFCBT (see Chapter 10 and Handout 10). In the group, participants are asked to experiment by recalling two instances of an activity that they do frequently: one instance in which they were absorbed in the activity and another in which they were less absorbed. The therapists then guide the group to vividly imagine each of the examples. Prompts about feelings, focus of attention, and sensory experience are used in the exercise to strengthen the effect (see Chapter 10). The therapists then facilitate a group discussion of what the patients noticed during the time they were absorbed versus the time they were not absorbed. The discussion is aimed at highlighting the benefits of being absorbed and the factors that increase absorption, such as the elements involved in "flow," as described in Chapter 10. The group discusses the questions "What can we learn from absorbing experiences?" and "How can we use what we know about these experiences to help us become more absorbed in other activities?" The point for therapists to convey is that absorption is an active coping response that can replace rumination. The therapist might say:

> "You can't ruminate if you're absorbed in the task at hand, no matter how simple that task is. The first step to using absorption is the simplest—simply imagining an absorbing thought instead of ruminating. The next step is to practice absorbing activities. The third step is trying to do the activity you're ruminating about in an absorbing way."

Plans are then made to build up absorbing activities, with patients completing individual plans by identifying potential absorbing activities to do, and then breaking these down into smaller steps and working out when, where, and how they will be done. Plans are also made to repeatedly practice the absorbing mental exercise, specifying when and where this is to be done.

Session 5

Compassion

The group RFCBT session on self-compassion is similar in content to individual RFCBT, although the approach is slightly simplified, and is less reliant on working through detailed memories (see Chapter 11). The group format moves away from the memory-based approach because it would be difficult and potentially counterproductive to ask patients to find compassionate memories without the time and scope for detailed individualized guidance. Instead, we adopt a more structured and scaffolded approach, in which patients are guided to generate self-compassionate statements and practice saying them in a compassionate tone of voice.

The therapists ask group members to imagine a time with a bad outcome for them, such as a setback, failure, or rejection, and to notice what their inner voice is saying and its tone of voice. The group members are then asked to imagine supporting a good friend who is experiencing a similar difficulty and to note what they say and how they say it. The group is then asked to compare these two examples. The therapists highlight the benefits of being compassionate, encouraging, and tolerant to the self. They draw out and share with the group the best examples of compassionate responses across the group. As these examples are discussed, therapists draw out examples of what one could say to oneself to build self-compassion (i.e., normalize the situation, focus on progress made, highlight success and strengths, put the situation in perspective, encourage yourself to go on to the next step; see Chapter 11). This should include a helpful tone of voice and nonverbal cues (e.g., warmth, calmness, firmness, being relaxed and open). Patients are encouraged to generate key phrases that help them to be self-compassionate and to write these suggestions down in the session. Group members are also encouraged to write down any examples generated by other group members that seem particularly pertinent for themselves.

The therapists then ask patients to work in pairs in a compassion practice exercise. One person selects and explains a difficult situation he or she is likely to face in the coming week. The second person in the pair then speaks to the first as a friend, encouraging and supporting him or her. The roles are then swapped and repeated. This exercise helps to strengthen and rehearse the compassion approach, as well as identify any difficulties.

The therapists then discuss potential barriers to self-compassion and how to overcome them. Typical barriers include not knowing what to say; fears about what will happen if one is more self-compassionate; fears that one will be less effective and less motivated; feeling uncomfortable and undeserving of being kind to oneself. The therapists encourage the group to brainstorm and problem-solve these barriers. We have found a number of potential solutions to look for from the group or, if necessary, for the therapists to suggest. First, it is helpful to ask each patient if there are a couple of key phrases he or she can use that keep the gentle tone of voice, and allow a first try at being compassionate. Second, there is value in encouraging patients to weigh how effective self-compassion is compared to talking to the self in a critical way. Have patients look at the pros and cons of each. Third, it often helps to break down the practice of self-compassion into smaller steps, for example, asking "What is the smallest bit of compassion you would be prepared to try?" An important option here is to introduce a graded hierarchy starting with easier and less discomforting steps. The homework emerging from this session is for patients to put into action their own individualized plans to speak to themselves compassionately in upcoming difficult situations. They are then to evaluate the effects of doing that over the next sessions.

People with a tendency to ruminate often have difficulty being self-compassionate because they experience this as "artificial" and as lying to themselves. This can be solved by combining self-compassion with concrete thinking. For example, instead of having patients say, "I am a good person," they can say, "I have done this particular task before and I remember from the feedback I got that I did well, so this time will probably be fine if I try to take a similar approach consisting of . . . ." A key message to reinforce is the importance of repeated practice to establish a new habit.

The therapists also ask participants to generate ideas about possible things they could do differently to be more self-compassionate, to think of ways they could act in a more caring ways toward themselves, by asking what activities they would increase or decrease to care for themselves. Examples are discussed and shared within the group. As part of their homework, participants identify one activity to increase and one activity to decrease over the weeks until the next session.

Session 6

Session 6 begins by reviewing progress on monitoring rumination, changing habits, and the use of If–Then plans that include concreteness, absorption, and compassion. The therapists highlight any successes from the previous week to the group and trouble-shoot any difficulties.

Interpersonal Effectiveness

After reviewing which strategies have been effective and ineffective over the previous weeks, the therapists introduce a further strategy of being assertive. The therapists note how many situations that trigger rumination involve other people, and how finding good ways to interact with others will reduce rumination. Relevant examples from the group members are highlighted, if useful. The therapists discuss how often people who ruminate lack self-confidence and are not good at standing up for themselves, expressing their opinion, or saying no, and how this lack of assertiveness can lead to problems, such as feeling undervalued or taken advantage of, and leaving difficulties unresolved. The therapists seek examples from the group members and use these to illustrate the potential disadvantages of not being assertive. The therapists introduce key principles about ways to be more assertive, including being calm and clear; repetition; valuing oneself; pointing out the effects of actions; taking another's perspective. The therapists can role-play examples of being assertive that are pertinent to the difficulties raised by the participants. Participants are then asked to generate plans for different ways to respond to the situations they identified. These plans are then discussed and refined in the group. Participants make homework plans for how they could act differently in the future. The therapists link the consideration of interpersonal effectiveness back to earlier themes, including the importance of tacking problems through approach rather than through avoidance, the use of concreteness, and being compassionate toward oneself.

Resilience and Relapse Prevention

The therapists return to looking at warning signs and stress, check If–Then plans, and review what was helpful or not helpful for the patients. Key questions that the therapists ask the group members to consider are: "What do I need to keep doing, regardless of my mood state, to live a fulfilling life?" and "What do I need to hold in mind if I face challenges or become depressed in the future?" In particular, the therapists ask the group to think of times over the course of the treatment when they have felt effective, fulfilled, or absorbed in what they were doing, and to compare what was different about these times compared to times when they did not feel effective, fulfilled, or absorbed. Comparing these situations can help to clarify what would be useful to include in future plans. The group members then explicitly discuss their warning signs for depression, stress, and rumination, and jointly plan the strategies they could use in response to these warning signs. The therapists encourage patients to brainstorm possible hurdles or difficulties in implementing these plans, and ways around these.

This session also includes some discussion of the group process itself and what patients can take from the experience of being in the group. Typical questions asked for group discussion include "What has been effective about the group?" with a FA of the circumstances that made the group effective. The therapists encourage patients to think about which aspects of the group have been most helpful to them, and how this can be carried on in the patient's everyday life. The therapists draw out how the group itself provided support; how individuals learned from each other; how the group may have normalized and validated each participant's experience because other people presented with similar difficulties; and how the group may have increased hope because patients saw how other people were successfully tackling problems.

Advantages of the Group Format

The group format has several advantages. First, it is cost-effective for delivery of treatment. In one hour, up to 12 patients can be treated. Second, if the group runs well, the members provide support and reinforcement to each other. The processes of normalization and self-empowerment emphasized in RFCBT can be readily facilitated in a group as each patient discovers that other people are experiencing the same difficulties, and each can also see examples of success in others (Principle 1: Normalize the Patient's Experience of Rumination). With skillful facilitation, the group members' participation can be used to generate a range of helpful versus unhelpful strategies and to distinguish between different processing modes. The therapists have more opportunities to draw out factors influencing rumination consistent with the RFCBT model. The trick here is to be on the lookout for these examples and to directly link them to the focus of the therapy.

Limitations of the Group Format

The nature of the group format means that there is less opportunity for detailed attention to individual patients than in one-to-one therapy. The main limitation is that it is not possible to conduct individualized FA for each problem for each patient, as we do in the one-to-one therapy. It is therefore not possible to tailor the treatment to the individual to the same degree, and to base the selection of interventions on the formulation derived from the FA. Nonetheless, in the treatment groups my colleagues and I have conducted, we have found successful ways to convey the key ideas and principles of RFCBT by stressing the rationale that rumination is a habit and by explicitly introducing new alternative strategies to try each week.

Addressing Limitations and Problems in Group RFCBT

There are several ways to tackle the potential limitations of a group. It is useful to try to work through at least one individual's problem in detail each week, relevant to the theme being covered. Conducting the FA of one individual in detail illustrates the process and gives pointers and ideas to others (Principle 4: Take a functional-analytic approach). It is important to ensure that detailed discussion of an issue is spread equitably among the patients across sessions, while also ensuring that examples are relevant to the goals of each session. We want each patient to have an opportunity for his or her particular difficulties to be addressed. Some patients will be shy and reluctant to volunteer details on a recent difficulty; others will be much more forward, and care needs to be taken that they do not overwhelm the session.

Within a group context, it is useful to have the occasional individual session. An individual session before the first group session can be particularly useful to orient and prepare the patient for what the group will involve and how it will work, as well as to begin a FA of the key issues for that patient. Similarly, an individual session midway through the group can be useful to review progress, pick up on any hurdles or problems, and, if necessary, use FA to address difficulties. In the same vein, a 10- to 15-minute catch-up with each individual at the beginning or end of group sessions, interspersed throughout the treatment course, is helpful to address any problems or difficulties. One advantage of having multiple therapists is that it makes such individual catch-ups feasible.

The group treatment takes a more experimental and psychoeducational approach to finding the right strategy for each patient. We explicitly inform patients that each week will involve learning a different strategy to tackle rumination, that different strategies work differently for different people, and that no single strategy will work for everyone (Principle 1: Normalize the patient's experience of rumination). The key message is that the best thing for each patient is to keep trying until she finds one or more strategies that work for her (Principle 6: Emphasize the importance of repetition and practice). A central focus, which serves as a refrain throughout the sessions, is the development of If–Then plans to tackle unhelpful habits. The initial sessions set up the importance of developing alternative responses to the triggering cues for rumination (If–Then plans) and map out the warning signs (Principle 5: Link behaviors to triggers and warning signs). The following sessions introduce and provide practice with potential alternative coping strategies to use as the "Then" part of the plan (i.e., concreteness, approach, absorption, compassion, assertiveness) (Principle 7: Shift to an adaptive style of thinking). Thus, rather than having the therapist work with each patient to select strategies based on the FA, the group setting gives patients a menu of options to consider and encourages patient experimentation from week to week to find the best one(s) to use. While not as focused as the FA in the one-to-one therapy, this approach does ensure that patients are exposed to the key ideas and techniques within RFCBT and learn which coping strategies to use based on personal experience and preference.

Group RFCBT is a combination of this menu approach and a more guided selection based on functional analyses. Within each session, examples of warning signs, consequences, and functions are discussed and potential alternatives highlighted. Patients with relevant issues are guided in a more targeted way toward which strategies to try when possible. Moreover, individual chats with patients help to narrow down options.

The key principles for RFCBT continue to apply for group-format RFCBT and, in some cases, need to be applied with even greater vigor. We have observed that a common problem when running group sessions is that they become too much like psychoeducation and move into conceptual discussion rather than focusing on specific details and experiential change (Principle 3: Encourage active, concrete, experiential, and specific behavior—the ACES rule). There can easily be lots of talking by the therapists but not much doing. Patients who ruminate have a tendency toward avoidance and abstraction. Group sessions can easily be deflected in these directions. Therapists therefore need to keep in mind the ACES principle and concentrate on spotting and naming avoidance and replacing it with approach behaviors. Thus, when discussing an example in the group, the therapist needs to drill down for detailed, specific, concrete, contextual descriptions and not rely on vague descriptions.

Any introduction of ideas or principles needs to be followed up with concrete and readily imagined examples, ideally taken from patients within the group. Questions need to be direct and concrete and push group participants toward direct experience. When patients generate their own examples and alternatives, therapists push them to describe behaviors in detail (see Chapters 2 and 9).

The group needs to avoid just talking, and rather to practice new ways of tackling difficulties. If in doubt, an experiential exercise or behavioral experiment within the group is advised, consistent with the ACES principle. Many RFCBT exercises and experiments can be done in a group setting, albeit with more generic instructions and less room for individual guidance. Although this diminishes their impact, these exercises can still be effective and illustrate the key points of RFCBT. Engaging patients in trying out new approaches and experiencing change is a key part of the therapy. As a general rule, each group session needs to include some psychoeducation for introduction of new ideas but also some direct experiential practice with new coping approaches.

Blocks to progress often reflect avoidance by the patient. This can be usefully tackled by considering the function of such avoidance and looking for alternative approach behaviors. Look out for patients who do not respond to questions, or who show other repetitive avoidant behaviors, such as suggesting reasons for not doing things ("Yes, buts") and shifting discussion onto different topics. Such repeated behaviors, once observed, need to be explicitly shared with the patients, considered functionally, their helpfulness questioned, and alternative responses by the patient encouraged and practiced (see Chapter 8).

Internet RFCBT (MindReSolve)

My research group has also developed an Internet variant of RFCBT for delivery in an online format, which we are currently investigating in a number of research trials. The background, content, principles, and techniques within the English-language version of this Internet RFCBT are branded under the name ©MindReSolve. This treatment follows closely the precepts, techniques, and principles of one-to-one face-to-face RFCBT but adapted for Internet delivery. Using this treatment requires access to the MindReSolve treatment platform (*www.mindresolve.minddistrict.co.uk*), which is currently limited to my research group and collaborators because we are still exploring and testing its efficacy. It is not yet an alternative form of RFCBT that is available for the reader to use directly with a patient. I include a brief description here because I believe that the development of Internet-delivered interventions is necessary in order to tackle the global burden of depression. I further anticipate that familiarity with e-mental health will become more common and more essential for therapists over the next decade. A brief introduction to the Internet RFCBT approach therefore seems timely.

We developed an Internet variant of RFCBT for several reasons. The primary one was to increase accessibility, availability, convenience, and coverage of psychological treatments. E-mental health has the potential to deliver increased treatment reach, scalability, and coverage (Kazdin & Blase, 2011). Depression is a major global health challenge (Collins et al., 2011), a highly prevalent, chronic, disabling, and recurrent disorder (Judd, 1997) with an enormous individual, societal, and economic burden (Lopez, Mathers, Ezzati, Jamison, & Murray, 2006). However, because of its prevalence and recurrent nature, traditional face-to-face psychotherapy can never be widely available enough to reduce the global burden of depression (Andrews, Issakidis, Sanderson, Corry, & Lapsley, 2004; Hollon et al., 2002; Kazdin & Blase, 2011). There is a need for alternative ways to deliver therapy, and Internet therapy offers a way to meet that need (National Institute for Health and Clinical Excellence, 2009). The effectiveness of Internet-based treatments for depression and anxiety is comparable to that of face-to-face treatment (Andrews et al., 2004) and permits increased access to therapy for those who may not wish to interact face to face with a therapist or who find this difficult because of stigma, physical access, time, or geographical constraints. Internet CBT has the potential to increase access to therapy by removing both time constraints and geographical restrictions (Andrews, Cuijpers, Craske, McEvoy, & Titov, 2010), which may be a cause of the attrition from existing services for anxiety and depression (Richards & Borglin, 2011). Internet therapy is convenient and can be accessed anytime and anyplace, without the need for scheduling appointments. This increased access and coverage is particularly important when developing preventative interventions: any intervention designed to prevent depression needs to be able to reach a large number of people. This is why we included an Internet variant of RFCBT in our research trial evaluating whether targeting rumination in high ruminators prevents later depression and anxiety (Topper et al., 2016; see Chapter 1).

The second reason is that Internet therapy has the potential to increase cost-effectiveness (Leykin, Muñoz, & Contreras, 2012) by increasing self-management of recovery (Gellatly et al., 2007; Kaltenthaler, Parry, & Beverley, 2004) and by reducing the therapist time per patient, for example by using standardized response templates for written feedback. Well-elaborated templates for feedback, personalized by therapists for each individual patient, may enable more efficient and cost-effective delivery of evidence-based therapy. If an Internet variant of RFCBT can be as effective as the face-to-face version and only requires 30 minutes per treatment session because the website covers much of the therapeutic content, compared to 60 minutes per face-to-face treatment session, then many more patients can be helped by the same number of therapists and the same cost. There is also scope for more efficient therapy by adopting a "blended" therapy model, in which standard face-to-face therapy is combined with internet-delivered therapy, so that the same content can be covered in fewer face-to-face sessions.

The third reason is that the content of the Internet treatment can also be standardized, reducing unwanted therapist variance and "drift" from treatment protocols (Andrews et al., 2010). Therapist support is still recommended in Internet therapy for depression to maintain motivation and guidance and increase adherence to the treatment (Andersson & Cuijpers, 2009), but using written feedback, as we do in the Internet RFCBT package, means that checking adherence and competence in supervising the therapy is enhanced. Feedback is screened so only responses that meet high levels of fidelity and competence are sent to patients. Thus, Internet therapy enables tighter control of what therapy is delivered, which is essential for conducting research on the active ingredients and mechanisms of therapy, an ongoing focus of my research. My colleagues and I are using an Internet variant of RFCBT to investigate the active mechanisms of RFCBT. Using a fractional factorial design, we have just completed our first feasibility study of Internet therapy to determine which modules within CBT and RFCBT are most effective at changing symptoms, and whether particular modules interact (the IMPROVE-1 trial).

The Internet version of RFCBT falls between individual RFCBT and group RFCBT in the degree to which it facilitates flexible and individualized formulation and FA. Like group RFCBT, Internet RFCBT does not have as much flexibility as face-to-face individual RFCBT to adapt plans and strategies and to personalize the therapy. There is less flexibility with regard to the content of the session and less opportunity for individual FA and formulations derived for each patient than individual face-to-face therapy. Instead, the content and structure of the treatment sessions (i.e., the web pages viewed by patients) are fixed in advance. Like group treatment, Internet RFCBT provides a range of alternative strategies to rumination, encouraging the patient to try each one out and to then select those that best work for him or her. Nonetheless, there is scope to individualize therapy because all of the patient's comments, responses, scores, and exercises are available to the online therapist, who adapts his or her written feedback to the specific concerns and comments of each patient. This enables more detailed functional analyses and informed selection of strategies. There is also detailed feedback to tighten up plans and strategies, in addition to general support, monitoring, and encouragement.

The Internet RFCBT treatment is accessed through a secure and password- protected website. Both patients and therapists can access the website only if they are already set up on it by the website manager, and then set their own personalized passwords to access the treatment site. At this time, the Internet RFCBT treatment is therefore not open access—at the moment, it is accessible only to patients invited to participate in our research trials and to our trial-approved therapists. We want to determine the efficacy and safety of the Internet RFCBT platform, and any limitations it may have, before making it more widely available. For example, the prevention trial suggests that Internet RFCBT may work well for preventing depression in young adults (see Chapter 1), and we are still investigating whether it is also effective for adults who currently have depression.

The current treatment package consists of six modules, each designed to be completed weekly or fortnightly by patients, with each in turn split into two to five smaller sessions. Each session consists of a single web page, which is designed to take 15 to 20 minutes for the patient to scroll down and complete. This organizes the treatment into easy-to-use, bite-size chunks that are not too taxing. The contents of the web pages include text providing psychoeducation and advice; pictures and photographs; written vignettes about individuals with depression; and talking-head videos of actors providing patients' testimonials, reflecting the experience of patients who completed the intervention and giving information about the treatment and explaining coping strategies, with some tailoring of examples based on participant gender and age. There are also online questionnaires, rating scales, exercises, behavioral experiments, and audio recordings that can be downloaded for practice in daily life. Audio recordings include versions of the experiential exercises used in individual RFCBT, such as the relaxation, compassion, concreteness, and absorption exercises. A number of questionnaires and exercises automatically provide feedback if an approach looks helpful (i.e., negative mood ratings decrease compared to scores obtained before the exercise). The components chosen reflect all the elements within

RFCBT, including BA, plus the work on FA, concreteness training, absorption, and compassion (Watkins et al., 2007, 2011).

In the Internet RFCBT used to date, all components involve brief prescribed therapist online support because supported Internet interventions outperform unsupported ones, with improved retention and adherence (Andrews et al., 2010). It is important to be aware that the support takes the form of the therapist reading the answers, exercises, and plans from the patient at the end of each module and then writing an online response to the patient that provides encouragement, support, guidance on plans and exercises, and feedback. This written support is then accessed by the patient when he or she next logs on to the treatment platform, making it secure and private. The patient is not able to progress to the next session without completing a module and reading the feedback. Patients receive an e-mail whenever there is feedback for them to read, and therapists receive an e-mail when a session has been completed by the patient.

The written online feedback takes an experienced therapist approximately 20–30 minutes per module per patient. The feedback is a mixture of scripted and free-form writing. The therapist follows a standardized template that reflects the responses made by the patient to the questions built into the Internet platform. There is a template for each therapy module, although therapists have room to respond within the principles of the therapy and their knowledge of the patient. The template consists of a structured form with several potential options for each section of the feedback.

This feedback is very different from the traditional therapeutic interaction in face-to-face RFCBT. First, the interaction between therapist and patient is asymmetric—the therapist and patient do not have to both be at the same place at the same time to communicate. Unlike face-to-face therapy, where patient and therapist directly and immediately respond to each other, in the Internet RFCBT package the therapist writes his or her feedback at one time, and the patient reads and responds at a different time. This has the disadvantage of reducing immediacy and flexibility in how each responds to the other. On the other hand, the asymmetric nature of written feedback has the advantage that therapist and patient do not have to schedule an appointment when both are available at the same time. This gives patients more flexibility in working through the platform, gives therapists time to work on responses, and gives patients more time to reflect on feedback.

Second, because all communication between patient and therapist is via written feedback in the current version of Internet RFCBT, interactions between therapist and patient do not include the nonverbal cues that can be so important in face-to-face or telephone contact, such as tone of voice and body language. Therapists cannot see or hear the patient's nonverbal cues during therapy, which makes it harder to interpret the patient's emotional and mental state and to judge how he or she is responding to any therapeutic action. Likewise, patients are not aware of the therapist's communication of warmth, support, and understanding through voice, facial expression, or posture. As a consequence, our research experience is that therapists need further special training when using the Internet RFCBT package in order to find ways to convey positive emotions, empathy, and warmth through just their written words. It takes particular skill to adhere to the principles of RFCBT, including being supportive, understanding, empathic, and motivating (Principle 8: Focus on nonspecific factors) when all communication is written. Therapists need to make a deliberate effort to convey their empathy, understanding, and support for the patient when writing. For example, it is important to acknowledge the patient's difficulties, reinforce his efforts and successes, highlight what he is doing well, empathize with him, and share emotional feelings in writing to enhance motivation and support.

All patients start with a module consisting of the welcome session, which includes an introduction to the treatment platform, an explanation of the importance of finding better ways to address stress, an introduction to a self-monitoring form and to the idea of unhelpful habits, and a brief explanation of making If–Then plans. All participants are also introduced to the concept of worry and rumination as risk factors.

Patients then work through the rest of the modules. Each module introduces different strategies and techniques from RFCBT designed to reduce rumination. The patient then practices these strategies in experiential exercises in the module and as homework following the module. The content of Internet RFCBT closely follows the content and strategies of face-to-face RFCBT.

Explicit themes running through the package are the importance of spotting warning signs for rumination, developing If–Then plans, and the repeated practice of alternative strategies (Principle 5: Link behaviors to triggers and warning signs; Principle 6: Emphasize the importance of repetition and practice). Therapists are able to reorder the presentation of modules if this seems useful for a particular patient. The first session in each module checks on progress on the homework from the last module and asks for any feedback or questions from the patient. The final session in each module provides a summary of what has been covered in the module, includes the making of a homework plan, and assesses the patient's anxiety, depression, and rumination symptoms through standardized questionnaires. The final session of the therapy includes reflection on the therapy and on what was helpful, a relapse prevention plan, and congratulations on completing the program.

My research lab is continuing to investigate Internet RFCBT with a view to making it more available in the future. If you are interested in finding out more about Internet RFCBT, please contact me.

APPENDIX

HANDOUTS

Handout 1. Key Facts about Rumination

What Is Rumination?

Do you ever find yourself dwelling on a problem over and over again without getting anywhere? Do you spend a lot of time thinking about yourself and how you feel? Do you get stuck thinking over why you feel depressed or reviewing your failings and mistakes? Do you often worry about things? Are you often asking "Why me?" Do you find yourself recalling a series of negative memories, with each upsetting memory leading on to another sad memory? Are you constantly judging and evaluating yourself, checking up on how well you are doing things, focusing on where you don't meet your expectations? All of these forms of repetitive thinking are what we call **RUMINATION**.

Rumination involves going round and round the same thoughts in your mind—getting stuck in an upsetting groove.

This handout explains why we want to reduce rumination and some of the important facts we know about rumination.

Let's start by looking at your own experience of rumination. Spend a few moments reflecting on the effects that this kind of thinking has on you. Note down your answers to the following questions.

Does it make you feel better or worse?

_____

Does it increase or reduce your energy levels?

_____

Does it increase or reduce the chances that you will get on with your plans and activities?

_____

Effects of Rumination

Most people find that much of the time rumination makes them feel worse and reduces their motivation to do things. In fact, there is a lot of scientific evidence now that rumination is a major factor contributing to the risk of getting depressed and to the maintenance of depression. People who ruminate more tend to get depressed more often and for longer. Furthermore, we know that rumination makes people more negative and less effective at solving problems. Rumination is considered to be a central engine driving the depression forward.

Spend a few moments thinking about how different you might feel if you reduced all the thinking we described at the beginning of this handout—imagine how your life would be without all that rumination. **This is what we hope to achieve within this therapy—helping you to find better ways to knock out the rumination.**

Learning about Rumination

A good start to dealing with rumination is to know a bit more about it. Here are some key facts about rumination.

1. Rumination is a common and normal response to difficulties. We all ruminate about things some of the time. When there is a problem, it is natural to try and solve it, work it through, make sense of it by thinking about it. Indeed, thinking about things can be helpful, for example, look at how analysis has helped us to solve practical problems. Indeed, this way of thinking has led to many of the scientific and technological advances humans have made.

However, dwelling on problems can become unhelpful if you get stuck, and it goes on too long and does not seem to reach any kind of resolution—this is the kind of thinking we are focusing on when we talk about depressive rumination. One important thing we will do in this therapy is to try and find the difference between helpful thinking that leads to solutions to problems versus rumination that gets stuck and does not find a solution.

2. Thinking about problems and difficulties can sometimes be helpful and sometimes be unhelpful. The way that we think about things is important in determining whether we get stuck or solve problems. We will spend time in this therapy learning how to increase the more helpful style of thinking. Thus, the second thing to remember about rumination is that the style of thinking is important in determining how things turn out. In particular, people seem to get stuck in rumination if they try and think about **the wrong things**, for example, if they ask questions that are not answerable or if the balance of their thinking is not quite right.

3. Useful thinking about upsetting events and problems has a good balance between thought and action. For thinking about problems and difficulties to be useful, the balance between thinking and action needs to be about right. If there is too much thinking that does not lead to action, then people often get stuck—just as it is unhelpful to have action without any thinking. Thinking is useful if it acts as a guide to action, and action then informs further thinking so that one feeds back into the other—however, if thinking becomes much more frequent than action or replaces action, then we end up with procrastination and avoidance, and problems are not solved.

Imagine that your car does not start. It is helpful to dwell on why it might not be starting and generate possible reasons for it not starting—problems with spark plugs, engine too cold, battery too low, and so forth—and thinking this through will help you to solve the problem. But for your thinking to be helpful you also need to actively investigate, for example, look under the hood, try different things—just thinking won't solve the problem. Likewise, just trying an action without dwelling on the problem probably won't solve the problem (e.g., repeatedly turning the key in the ignition). So a balance is important.

Imagine the difference between asking:

Why isn't the car starting? How can I fix it?

versus

Why is this happening to me?

What was the effect of asking these two different questions?

Did you find that "Why isn't the car starting? How can I fix it?" helped to focus you on what was happening, how the car had been acting and how you might fix the problem?

Did you notice that "Why is this happening to me?" led you to focus more on yourself and perhaps think about the meaning of the car not starting (e.g., how inconvenient the car not starting may be or how things like this keep happening to me or that this is my fault)? Did you think about other bad things that happen to you?

In general we find that questions that ask "why?" and look at evaluating meanings are unhelpful, while thinking about how to fix things and get things done is helpful. We will focus more on this distinction between thinking about the concrete details and thinking about the meaning of events as therapy progresses, using your own experience to fine-tune your skills at this.

4. Rumination is a learned habit, and old habits can be replaced with new habits. Rumination is learned because it was taught to us, or because at some point in our past there was some kind of payoff or reward for ruminating. Many people who ruminate talk about how they learned to think like this from one or both of their parents. For some people, rumination may have been a helpful response during their childhood, even though it is not helpful anymore. For example, for someone with a very critical, easily angered parent, spending a lot of time dwelling on whether the parent is upset and thinking about how to get everything right might be a good strategy to avoid criticism or punishment. However, if overlearned and applied to other situations, this strategy could then become problematic as everyone's behavior becomes overanalyzed.

313

The main message is that any learned behavior or habit can be replaced with a new, more helpful habit—repeated attempts at doing different things can help us learn a new set of responses. Thus we can be hopeful about the possibility of changing the rumination habit. One of the first things the therapy will ask you to do is to keep a record of your rumination—this is designed to help make you more aware of this habit. Increased awareness of a habit is the first step in changing it.

Key Points

1. Rumination is a major factor in causing and maintaining depression.
2. Rumination is a normal and common response to problems.
3. Rumination becomes unhelpful when the balance between thinking and action is lost.
4. Rumination is a learned habit.
5. This therapy will focus on unlearning unhelpful rumination and learning new habits of more effective thinking.

Things to Do

1. Try to become more aware of your rumination using the rumination diary forms (Handouts 5 and 6) each week.
2. Try to notice the differences between helpful and unhelpful thinking—look out for those times when your thinking helps to solve a problem or make a plan, and compare them to times when your thinking gets stuck and makes you feel worse. Compare the two situations and see what is different between them.

Handout 2. Avoidance

What Is Avoidance?

A common element that helps to maintain many people's depression is avoidance. Avoidance can take many forms, including:

1. Procrastination—putting things off, going over and over things in your head without making a decision
2. Trying to avoid thinking about upsetting or emotional events
3. Suppressing feelings
4. Not trying new challenges and not taking risks
5. Withdrawal from other people and hiding away
6. Giving up activities that you used to enjoy or be good at
7. Not being assertive or expressing feelings to other people
8. Preferring to think about things rather than doing things
9. Numbing oneself with drugs or alcohol

Spend a few moments reflecting on which of these forms of avoidance (or other types of avoidance not listed here) you might be using.

Use the lines below to write down the main things that you avoid. Try to be as specific and detailed as possible:

_____
_____
_____
_____
_____
_____

Key Messages about Avoidance

1. Avoidance is a normal response to threats and difficulties. It is useful for short-lived problems. For acute or short-term difficulties, avoidance can be a very effective strategy. When faced with an immediate threat, such as being attacked, getting away and escaping is the most sensible thing to do.

Likewise, when working on an important job, it may be useful to push away interfering upsetting thoughts until the job is finished. However, avoidance is less helpful when applied to longer-term problems that do not resolve themselves quickly.

2. Avoidance is less helpful in the longer term. There are several disadvantages to avoidance over the longer term.

Avoidance leads to not coming into direct contact with an ongoing problem. When you avoid facing the problem, there is no chance of fixing it, and it will continue, leading to more distress and difficulty. For example, not telling someone else about how they act in a way that upsets you is likely to lead to their behavior continuing, which leads to more distress for you.

Avoidance closes life down. Avoidance tends to spread out and generalize to more and more things, leading to a closed, not very fulfilled life. By trying to avoid bad things, we often curtail our activities so that there are fewer positive things as well. To avoid the risk of failure, a person stops doing things where there is also the chance of success, or of learning something new. Avoidance can expand and expand until there are very few activities where there is any chance of feeling alive or fulfilled, further fueling the depressed mood. To reduce depression, you need to open up your options and possibilities and introduce the chance of doing exciting and rewarding activities—avoidance prevents and limits this.

Your Own Experience of Avoidance

Reflect on your own experience of avoidance—while it may have helped in the short term to avoid pain and upset, have things in the longer term gotten better or worse?

_____

_____

_____

Once you start avoiding things, have you noticed that the avoidance has increased or decreased over time?

_____

_____

_____

Reducing Avoidance

1. Replace avoidance with approach—try new things. It can be difficult to reduce avoidance. Avoidance has become a habit and feels safe. The fear of things getting worse or of failure and humiliation or of people responding badly makes it hard to try and change. However, this therapy will focus on reducing avoidance and replacing it with approach behaviors—on trying to embrace life and what you can get out of it, rather than trying to get through it with as little pain as possible.

2. Start by trying small steps first. Identify things you used to do and enjoy and work on building them up first.

> Break each task down into smaller manageable steps—don't try to do it all at once.

3. Look at the pros and cons of avoidance. For each activity you avoid, weigh up the advantages and disadvantages of not doing versus doing that activity. Will you feel better once you have done it rather than putting it off?

4. Focus on what is good about doing something for its own sake rather than whether you are doing it well enough. A lot of avoidance is concerned with fear of not doing things well enough, of not being good enough. Instead of concentrating on the outcome of what you are doing (did it work or not?), as best you can, focus on the process of what you are doing—get absorbed in how you do it and focus on the intrinsic pleasure of doing it. For example, when playing sports you can focus on improving your technique and on the pleasure of taking part, rather than on whether you win or lose.

5. Remember that getting better at things takes practice.

6. The anticipation of things is often more frightening than the reality. It is therefore useful to try things out and see whether they go as badly as you expected.

7. Good preparation can help make it easier to try new things. Imagining how something might turn out in advance can be helpful. Imagine as vividly as you can how you will feel when you do an activity (or how you used to feel when you did it)—this can help motivate you to do it.

8. Have a good routine. Doing the same activities at the same time and place can help reduce avoidance.

9. When planning to do things, it is useful to say when and where and how you will do them. For example, you might say, "I will go swimming at 10:00 A.M. on Saturday, and I will prepare my bag with my swimsuit and towel the night before." Saying when and where you will do something makes it more likely that you will do it, rather than putting it off to do another day.

Things to Do

1. Look at your list of things that you are avoiding. Reflect on the pros and cons of not doing these things.
2. Keep monitoring your avoidance in the weekly diary record (Handout 5).
3. Choose one activity that you are avoiding and plan how to start doing it again. The best activities to choose are those that seem easiest to get back into and those that you know will improve how you feel when you do them.
4. Explore with the therapist how you can start on the new activity.

Handout 3. Goal Setting

When people are depressed, they often find it difficult to set goals for themselves. In particular, rumination can be associated with having **unrealistic or unattainable** goals. It is therefore important to consider carefully the goals you set for yourself.

When considering goals and plans, it is useful to use the mnemonic **SMART**, which stands for:

Specific
Measurable
Achievable
Realistic
Time-Limited

Specific

The goal or plan is focused and concrete, broken down into small steps, and laid out in terms of how, when, where, and with whom you will do it.

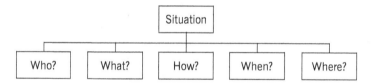

Measurable

The goal can be described in sufficient detail in terms of what you would actually do so that you (and other people) can determine whether you did it or not. Making a goal measurable ensures that it is not too abstract. One way to make a goal measurable is to have a clear physical marker of the success you are trying to achieve.

It is better to avoid goals that involve the absence of an outcome (e.g., not failing, not upsetting people, not being depressed). Such goals do not have a clear point of completion. Rather, have goals that set out what you want to move toward and achieve.

Achievable: Can Someone Succeed at This Goal?

The goal needs to be achievable at some point. Goals that are impossible are not achievable. Ideally it should be something that could happen assuming that you had the skills and abilities to do the right thing. If the outcome is not likely to occur even if you do everything right, then the goal may be considered to not be achievable.

Goals are often not directly achievable because the goal or plan requires something out of your control to occur (e.g., for someone else to agree to a request when all the evidence points to the fact that they are not likely to agree to any requests, whether reasonable or unreasonable). In situations where one aspect of the environment (e.g., a particular person) is unlikely to provide the desired outcome, the goal may be usefully reframed by focusing on either changing the environment (e.g., leaving a relationship) or concentrating on other aspects of the environment (e.g., could someone else provide help and support?).

Realistic: Are You Ready and Able for This Goal?

Can you realistically do something to achieve the goal? Is it realistic for you to try and solve the goal right now? Assuming that the goal is achievable, do you have the skills, abilities, and background to succeed? Ideally, a goal should be just ahead of where you are now (i.e., a small step forward). If the goal is not immediately realistic, look for what stops the goal from being realistic and adjust it to deal with the obstacles, or set a new smaller goal to build toward that point.

Time-Limited

The goal or plan has a time sequence to be achieved and has a time set for when it will be implemented. Having a timeline is critical for focusing your plans to achieve the goal.

It is useful to review the **SMART** mnemonic whenever your plans succeed or fail so that you can learn from your experiences and build on the more useful aspects of the **SMART** approach for future situations.

Goal Conflict

It is also useful to check whether any of your goals are in conflict with each other, as having conflicting goals is a good way to get stressed and start ruminating.

For example, to want people to do things properly and to want to never disagree with people are likely to be goals that are in conflict.

If any goals are in conflict, it is useful to weigh up the goals, consider their advantages and disadvantages so as to prioritize one of them, and to put one of the goals first.

Handout 4. Self-Monitoring

An important aspect of this therapy approach is self-monitoring of rumination and avoidance, so you can practice **spotting them as early as possible**.

Self-monitoring is an important part of therapy because both rumination and avoidance are **automatic habits** that happen without thinking, so that they can often happen without you noticing.

Key Aspects of Self-Monitoring

1. The first step in changing a habit is to notice that you are doing it. Once you are aware of the habit and when it happens, then you can start to change it. Much of what we will do in therapy depends on you noticing your thinking—without awareness it is almost impossible to change a habit.

2. The more often and the earlier you spot a habit, the better. The longer avoidance or rumination continues, the worse it gets, the harder it is to stop, and the more it becomes learned, strengthened, and automatic. Conversely, the more you can spot it, the more you are aware of it, the less habitual it becomes, and the weaker it becomes. Likewise, the earlier you can spot the early signs or triggers for dwelling on negative things, the earlier you can stop it, and the earlier you can replace the rumination with a new response.

Spotting rumination as early as possible and then intervening as quickly as possible also has the benefit of extending the period of time without rumination. Furthermore, if you repeatedly use a new response when the early signs for rumination occur, then these triggers become linked to the positive response, rather than to the rumination. Thus there are many advantages to becoming more aware of the triggers for rumination. Becoming more aware of the early signs will help you to "nip rumination in the bud."

3. Look out for warning signs of rumination and avoidance.

> **When trying to spot rumination and avoidance, it is important to notice the signs and triggers associated with the onset of these behaviors. Recognizing these early warning signs gives you further points where you can intervene and introduce new, more helpful responses instead of rumination.**

Triggers can include:
1. Feelings and emotions (e.g., feeling sad, angry, or anxious)—paying attention to your facial expression, posture, and internal sensations can help you to notice changes in your emotions.

2. Physical sensations (e.g., tiredness, pain, tension, headaches).
3. Thoughts and images (e.g., imagining a negative experience, making a comparison between yourself and someone else).
4. Behaviors (e.g., confronting someone).
5. Cues in the world around you (e.g., going to a particular place, a time of day).
6. How other people act toward you.

When looking for cues to rumination and avoidance it is useful to consider all of these different possibilities.

4. Hunt for clues. It is useful to take a **"treasure hunt"** approach, where each week you search for earlier and earlier cues to rumination and avoidance. Keep asking yourself, "What new, earlier cues did I discover this week?"

> **The earlier you can spot the signs that you are about to ruminate or avoid a situation, the more you will be able to stop the rumination or avoidance. To do this, I recommend that you keep looking to see if an earlier sign can be identified.**

5. Use the tracking forms. The therapy builds self-monitoring into the plan between sessions by asking you to complete the rumination tracking forms, noting down key episodes of rumination and avoidance and how frequently they occur.

These forms, which you fill in every week, are designed to help you become more aware of rumination and avoidance and their triggers. It is important to complete each form each week—every session we will review the forms to see how self-monitoring is going and to see whether any new signs are being observed.

Key Points

1. The first step in changing a habit is to notice that you are doing it.
2. The more often and the earlier you spot a habit, the better the outcome.
3. Look out for warning signs of rumination and avoidance.
4. Hunt for clues.
5. Use the tracking forms.

Things to Do

1. Complete a rumination and avoidance tracking form each week (see Handout 5).
2. It may also be helpful to keep and update a list of signs and cues noticed (a trigger/sign list).

Handout 5. Tracking Rumination and Avoidance

Name: _____ **Date completed:** _____

It will be very helpful if you can keep a record of how much you are repeatedly thinking about, dwelling on, worrying about, or being preoccupied by your feelings, past upsetting events, current problems, and things about yourself or the future. We call this **"rumination."** Also keep track of how much you **avoid** things (e.g., not asserting yourself with other people, not going certain places, not trying new or difficult activities, not following through with plans, withdrawing from activities, procrastinating about things). It would really help if **every week** before the therapy starts you complete the following questions, which will help your therapist to understand how much you are dwelling on negative things.

In the last week, what percentage of time were you repeatedly dwelling on or preoccupied with negative thoughts about an upsetting issue, event or problem, from 0, not at all, to 100, all the time? _____/100

In the last week, how much control did you feel you had over this repeated worrying, from 0, no control at all, to 100, totally in control of it? _____/100

In the last week, how much did the dwelling on negative things interfere with your plans or stop you from doing what you wanted, from 0, no effect at all, to 100, completely stopped me from doing everything I wanted? _____/100

How long did the worst period of rumination last? _____ minutes/hours.

How long did the rumination last in total across the whole week? _____ hours.

In the last week, how often did you avoid or put off doing things, from 0, none of the time, to 100, all of the time? _____/100

In the last week, how much control did you feel you had over your avoidance—how much could you control whether you did something even if you did not feel like doing it—from 0, no control at all, to 100, totally in control? _____/100

In the last week, how much did avoiding things interfere with or stop you from doing what you wanted, from 0, no interference, to 100, completely stopped me from doing everything I wanted? _____/100

THANK YOU!

Handout 6. Rumination Episodes Recording Form

Fill in details about **TWO** episodes when you worried or dwelled on something upsetting **Each Week.** Use the form below. This information will help the therapist to understand what you are bothered about and how to help you. By **"rumination"** we mean repeatedly thinking about, dwelling on, worrying about, or being preoccupied by your feelings, past upsetting events, current problems, things about yourself, or the future. For each example, please note when it happened, what happened just before it started, how you felt before, how long it lasted, what it was about, what effect it had on you, and what stopped it. Don't be concerned about how you are filling in the form—there are no right or wrong answers and spelling, grammar, and neatness are not important—the form is just a way of gathering helpful information about your thinking.

Date	Time	What happened just before the rumination started?	How did you feel before?	Duration	What were you thinking about?	What were the consequences of rumination—for mood and actions?	What stopped the rumination? What did you try to stop it? Was it useful?
10/5/15	10 P.M.	Went to bed.	Anxious, sad	2 hours	Why do I feel so bad? Why can't I sleep? All the things I didn't do today.	Could not sleep. Felt worse.	Eventually fell asleep after taking sleeping pills.

From *Rumination-Focused Cognitive-Behavioral Therapy for Depression* by Edward R. Watkins. Copyright © 2016 The Guilford Press. Permission to photocopy this handout is granted to purchasers of this book for personal use or use with individual patients (see copyright page for details). Purchasers can download enlarged versions of this handout (see the box at the end of the table of contents).

Handout 7. Antecedent–Behavior–Consequence (ABC) Form

This ABC form is designed to help spot the warning signs and effects of rumination. Identify a recent example of when you ruminated and then fill in the boxes below, answering the questions within each box, initially with the help of your therapist.

Antecedent	What precedes B? What triggers B: event, feeling, thought, person, place, time, activity? Determine context: where?, when?, who?, what?, how?
Behavior	What you did: the target behavior to understand, and increase or decrease. Provide details on how the behavior occurs (e.g., content and style of rumination).
Consequence	What is the consequence of B—positive/negative, short-term/long-term, for self, for others—on valued goals? What effect does it have? What does it increase/decrease? What are its pros/cons? What does it avoid? What would happen if you didn't do B? What is the effect of not doing B? What would you be doing instead? What has the consequence of B been in the past?

Handout 8. Being More Effective

Becoming more effective in thinking and actions involves learning to direct your thoughts and actions so that you can be more successful at achieving your desired goals. We have already seen how **rumination often involves thinking that does not lead to helpful action**—learning to be more effective will reduce rumination.

Remember too that we have observed that you can think about problems in different ways:

1. Sometimes thinking about problems is helpful and solves the problem, making you feel better.	**2. Sometimes you can become stuck, ruminating over and over in a way that just makes you feel worse, without making any progress.**

We are going to focus on how you can learn from your own experience to increase the helpful thinking while reducing unhelpful thinking, and reduce rumination.

> **The key to being more effective is to use your own experience to learn what works and then change your thinking and behavior for the better.**

Learning from Your Own Experience

Being more effective means learning what works and what does not work. Being more effective involves learning as much as we can from our own experience—by paying attention to what worked and what did not work in the past, and noticing the differences between these situations.

We all learn from our own experience to get more effective. Look back over your life and think of skills that you have gotten better at. Consider how you have learned both from your successes and your failures.

Depression and rumination can reduce the ability to learn from experience. When people are depressed, they tend to not notice changes and to think that everything stays the same and cannot improve, making it hard to learn from success and failure. Likewise, rumination involves a tendency to look at the similarities across situations and see common and general abstract themes across different events, often relating to personal inadequacy, such as "I am a failure." During rumination, one negative thought or memory is often linked with other negative memories, rapidly leading to a spiral of negative memories.

To be more effective, you need a systematic approach that fights off the effects of depression and rumination. We call this approach "functional analysis," and it is an approach you have been practicing with your therapist.

Key Aspects of Functional Analysis

Pay Attention to Change: Look Out for Differences between Situations and How Things Change across Time

Noticing that sometimes we succeed and sometimes we fail and looking for what is different between success and failure is a key step in altering our thinking and behavior to become more successful. Deliberately looking out for how situations and actions vary is important to overcome the sense that nothing changes, which is often produced by depression.

For example, imagine that Jill wants to do some important writing (deal with bills, catch up on letters, get on with work, etc.) but finds it difficult to start and keeps putting the job off. Jill then starts to dwell on not getting it done, feeling down on herself and thinking "Why can't I do this?"

To be more effective, Jill could reflect on whether there have been differences in how well she has been able to get her writing done on different occasions. In fact, she remembers that there have been times when she has gotten going on her writing quite well and times when she has found it more difficult.

Looking at the differences between those times we can see the following:

GOOD AT WRITING
Jill has a tidy space away from distractions.
Jill is focusing on the step by step details of what she is doing.

BAD AT WRITING
Jill's writing area is a mess.
Jill is focused on evaluating how well she is doing—will the writing be good enough?

So to find writing easier, Jill may need to plan to work in an undisturbed, neat place and to focus on each item she is working on one at a time rather than checking up on her performance.

Differences in the world around us, how people are thinking, and what people are doing can all determine whether thinking about problems is helpful (problem solving) or unhelpful (rumination). Consider what happens when you start thinking about a problem. Think of a time when you thought about a problem and reached a plan or decision quickly, within 15 minutes.

Remember the situation as vividly as possible. Note down what you were doing, what you were thinking, where you were, and how you approached the problem.

Now, think of a time when you thought about a problem and found it difficult to reach a plan or decision, going over and over the problem for hours and hours without success. Remember the situation as vividly as possible. Note down what you were doing, what you were thinking, where you were, and how you approached the problem.

What was different between the two situations? How were the problems different? Was the way that you thought about them different? What can you learn from this experience?

Pay Attention to What Is Unique about Each Situation: Note the Particular Circumstances

Every attempt at thinking and action occurs in a different context and set of circumstances—a unique and different combination of what you do, how you do it, when you do it, where you do it, why you do it, who else is involved, your physical and mental state, the conditions in which you do it. Fully describing all these elements is essential to learning what factors influence success.

For example, Jill needs to remember the details of each time she tries to write in order to notice what differences there may be between when she is effective and not effective.

A quick review of useful questions:

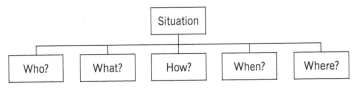

For Jill, these questions might provide the following information:

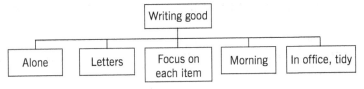

327

Focusing on the particular, unique aspects of a situation works against the tendency of rumination to generalize one situation to many situations. It is more useful to think "I failed because I was tired and unprepared" than to think "I am a failure." The explanation that involves information specific to the situation is less general and gives clues as to what to do next time to improve performance.

Notice the Consequences of Any Action

Does the action have any benefits or rewards that increase the likelihood of doing the action again? What purposes does the action serve? Understanding the consequences of an action can determine whether it is useful (does it get what I want?) and whether there are alternatives (are there other ways to achieve the same ends?).

For example, for Jill, putting off writing may be a way to avoid a situation that involves judging herself. To get back to writing, Jill may need to find a way to write without always evaluating herself. Yet, when Jill does write she begins to feel more in control and more productive.

Practicing Functional Analysis

For each situation, thinking about differences, particular circumstances, and consequences will help to produce a more useful view of what might be going on, reduce rumination, and guide future plans.

We have a specific form to help—the Being More Effective Form. Handout 9 is an example of a blank form. Look at the form and consider how you would use it. Your therapist will discuss with you how to use this form day to day.

Over time, a collection of these forms will provide information about what increases the chances of helpful thinking and useful action. This information can then be used to make better plans.

Key Points

1. Being more effective means learning what works and what does not work.
2. We all learn from our own experience to become more effective.
3. Depression and rumination can reduce the ability to learn from experience.
4. Therefore, to be more effective, you need a systematic approach that fights off the effects of depression and rumination. We call this "functional analysis."
5. The key aspects of functional analysis are:
    Pay attention to change—look out for differences between situations and how things change across time.

328

Pay attention to what is unique about each situation—note the particular circumstances.

Notice the consequences of any action.

Things to Do

1. Complete the *Being More Effective Form* regularly as a response to difficulties and warning signs for rumination and avoidance.

2. Review what is learned as you complete a number of these forms. What approaches are more helpful than others? Change how you handle situations in response to this information.

Handout 9. Being More Effective Form

Complete this form after every success or failure. Use the questions below the form to complete each column and then note down your plan/decision.

Detailed questions	Current situation[a] (success/failure) (e.g., intended to do something and did it)	Similar situation with opposite outcome[b] (failure/success) (e.g., intended to do something and did not do it)
What? Include goal, events, actions, feelings, physical state, outcome		
Where? Location, setting, state		
When? Time, day, what preceded the situation		
How? Step by step how the event unfolded, your approach during the situation		
Who?		

[a]What was unique about this situation? Describe in detail the context of the event in response to each question. Was the event a success or failure?
[b]Describe a similar situation or task that had a different outcome (e.g., success or failure), and that happened either this week or earlier. How do the situations differ? What can you learn from this?

Plan/decision for the future:

Handout 10. Engaging with Life through Concreteness

Not Connecting with Experience

You're there but not there!

Depression often makes it hard for people to fully connect with experience, to fully *engage* with life. You can be doing something you might usually enjoy but not feel anything, or feel disconnected. You can be physically present but not mentally or emotionally there. For example, you could be talking to a friend or playing with your children but not feeling anything. You're there but you're not there—you are not *fully* attending to or connecting with experience.

Spend a few moments reflecting on those times when you don't fully connect or attend to the experience of what you are doing—those times when you are not fully there. These might be times when you feel a bit numb, or when you feel spaced out, or a bit distanced, or when you feel like you are going through the motions. Use the lines below to write down some examples of times when you have not fully experienced what you are doing.

Try to be as specific and detailed (concrete) as possible:

_____

_____

_____

Effects of Not Connecting with Experience

Let's start by looking at your own experience of not fully connecting with activities or other people. Spend a few moments reflecting on the effects this has on you and note down your answers to the following questions.

Does it make you **feel** better or worse?   ☐ **Better**   ☐ **Worse**

Does it increase or reduce your **energy levels**?   ☐ **Increase**   ☐ **Reduce**

Does it increase or reduce the chance that you will   ☐ **Increase**   ☐ **Reduce**
carry out your **plans and activities**?

Depression and Not Connecting with Experience

Not being connected to experience contributes to depression in two main ways:

- If you are not connecting with experience then you don't get the benefit of doing something enjoyable—you can do something that would normally be rewarding or pleasurable but it does not make you feel better. Thus, whatever you do, your mood will not improve.

- If you are not connecting with experience, you are not able to notice what is going on around you, notice any changes, or learn from success and failure. You are likely to keep repeating the same mistakes again and again, since there is no chance of realizing what you could do differently.

Abstract thinking and Not Connecting with Experience

Both **rumination** and **overgeneralization** contribute to not being able to connect directly with experience. When someone is ruminating, her mind is full of thoughts going round and round about her problems, and she is not really attending to what she is doing. Likewise, when someone is jumping to conclusions from an event and thinking about what it might mean about his future and himself (overgeneralizing), he is moving away from the direct experience of what is happening and moving into *abstract* thoughts *about* the experience. Too much abstract thinking can stop you from connecting with experience and prevents the benefits of directly connecting with the world around you.

Avoidance and Not Connecting with Experience

We can also lose connection with our direct experience because we are trying to avoid thinking about upsetting or emotional events, trying to avoid unpleasant feelings, or avoiding new challenges or risks. By trying to avoid threats or possible failure, we often reduce our activities, resulting in fewer positive experiences as well. To avoid any risk of failure, you might also stop doing things where there is at least a chance of success, or of learning something new. Therefore, avoidance can increase until there are very few activities where there is any chance of feeling alive or fulfilled, further fueling the depressed mood.

Avoidance can close life down, shutting out the chance of fully experiencing life. While this might be a way to reduce the risk of experiencing more pain, it also makes it hard to fully connect with all the good things in life. To reduce depression, you need to open up your options and possibilities and introduce the chance of doing exciting and rewarding activities—avoidance prevents and limits this.

Reconnecting with Experience

The way to reconnect with experience is to directly attend to what you are doing and to the world around you. A good way to do this is to focus your attention on an activity that you find interesting and in which you can become completely absorbed and immersed. You can do this via a mental exercise that re-creates the experience of being absorbed in an activity.

You can also reconnect with experience by deliberately increasing the activities that you find interesting and absorbing. When they are depressed, people often drop the activities that excite and absorb them, while carrying on with the chores and duties they feel they should do. The consequence of this is that you can end up doing all the dull and effortful activities that you find tiring and draining but not doing any of the interesting and fun activities that make you feel better and give you more energy. It is important to get the balance between chores and duties and positive activities right, because the former drain your batteries while the latter recharge your batteries. This means that if you are doing too many chores and not enough fun, engaging activities, you are going to wear yourself out.

Absorbing Activities

The kinds of experiences we are looking for are those where you feel completely absorbed, immersed, or caught up in the process and details of what you are doing; where you lose all sense of self and time; where you experience things coming together naturally without much conscious thought; where there is a deep and effortless involvement in the activity, a merging of action and awareness and a sense of being completely focused in the present moment. Such absorbing experiences are sometimes described as "flow" experiences or peak experiences—people who play sports refer to being "in the zone." Critically, such experiences involve concrete thinking, since attention is focused on the details of the task and on sensory experience, as you concentrate on the process and sequence of what is happening. Even more important, such experiences are a very strong antidote to rumination, overgeneralization, and inactivity, and act as a powerful antidepressant.

Different people find different activities absorbing. Absorbing activities can include doing something creative, musical, or artistic, focusing on the natural world, participating in sports, dance, or other challenging physical activities, and taking part in activities that involve intellectual stimulation and learning.

Specific examples include sensation-seeking, high-adrenaline activities like rock climbing, scuba diving, horseback riding, surfing, or sky diving, where you are completely focused on the experience of what you are doing (e.g., focusing on where to put your hands next when rock climbing).

Or absorbing activities could be creative activities like painting, where you are focused on the patterns of light and dark, the differences in color and texture on the canvas, and where you sense you should put the brush next.

Activities You Find Absorbing

There is no right or wrong way to become absorbed. Try and think of memories of when you have been completely absorbed in an activity. Use the lines below to write down several examples of times when you have been fully absorbed in what you are doing. **Try to be as specific and detailed (concrete) as possible:**

333

1. _____
2. _____
3. _____
4. _____
5. _____
6. _____

Common Themes in Absorbing Activities

As you look at these different examples, you might find that there are some elements in common between them. *Positive* absorption is more likely to occur under particular conditions, many of which are under your control:

- There is a balance between the challenge (difficulties and opportunities) of the task and your skills—if the task is too difficult, it is hard to get absorbed, but if it is too easy it will be boring. Ideally, you need to try tasks that are within the reach of your skills while slightly stretching you.
- Your attention is focused on the task at hand—the more you attend directly to what you are doing, the more absorbed and connected you become.
- The activity involves a narrow temporal focus—your attention is focused on the immediate, present moment, on what is happening in the moment right now, rather than on the past and the future.
- There are clear goals, rules, and immediate feedback. It is easier to get absorbed when you know what you are trying to do and for every action you take there is an immediate and direct response—for example, when playing a musical instrument, you immediately hear what note was played; when painting you can directly see the effect of the brush on the canvas.
- The activity is rewarding in itself—what you are doing is valued as an end in itself because the *process* of doing it is interesting, rather than because of what you might achieve *as a result* of doing the activity. For example, playing a sport might feel good as you are doing it because of the feeling in your body, whether you win or lose.
- There is a focus on discovery, learning, growth—you are doing the activity out of curiosity, to see what happens or to learn and improve.
- The activity is consistent with what you value—it reflects what is important and meaningful to you. For example, if you appreciate the natural world, then you might find walking in the country and paying attention to nature absorbing. If you value learning and curiosity, you will be find activities that involve learning more absorbing, for example, learning to play a musical instrument.

334

Your Examples of Absorbing Activities Are an Important Starting Point

The examples you listed above provide memories you can use for **the mental exercise of imagining and re-creating absorbing activities.** During these mental self-help exercises, you will imagine one of these absorbing situations as vividly and as concretely as you can. You imagine that you are there right now, looking out onto the scene, seeing through your own eyes, experiencing the sensations of being in your own body, using all of your senses to become fully aware of your experience in the moment. You can use these exercises to get yourself into a frame of mind where you are more directly connected to experience, in order to practice this skill and as a means to fully experience what you are doing. In addition, the state of mind you have when you are absorbed makes you more motivated to do things and makes it easier to fully experience what you are doing and get more enjoyment from it. It can therefore be helpful to practice the absorption exercise to get yourself into the right frame of mind before starting an activity, to increase your chance of getting started and to increase your enjoyment of what you are doing.

   Your examples give you clues as to activities that you can find absorbing and beneficial. Take a look at the examples you listed. How many of these activities have you stopped doing or are you doing less frequently? Write down which of these activities that you would like to do more often below:

1. _____
2. _____
3. _____

Choose one of these activities and plan how you would start doing it again over the next few weeks. Note down the steps of your plan here:

Activity:

Step 1. _____
Step 2. _____
Step 3. _____
Step 4. _____

Often people find that making a written commitment increases the likelihood that they will do something. Are you happy to commit to your plan?

I, *(insert name)* _____, commit to *(insert activity)* _____ at *(insert times)* _____ on *(insert dates)* _____
Signed: _____ Date: _____

You can talk about this plan with your therapist at your next session.

References

Abela, J. R., Brozina, K., & Haigh, E. P. (2002). An examination of the response styles theory of depression in third- and seventh-grade children: A short-term longitudinal study. *Journal of Abnormal Child Psychology, 30*(5), 515–527.

Addis, M., & Martell, C. (2004). *Overcoming depression one step at a time: The new behavioral activation approach to getting your life back.* Oakland, CA: New Harbinger Press.

Aldao, A., Nolen-Hoeksema, S., & Schweizer, S. (2010). Emotion-regulation strategies across psychopathology: A meta-analytic review. *Clinical Psychology Review, 30*(2), 217–237.

American Psychiatric Association. (2013). *Diagnostic and statistical manual of mental disorders* (5th ed.). Arlington, VA: Author.

Andersson, G., & Cuijpers, P. (2009). Internet-based and other computerized psychological treatments for adult depression: A meta-analysis. *Cognitive Behavior Therapy, 38*(4), 196–205.

Andrews, G., Cuijpers, P., Craske, M. G., McEvoy, P., & Titov, N. (2010). Computer therapy for the anxiety and depressive disorders is effective, acceptable and practical health care: A meta-analysis. *PloS ONE, 5*(10), 1–6.

Andrews, G., Issakidis, C., Sanderson, K., Corry, J., & Lapsley, H. (2004). Utilising survey data to inform public policy: Comparison of the cost-effectiveness of treatment of ten mental disorders. *British Journal of Psychiatry, 184*(6), 526–533.

Bargh, J. (1994). The four horsemen of automaticity: Awareness, intention, efficiency, and control in social cognition. In R. S. Wyer, Jr., & T. K. Srull (Eds.), *Handbook of social cognition* (2nd ed., Vol. 1, pp. 1–40). Hillsdale, NJ: Erlbaum.

Barlow, D. H. (2004). Psychological treatments. *American Psychologist, 59*(9), 869–878.

Barlow, D. H., Allen, L. B., & Choate, M. L. (2004). Toward a unified treatment for emotional disorders. *Behavior Therapy, 35*(2), 205–230.

Beck, A. T., Rush, A. J., Shaw, B. F., & Emery, G. (1979). *Cognitive therapy of depression.* New York: Guilford Press.

Bernstein, D. A., & Borkovec, T. D. (1973). *Progressive relaxation training: A manual for the helping professions.* Champaign, IL: Research Press.

Blagden, J. C., & Craske, M. G. (1996). Effects of active and passive rumination and distraction: A pilot replication with anxious mood. *Journal of Anxiety Disorders, 10*(4), 243–252.

Borkovec, T. D., & Costello, E. (1993). Efficacy of applied relaxation and cognitive-behavioral therapy in the treatment of generalized anxiety disorder. *Journal of Consulting and Clinical Psychology, 61*(4), 611–619.

Borkovec, T. D., & Newman, M. G. (1998). Worry and generalized anxiety disorder. *Comprehensive Clinical Psychology, 6*, 439–459.

Borkovec, T. D., Ray, W. J., & Stober, J. (1998). Worry: A cognitive phenomenon intimately linked to affective, physiological, and interpersonal behavioral processes. *Cognitive Therapy and Research, 22*(6), 561–576.

Borkovec, T. D., & Roemer, L. (1995). Perceived functions of worry among generalized anxiety disorder subjects: Distraction from more emotionally distressing topics? *Journal of Behavior Therapy and Experimental Psychiatry, 26*(1), 25–30.

Brandstätter, V., Lengfelder, A., & Gollwitzer, P. M. (2001). Implementation intentions and efficient action initiation. *Journal of Personality and Social Psychology, 81*(5), 946–960.

Bruce, S. E., Yonkers, K. A., Otto, M. W., Eisen, J. L., Weisberg, R. B., Pagano, M., et al. (2005). Influence of psychiatric comorbidity on recovery and recurrence in generalized anxiety disorder, social phobia, and panic disorder: A 12-year prospective study. *American Journal of Psychiatry, 162*(6), 1179–1187.

Butler, L. D., & Nolen-Hoeksema, S. (1994). Gender differences in responses to depressed mood in a college sample. *Sex Roles, 30*(5–6), 331–346.

Carver, C. S. (1998). Generalization, adverse events, and development of depressive symptoms. *Journal of Personality, 66*(4), 607–619.

Carver, C. S., & Scheier, M. F. (1982). Control theory: A useful conceptual framework for personality—social, clinical, and health psychology. *Psychological Bulletin, 92*(1), 111–135.

Carver, C. S., & Scheier, M. F. (1990). Origins and functions of positive and negative affect: A control-process view. *Psychological Review, 97*(1), 19–35.

Carver, C. S., & Scheier, M. F. (1998). *On the self-regulation of behavior.* New York: Cambridge University Press.

Caselli, G., Ferretti, C., Leoni, M., Rebecchi, D., Rovetto, F., & Spada, M. M. (2010). Rumination as a predictor of drinking behavior in alcohol abusers: A prospective study. *Addiction, 105*(6), 1041–1048.

Chambers, R., Lo, B. C. Y., & Allen, N. B. (2008). The impact of intensive mindfulness training on attentional control, cognitive style, and affect. *Cognitive Therapy and Research, 32*(3), 303–322.

Ciesla, J. A., & Roberts, J. E. (2002). Self-directed thought and response to treatment for depression: A preliminary investigation. *Journal of Cognitive Psychotherapy: An International Quarterly, 16*, 435–453

Ciesla, J. A., & Roberts, J. E. (2007). Rumination, negative cognition, and their interactive effects on depressed mood. *Emotion, 7*(3), 555–565.

Collins, P. Y., Patel, V., Joestl, S. S., March, D., Insel, T. R., Daar, A. S., et al. (2011). Grand challenges in global mental health. *Nature, 475*(7354), 27–30.

Conway, M., Mendelson, M., Giannopoulos, C., Csank, P. A., & Holm, S. L. (2004). Childhood and adult sexual abuse, rumination on sadness, and dysphoria. *Child Abuse and Neglect, 28*(4), 393–410.

Cornwall, P., & Scott, J. (1997). Partial remission in depressive disorders. *Acta Psychiatrica Scandinavica, 95*(4), 265–271.

Cribb, G., Moulds, M. L., & Carter, S. (2006). Rumination and experiential avoidance in depression. *Behavior Change, 23*(3), 165–176.

Csikszentmihalyi, M. (2002). *Flow: The classic work on how to achieve happiness.* London: Rider.

Dimidjian, S., Hollon, S. D., Dobson, K. S., Schmaling, K. B., Kohlenberg, R. J., Addis, M. E., et al. (2006). Randomized trial of behavioral activation, cognitive therapy, and antidepressant medication in the acute treatment of adults with major depression. *Journal of Consulting and Clinical Psychology, 74*(4), 658–670.

Donaldson, C., & Lam, D. (2004). Rumination, mood and social problem-solving in major depression. *Psychological Medicine, 34*(7), 1309–1318.

Dykman, B. M. (1998). Integrating cognitive and motivational factors in depression: Initial tests of a goal-orientation approach. *Journal of Personality and Social Psychology, 74*(1), 139–158.

D'Zurilla, T. J., & Nezu, A. M. (1999). *Problem-solving therapy: A social competence approach to clinical* (2nd ed.). New York: Springer.

Ehring, T., Szeimies, A.-K., & Schaffrick, C. (2009). An experimental analogue study into the role of abstract thinking in trauma-related rumination. *Behaviour Research and Therapy, 47*(4), 285–293.

Ehring, T., & Watkins, E. R. (2008). Repetitive negative thinking as a transdiagnostic process. *International Journal of Cognitive Therapy, 1*(3), 192–205.

Fairburn, C. G., Cooper, Z., & Shafran, R. (2003). Cognitive behavior therapy for eating disorders: A "transdiagnostic" theory and treatment. *Behaviour Research and Therapy, 41*(5), 509–528.

Fava, G. A. (1999). Subclinical symptoms in mood disorders: Pathophysiological and therapeutic implications. *Psychological Medicine, 29*(1), 47–61.

Fava, G. A., Zielezny, M., Savron, G., & Grandi, S. (1995). Long-term effects of behavioral treatment for panic disorder with agoraphobia. *British Journal of Psychiatry, 166*(1), 87–92.

Feldman, G., Greeson, J., & Senville, J. (2010). Differential effects of mindful breathing, progressive muscle relaxation, and loving-kindness meditation on decentering and negative reactions to repetitive thoughts. *Behaviour Research and Therapy, 48*(10), 1002–1011.

Ferster, C. B. (1973). A functional analysis of depression. *American Psychologist, 28*(10), 857–870.

Freeston, M. H., Rhéaume, J., Letarte, H., Dugas, M. J., & Ladouceur, R. (1994). Why do people worry? *Personality and Individual Differences, 17*(6), 791–802.

Fresco, D. M., Frankel, A. N., Mennin, D. S., Turk, C. L., & Heimberg, R. G. (2002). Distinct and overlapping features of rumination and worry: The relationship of cognitive production to negative affective states. *Cognitive Therapy and Research, 26*(2), 179–188.

Gellatly, J., Bower, P., Hennessy, S., Richards, D., Gilbody, S., & Lovell, K. (2007). What makes self-help interventions effective in the management of depressive symptoms? Meta-analysis and meta-regression. *Psychological Medicine, 37*(9), 1217–1228.

Geschwind, N., Peeters, F., Drukker, M., van Os, J., & Wichers, M. (2011). Mindfulness training increases momentary positive emotions and reward experience in adults vulnerable to depression: A randomized controlled trial. *Journal of Consulting and Clinical Psychology, 79*(5), 618.

Gilbert, P. (2009). Introducing compassion-focused therapy. *Advances in Psychiatric Treatment, 15*(3), 199–208.

Gilbert, P. (2010). *Compassion focused therapy: Distinctive features.* New York: Routledge.

Gilbert, P., & Irons, C. (2004). A pilot exploration of the use of compassionate images in a group of self-critical people. *Memory, 12*, 507–516.

Gilbert, P., & Proctor, S. (2006). Compassionate mind training for people with high shame and self-criticism: Overview and pilot study of a group therapy approach. *Clinical Psychology and Psychotherapy, 13*, 353–379.

Giorgio, J. M., Sanflippo, J., Kleiman, E., Reilly, D., Bender, R. E., Wagner, C. A., et al. (2010). An experiential avoidance conceptualization of depressive rumination: Three tests of the model. *Behaviour Research and Therapy, 48*(10), 1021–1031.

Gollwitzer, P. M. (1999). Implementation intentions: Strong effects of simple plans. *American Psychologist, 54*(7), 493–503.

Gollwitzer, P. M., & Sheeran, P. (2006). Implementation intentions and goal achievement: A meta-analysis of effects and processes. *Advances in Experimental Social Psychology, 38*, 69–119.

Gortner, E. T., Gollan, J. K., Dobson, K. S., & Jacobson, N. S. (1998). Cognitive–behavioral treatment for depression: Relapse prevention. *Journal of Consulting and Clinical Psychology, 66*(2), 377–384.

Grant, K. E., Lyons, A. L., Finkelstein, J.-A. S., Conway, K. M., Reynolds, L. K., O'Koon, J. H., et al. (2004). Gender differences in rates of depressive symptoms among low-income, urban, African American youth: A test of two mediational hypotheses. *Journal of Youth and Adolescence, 33*(6), 523–533.

Harvey, A., Watkins, E., Mansell, W., & Shafran, R. (2004). *Cognitive behavioral processes across psychological disorders: A transdiagnostic approach to research and treatment.* Oxford, UK: Oxford University Press.

Hawton, K. E., Salkovskis, P. M., Kirk, J. E., & Clark, D. M. (1989). *Cognitive behavior therapy for psychiatric problems: A practical guide.* New York: Oxford University Press.

Hertel, P. T. (1998). Relation between rumination and impaired memory in dysphoric moods. *Journal of Abnormal Psychology, 107*(1), 166–172.

Hertel, P. T. (2004). Memory for emotional and nonemotional events in depression: A question of habit? In D. Reisberg & P. Hertel (Eds.), *Memory and emotion* (pp. 186–216). New York: Oxford University Press.

Hvenegaard, M., Watkins, E., Gondan, M., Grafton, B., & Moeller, S. B. (2015, November 13). *Rumination-focused CBT versus CBT for depression (RuCoD-trial): A randomised controlled trial.* Presented at the annual convention of the Association for Behavioral and Cognitive Therapies, Chicago.

Holland, R. W., Aarts, H., & Langendam, D. (2006). Breaking and creating habits on the working floor: A field-experiment on the power of implementation intentions. *Journal of Experimental Social Psychology, 42*(6), 776–783.

Hollon, S. D., DeRubeis, R. J., Shelton, R. C., Amsterdam, J. D., Salomon, R. M., O'Reardon, J. P., et al. (2005). Prevention of relapse following cognitive therapy vs medications in moderate to severe depression. *Archives of General Psychiatry, 62*(4), 417–422.

Hollon, S. D., Muñoz, R. F., Barlow, D. H., Beardslee, W. R., Bell, C. C., Bernal, G., et al. (2002). Psychosocial intervention development for the prevention and treatment of depression: Promoting innovation and increasing access. *Biological Psychiatry, 52*(6), 610–630.

Holm-Denoma, J. M., & Hankin, B. L. (2010). Perceived physical appearance mediates the rumination and bulimic symptom link in adolescent girls. *Journal of Clinical Child and Adolescent Psychology, 39*(4), 537–544.

Hong, R. Y. (2007). Worry and rumination: Differential associations with anxious and depressive symptoms and coping behavior. *Behaviour Research and Therapy, 45*(2), 277–290.

Jacobson, N. S., Dobson, K. S., Truax, P. A., Addis, M. E., Koerner, K., Gollan, J. K., et al. (1996). A component analysis of cognitive-behavioral treatment for depression. *Journal of Consulting and Clinical Psychology, 64*(2), 295–304.

Jacobson, N. S., Martell, C. R., & Dimidjian, S. (2001). Behavioral activation treatment for depression: Returning to contextual roots. *Clinical Psychology: Science and Practice, 8*(3), 255–270.

Jain, S., Shapiro, S. L., Swanick, S., Roesch, S. C., Mills, P. J., Bell, I., et al. (2007). A randomized controlled trial of mindfulness meditation versus relaxation training: Effects on distress, positive states of mind, rumination, and distraction. *Annals of Behavioral Medicine, 33*(1), 11–21.

Ji, M. F., & Wood, W. (2007). Purchase and consumption habits: Not necessarily what you intend. *Journal of Consumer Psychology, 17*(4), 261–276.

Judd, L. L. (1997). The clinical course of unipolar major depressive disorders. *Archives of General Psychiatry, 54*(11), 989–991.

Judd, L. L., Paulus, M. P., & Zeller, P. (1999). The role of residual subthreshold depressive symptoms in early episode relapse in unipolar major depressive disorder. *Archives of General Psychiatry, 56*(8), 764–765.

Just, N., & Alloy, L. B. (1997). The response styles theory of depression: Tests and an extension of the theory. *Journal of Abnormal Psychology, 106*(2), 221–229.

Kabat-Zinn, J. (1990). *Full catastrophe living: Using the wisdom of your body and mind to face stress, pain and illness.* New York: Delacorte.

Kaltenthaler, E., Parry, G., & Beverley, C. (2004). Computerized cognitive behavior therapy: A systematic review. *Behavioral and Cognitive Psychotherapy, 32*(1), 31–55.

Kao, C. M., Dritschel, B. H., & Astell, A. (2006). The effects of rumination and distraction on over-general autobiographical memory retrieval during social problem solving. *British Journal of Clinical Psychology, 45*(2), 267–272.

Kazdin, A. E., & Blase, S. L. (2011). Rebooting psychotherapy research and practice to reduce the burden of mental illness. *Perspectives on Psychological Science, 6*(1), 21–37.

Kessler, R. C., Chiu, W. T., Demler, O., & Walters, E. E. (2005). Prevalence, severity, and comorbidity of 12-month DSM-IV disorders in the National Comorbidity Survey Replication. *Archives of General Psychiatry, 62*(6), 617–627.

Kessler, R. C., McGonagle, K. A., Zhao, S., Nelson, C. B., Hughes, M., Eshleman, S., et al. (1994). Lifetime and 12-month prevalence of DSM-III-R psychiatric disorders in the United States: Results from the National Comorbidity Survey. *Archives of General Psychiatry, 51*(1), 8–9.

Killingsworth, M. A., & Gilbert, D. T. (2010). A wandering mind is an unhappy mind. *Science, 330*(6006), 932.

Kingston, R. E. F., & Watkins, E. R. (2015). *Positive metacognitive beliefs about rumination and worry increase repetitive negative thinking after a stressful event.* Conference paper at NHMRC Centre for Research Excellence in Mental Health and Substance Use Annual Colloquium, Canberra, Australia.

Kingston, R. E. F., Watkins, E. R., & Nolen-Hoeksema, S. (2015). Investigating functional properties of depressive rumination. *Journal of Experimental Psychopathology, 5*(3), 244–258.

Kingston, R., Watkins, E. R., & O'Mahen, H. (2013). An integrated examination of risk factors for repetitive negative thought. *Journal of Experimental Psychopathology, 4*, 161–181.

Kocsis, J. H., Leon, A. C., Markowitz, J. C., Manber, R., Arnow, B., Klein, D. N., et al. (2009). Patient preference as a moderator of outcome for chronic forms of major depressive disorder treated with nefazodone, cognitive behavioral analysis system of psychotherapy, or their combination. *Journal of Clinical Psychiatry, 70*(3), 354–361.

Kuehner, C., & Weber, I. (1999). Responses to depression in unipolar depressed patients: An investigation of Nolen-Hoeksema's response styles theory. *Psychological Medicine, 29*(06), 1323–1333.

Kuyken, W., Byford, S., Taylor, R. S., Watkins, E., Holden, E., White, K., et al. (2008). Mindfulness-based cognitive therapy to prevent relapse in recurrent depression. *Journal of Consulting and Clinical Psychology, 76*(6), 966–978.

Kuyken, W., Watkins, E., Holden, E., White, K., Taylor, R. S., Byford, S., et al. (2010). How does mindfulness-based cognitive therapy work? *Behaviour Research and Therapy, 48*(11), 1105–1112.

Lavender, A., & Watkins, E. (2004). Rumination and future thinking in depression. *British Journal of Clinical Psychology, 43*(2), 129–142.

Leary, M. R., Adams, C. E., & Tate, E. B. (2006). Hypo-egoic self-regulation: Exercising self-control by diminishing the influence of the self. *Journal of Personality, 74*(6), 1803–1832.

Leykin, Y., Muñoz, R. F., & Contreras, O. (2012). Are consumers of Internet health information "cyberchondriacs"? Characteristics of 24,965 users of a depression screening site. *Depression and Anxiety, 29*(1), 71–77.

Lopez, A. D., Mathers, C. D., Ezzati, M., Jamison, D. T., & Murray, C. J. (2006). Global and regional burden of disease and risk factors, 2001: Systematic analysis of population health data. *Lancet, 367*(9524), 1747–1757.

Lyubomirsky, S., Caldwell, N. D., & Nolen-Hoeksema, S. (1998). Effects of ruminative and distracting responses to depressed mood on retrieval of autobiographical memories. *Journal of Personality and Social Psychology, 75*(1), 166–177.

Lyubomirsky, S., Kasri, F., & Zehm, K. (2003). Dysphoric rumination impairs concentration on academic tasks. *Cognitive Therapy and Research, 27*(3), 309–330.

Lyubomirsky, S., & Nolen-Hoeksema, S. (1993). Self-perpetuating properties of dysphoric rumination. *Journal of Personality and Social Psychology, 65*(2), 339–349.

Lyubomirsky, S., & Nolen-Hoeksema, S. (1995). Effects of self-focused rumination on negative thinking and interpersonal problem solving. *Journal of Personality and Social Psychology, 69*(1), 176–190.

Lyubomirsky, S., Tucker, K. L., Caldwell, N. D., & Berg, K. (1999). Why ruminators are poor problem solvers: Clues from the phenomenology of dysphoric rumination. *Journal of Personality and Social Psychology, 77*(5), 1041–1060.

Ma, S. H., & Teasdale, J. D. (2004). Mindfulness-based cognitive therapy for depression: Replication and exploration of differential relapse prevention effects. *Journal of Consulting and Clinical Psychology, 72*(1), 31–40.

Mansell, W., Harvey, A., Watkins, E. R., & Shafran, R. (2008). Cognitive behavioral processes across psychological disorders: A review of the utility and validity of the transdiagnostic approach. *International Journal of Cognitive Therapy, 1*(3), 181–191.

Marteau, T. M., Hollands, G. J., & Fletcher, P. C. (2012). Changing human behavior to prevent disease: The importance of targeting automatic processes. *Science, 337,* 1492–1495.

Martell, C. R. (2003). Behavioral activation treatment for depression. In W. O'Donohue, J. Fisher, & S. Hayes (Eds.), *Cognitive behavior therapy: Applying empirically supported techniques in your practice* (pp. 28–32). New York: Wiley.

Martell, C. R., Addis, M. E., & Jacobson, N. S. (2001). *Depression in context: Strategies for guided action.* New York: Norton.

Martin, L. L., & Tesser, A. (1989). Toward a motivational and structural theory of ruminative thought. In J. S. Uleman & J. A. Bargh (Eds.), *Unintended thought* (pp. 306–326). New York: Guilford Press.

Martin, L. L., & Tesser, A. (1996a). Some ruminative thoughts. In R. S. Wyer (Ed.), *Advances in social cognition* (Vol. 9, pp. 1–47). Hillsdale, NJ: Erlbaum.

Martin, L. L., & Tesser, A. (1996b). *Striving and feeling: Interactions among goals, affect, and self-regulation.* Mahwah, NJ: Erlbaum.

McLaughlin, K. A., Borkovec, T. D., & Sibrava, N. J. (2007). The effects of worry and rumination on affect states and cognitive activity. *Behavior Therapy, 38*(1), 23–38.

McLaughlin, K. A., & Nolen-Hoeksema, S. (2011). Rumination as a transdiagnostic factor in depression and anxiety. *Behaviour Research and Therapy, 49*(3), 186–193.

Meyer, T. J., Miller, M. L., Metzger, R. L., & Borkovec, T. D. (1990). Development and validation of the Penn State worry questionnaire. *Behaviour Research and Therapy, 28*(6), 487–495.

Michael, T., Halligan, S. L., Clark, D. M., & Ehlers, A. (2007). Rumination in posttraumatic stress disorder. *Depression and Anxiety, 24*(5), 307–317.

Morrow, J., & Nolen-Hoeksema, S. (1990). Effects of responses to depression on the remediation of depressive affect. *Journal of Personality and Social Psychology,* *58*(3), 519–527.

Moulds, M. L., Kandris, E., Starr, S., & Wong, A. (2007). The relationship between rumination, avoidance and depression in a non-clinical sample. *Behaviour Research and Therapy, 45*(2), 251–261.

Murray, C. J., & Lopez, A. D. (1996). Evidence-based health policy: Lessons from the Global Burden of Disease Study. *Science, 274,* 740–743.

Nathan, P. E., & Gorman, J. M. (2007). *A guide to treatments that work* (3rd ed.). New York: Oxford University Press.

National Institute for Health and Clinical Excellence. (2009). *Depression: The treatment and management of depression in adults* (NICE Guidelines, CG90). London: Author.

Nolen-Hoeksema, S. (1991). Responses to depression and their effects on the duration of depressive episodes. *Journal of Abnormal Psychology, 100*(4), 569–582.

Nolen-Hoeksema, S. (2000). The role of rumination in depressive disorders and mixed anxiety/depressive symptoms. *Journal of Abnormal Psychology, 109*(3), 504–511.

Nolen-Hoeksema, S., Larson, J., & Grayson, C. (1999). Explaining the gender difference in depressive symptoms. *Journal of Personality and Social Psychology, 77*(5), 1061–1072.

Nolen-Hoeksema, S., McBride, A., & Larson, J. (1997). Rumination and psychological distress among bereaved partners. *Journal of Personality and Social Psychology, 72*(4), 855–862.

Nolen-Hoeksema, S., & Morrow, J. (1991). A prospective study of depression and posttraumatic stress symptoms after a natural disaster: The 1989 Loma Prieta earthquake. *Journal of Personality and Social Psychology, 61*(1), 115–121.

Nolen-Hoeksema, S., & Morrow, J. (1993). Effects of rumination and distraction on naturally occurring depressed mood. *Cognition and Emotion, 7*(6), 561–570.

Nolen-Hoeksema, S., Morrow, J., & Fredrickson, B. L. (1993). Response styles and the duration of episodes of depressed mood. *Journal of Abnormal Psychology, 102*(1), 20–28.

Nolen-Hoeksema, S., Parker, L. E., & Larson, J. (1994). Ruminative coping with depressed mood following loss. *Journal of Personality and Social Psychology, 67*(1), 92–104.

Nolen-Hoeksema, S., Stice, E., Wade, E., & Bohon, C. (2007). Reciprocal relations between rumination and bulimic, substance abuse, and depressive symptoms in female adolescents. *Journal of Abnormal Psychology, 116*(1), 198–207.

Nolen-Hoeksema, S., & Watkins, E. R. (2011). A heuristic for developing transdiagnostic models of psychopathology explaining multifinality and divergent trajectories. *Perspectives on Psychological Science, 6*(6), 589–609.

Nolen-Hoeksema, S., Wisco, B. E., & Lyubomirsky, S. (2008). Rethinking rumination. *Perspectives on Psychological Science, 3*(5), 400–424.

Nolen-Hoeksema, S., Wolfson, A., Mumme, D., & Guskin, K. (1995). Helplessness in children of depressed and nondepressed mothers. *Developmental Psychology, 31*(3), 377–387.

Papageorgiou, C., & Wells, A. (1999). Process and meta-cognitive dimensions of depressive and anxious thoughts and relationships with emotional intensity. *Clinical Psychology and Psychotherapy, 6*, 156–162.

Papageorgiou, C., & Wells, A. (2001). Metacognitive beliefs about rumination in recurrent major depression. *Cognitive and Behavioral Practice, 8*(2), 160–164.

Park, R. J., Goodyer, I., & Teasdale, J. D. (2004). Effects of induced rumination and distraction on mood and overgeneral autobiographical memory in adolescent major depressive disorder and controls. *Journal of Child Psychology and Psychiatry, 45*(5), 996–1006.

Paykel, E., Ramana, R., Cooper, Z., Hayhurst, H., Kerr, J., & Barocka, A. (1995). Residual symptoms after partial remission: An important outcome in depression. *Psychological Medicine, 25*(6), 1171–1180.

Paykel, E. S., Scott, J., Teasdale, J. D., Johnson, A. L., Garland, A., Moore, R., et al. (1999). Prevention of relapse in residual depression by cognitive therapy: A controlled trial. *Archives of General Psychiatry, 56*(9), 829–835.

Pyszczynski, T., & Greenberg, J. (1987). Self-regulatory perseveration and the depressive self-focusing style: A self-awareness theory of reactive depression. *Psychological Bulletin, 102*(1), 122–138.

Ramel, W., Goldin, P. R., Carmona, P. E., & McQuaid, J. R. (2004). The effects of mindfulness meditation on cognitive processes and affect in patients with past depression. *Cognitive Therapy and Research, 28*(4), 433–455.

Richards, D. A., & Borglin, G. (2011). Implementation of psychological therapies for anxiety and depression in routine practice: Two year prospective cohort study. *Journal of Affective Disorders, 133*(1), 51–60.

Rimes, K. A., & Watkins, E. (2005). The effects of self-focused rumination on global negative self-judgements in depression. *Behaviour Research and Therapy, 43*(12), 1673–1681.

Riso, L. P., Du Toit, P., Blandino, J. A., Penna, S., Dacey, S., Duin, J. S., et al. (2003). Cognitive aspects of chronic depression. *Journal of Abnormal Psychology, 112*(1), 72–80.

Roberts, J. E., Gilboa, E., & Gotlib, I. H. (1998). Ruminative response style and vulnerability to episodes of dysphoria: Gender, neuroticism, and episode duration. *Cognitive Therapy and Research, 22*(4), 401–423.

Rohan, K. J., Sigmon, S. T., & Dorhofer, D. M. (2003). Cognitive-behavioral factors in seasonal affective disorder. *Journal of Consulting and Clinical Psychology, 71*(1), 22–30.

Sakamoto, S., Kambara, M., & Tanno, Y. (2001). Response styles and cognitive and affective symptoms of depression. *Personality and Individual Differences, 31*(7), 1053–1065.

Sanislow, C. A., Pine, D. S., Quinn, K. J., Kozak, M. J., Garvey, M. A., Heinssen, et al. (2010). Developing constructs for psychopathology research: Research domain criteria. *Journal of Abnormal Psychology, 119*(4), 631–639.

Schmaling, K. B., Dimidjian, S., Katon, W., & Sullivan, M. (2002). Response styles among patients with minor depression and dysthymia in primary care. *Journal of Abnormal Psychology, 111*(2), 350–356.

Segerstrom, S. C., Tsao, J. C., Alden, L. E., & Craske, M. G. (2000). Worry and rumination: Repetitive thought as a concomitant and predictor of negative mood. *Cognitive Therapy and Research, 24*(6), 671–688.

Sezibera, V., Van Broeck, N., & Philippot, P. (2009). Intervening on persistent post-traumatic stress disorder: Rumination-focused cognitive and behavioral therapy in a population of young survivors of the 1994 genocide in Rwanda. *Journal of Cognitive Psychotherapy, 23*(2), 107–113.

Skitch, S. A., & Abela, J. R. (2008). Rumination in response to stress as a common vulnerability factor to depression and substance misuse in adolescence. *Journal of Abnormal Child Psychology, 36*(7), 1029–1045.

Smith, J. M., Alloy, L. B., & Abramson, L. Y. (2006). Cognitive vulnerability to depression, rumination, hopelessness, and suicidal ideation: Multiple pathways to self-injurious thinking. *Suicide and Life-Threatening Behavior, 36*(4), 443–454.

Spasojević, J., & Alloy, L. B. (2001). Rumination as a common mechanism relating depressive risk factors to depression. *Emotion, 1*(1), 25–37.

Spasojević, J., & Alloy, L. B. (2002). Who becomes a depressive ruminator? Developmental antecedents of ruminative response style. *Journal of Cognitive Psychotherapy, 16*(4), 405–419.

Stöber, J. (1998). Worry, problem elaboration and suppression of imagery: The role of concreteness. *Behaviour Research and Therapy, 36*(7), 751–756.

Stöber, J., & Borkovec, T. (2002). Reduced concreteness of worry in generalized anxiety disorder: Findings from a therapy study. *Cognitive Therapy and Research, 26*(1), 89–96.

Takano, K., & Tanno, Y. (2009). Self-rumination, self-reflection, and depression: Self-rumination counteracts the adaptive effect of self-reflection. *Behaviour Research and Therapy, 47*(3), 260–264.

Taylor, S. E., Pham, L. B., Rivkin, I. D., & Armor, D. A. (1998). Harnessing the imagination: Mental simulation, self-regulation, and coping. *American Psychologist, 53*(4), 429–439.

Teasdale, J. D., Segal, Z., & Williams, J. M. G. (1995). How does cognitive therapy prevent depressive relapse and why should attentional control (mindfulness) training help? *Behaviour Research and Therapy, 33*(1), 25–39.

Teasdale, J. D., Segal, Z. V., Williams, J. M. G., Ridgeway, V. A., Soulsby, J. M., & Lau, M. A. (2000). Prevention of relapse/recurrence in major depression by mindfulness-based cognitive therapy. *Journal of Consulting and Clinical Psychology, 68*(4), 615–623.

Teismann, T., von Brachel, R., Hanning, S., Grillenberger, M., Hebermehl, L., Hornstein, I., et al. (2014). A randomized controlled trial on the effectiveness of a rumination-focused group treatment for residual depression. *Psychotherapy Research, 24*, 80–90.

Topper, M., Emmelkamp, P. M., & Ehring, T. (2010). Improving prevention of depression and anxiety disorders: Repetitive negative thinking as a promising target. *Applied and Preventive Psychology, 14*(1), 57–71.

Topper, M., Emmelkamp, P. M., Watkins, E., & Ehring, T. (2014). Development and assessment of brief versions of the Penn State Worry Questionnaire and the Ruminative Response Scale. *British Journal of Clinical Psychology, 53*(4), 402–421.

Topper, M., Emmelkamp, P. M., Watkins, E. R., & Ehring, T. (2016). *Prevention of anxiety disorders and depression by targeting excessive worry and rumina-*

tion in adolescents: A randomized controlled trial. Manuscript submitted for publication.

Treynor, W., Gonzalez, R., & Nolen-Hoeksema, S. (2003). Rumination reconsidered: A psychometric analysis. *Cognitive Therapy and Research, 27*(3), 247–259.

Verplanken, B. (2006). Beyond frequency: Habit as mental construct. *British Journal of Social Psychology, 45*(3), 639–656.

Verplanken, B., Friborg, O., Wang, C. E., Trafimow, D., & Woolf, K. (2007). Mental habits: Metacognitive reflection on negative self-thinking. *Journal of Personality and Social Psychology, 92*(3), 526–541.

Verplanken, B., & Orbell, S. (2003). Reflections on past behavior: A self-report index of habit strength. *Journal of Applied Social Psychology, 33*(6), 1313–1330.

Verplanken, B., & Wood, W. (2006). Interventions to break and create consumer habits. *Journal of Public Policy and Marketing, 25*(1), 90–103.

Watkins, E. R. (2004a). Adaptive and maladaptive ruminative self-focus during emotional processing. *Behavior Research and Therapy, 42*(9), 1037–1052.

Watkins, E. R. (2004b). Appraisals and strategies associated with rumination and worry. *Personality and Individual Differences, 37*(4), 679–694.

Watkins, E. R. (2008). Constructive and unconstructive repetitive thought. *Psychological Bulletin, 134*(2), 163–206.

Watkins, E. R. (2011). Dysregulation in level of goal and action identification across psychological disorders. *Clinical Psychology Review, 31*(2), 260–278.

Watkins, E. R. (2013). Repetitive thought. In M. D. Robinson, E. R. Watkins, & E. Harmon-Jones (Eds.), *Handbook of cognition and emotion* (pp. 383–400). New York: Guilford Press.

Watkins, E. R., Baeyens, C. B., & Read, R. (2009). Concreteness training reduces dysphoria: Proof-of-principle for repeated cognitive bias modification in depression. *Journal of Abnormal Psychology, 118*(1), 55–64.

Watkins, E. R., & Baracaia, S. (2001). Why do people ruminate in dysphoric moods? *Personality and Individual Differences, 30*(5), 723–734.

Watkins, E. R., & Baracaia, S. (2002). Rumination and social problem-solving in depression. *Behaviour Research and Therapy, 40*(10), 1179–1189.

Watkins, E. R., & Brown, R. (2002). Rumination and executive function in depression: An experimental study. *Journal of Neurology, Neurosurgery and Psychiatry, 72*(3), 400–402.

Watkins, E. R., Moberly, N. J., & Moulds, M. L. (2008). Processing mode causally influences emotional reactivity: Distinct effects of abstract versus concrete construal on emotional response. *Emotion, 8*(3), 364–378.

Watkins, E. R., & Moulds, M. L. (2005). Distinct modes of ruminative self-focus: Impact of abstract versus concrete rumination on problem solving in depression. *Emotion, 5*(3), 319–328.

Watkins, E. R., & Moulds, M. L. (2007). Reduced concreteness of rumination in depression: A pilot study. *Personality and Individual Differences, 43*(6), 1386–1395.

Watkins, E. R., Moulds, M., & Mackintosh, B. (2005). Comparisons between rumination and worry in a non-clinical population. *Behaviour Research and Therapy, 43*(12), 1577–1585.

Watkins, E. R., Mullan, E., Wingrove, J., Rimes, K., Steiner, H., Bathurst, N., et al. (2011). Rumination-focused cognitive-behavioral therapy for residual depression: Phase II randomised controlled trial. *British Journal of Psychiatry, 199*(4), 317–322.

Watkins, E. R., & Nolen-Hoeksema, S. (2014). A habit-goal framework of depressive rumination. *Journal of Abnormal Psychology, 123*(1), 24–34.

Watkins, E. R., Scott, J., Wingrove, J., Rimes, K., Bathurst, N., Steiner, H., et al. (2007). Rumination-focused cognitive behavior therapy for residual depression: A case series. *Behaviour Research and Therapy, 45*(9), 2144–2154.

Watkins, E. R., Taylor, R., Byng, R., Baeyens, C., Read, R., Pearson, K., et al. (2012). Guided self-help concreteness training as an intervention for major depression in primary care: A Phase II randomized controlled trial. *Psychological Medicine, 42*(7), 1359–1371.

Watkins, E. R., & Teasdale, J. D. (2001). Rumination and overgeneral memory in depression: Effects of self-focus and analytic thinking. *Journal of Abnormal Psychology, 110*(2), 353–357.

Watkins, E. R., & Teasdale, J. D. (2004). Adaptive and maladaptive self-focus in depression. *Journal of Affective Disorders, 82*(1), 1–8.

Webb, T. L., & Sheeran, P. (2006). Does changing behavioral intentions engender behavior change?: A meta-analysis of the experimental evidence. *Psychological Bulletin, 132*(2), 249–268.

Wells, A. (1995). Meta-cognition and worry: A cognitive model of generalized anxiety disorder. *Behavioral and Cognitive Psychotherapy, 23*(03), 301–320.

Wilamowska, Z. A., Thompson-Hollands, J., Fairholme, C. P., Ellard, K. K., Farchione, T. J., & Barlow, D. H. (2010). Conceptual background, development, and preliminary data from the unified protocol for transdiagnostic treatment of emotional disorders. *Depression and Anxiety, 27*(10), 882–890.

Williams, J. M. G., Barnhofer, T., Crane, C., Herman, D., Raes, F., Watkins, E., et al. (2007). Autobiographical memory specificity and emotional disorder. *Psychological Bulletin, 133*(1), 122–148.

Wood, W., & Neal, D. T. (2007). A new look at habits and the habit–goal interface. *Psychological Review, 114*(4), 843–863.

Wood, W., Tam, L., & Witt, M. G. (2005). Changing circumstances, disrupting habits. *Journal of Personality and Social Psychology, 88*(6), 918–933.

World Health Organization. (1992). *The ICD-10 classification of mental and behavioural disorders: Clinical descriptions and diagnostic guidelines.* Geneva, Switzerland: Author.

World Health Organization. (2001). *The world health report 2001—Mental health: New understanding, new hope.* Geneva, Switzerland: Author.

World Health Organization. (2008). *The global burden of disease: 2004 update.* Geneva, Switzerland: Author.

Index

Note, f, n, or *t* following a page number indicates a figure, note, or a table.

E

Eating disorders, 9, 141–149
Effects of rumination. *See also* Consequences
  assessment and, 86
  case examples, 126–129, 280
  CUDOS (Context, Usefulness, Development,
    OptionS) analysis and, 42–43
  therapy rationale and, 91
  treatment planning and, 169–170
Elaborations, 30–31
E-mental health. *See* Internet-delivered RFCBT
Emotion regulation, 36–37
Emotional abuse, 24
Emotional exposure, 45–46. *See also* Exposure
  approaches
Emotions. *See also* Feelings
  concreteness training and, 200–203
  functional analysis (FA) and, 175, 179
  psychoeducation about, 97
  therapy rationale and, 97
  thinking style and, 208
  visualizations and imagery techniques and,
    215–216
Empathy, 57–58
Emphasize the Importance of Repetition
  and Practice (RFCBT Principle 6), 56,
  172–173, 178, 179, 193, 255, 302, 308.
  See also Practice; Principles of RFCBT;
  Repetition
Encourage Active, Concrete, Experiential,
  and Specific Behavior—The ACES Rule
  principle (RFCBT Principle 3), 50–53, 172,
  176, 178, 180, 193, 203, 245, 303. *See
  also* ACES (Active, Concrete, Experiential,
  Specific) rule; Principles of RFCBT
Encouragement, 196–199, 201–202
Environment. *See also* Altering environmental
  contingencies; Interventions
  altering environmental contingencies and,
    136–149
  assessment and, 86
  case examples, 125–126, 141–148, 280, 281
  concreteness training and, 205
  flow and, 226–227
  key aspects of, 136–140
  overview, 44, 134
  treatment planning and, 170
Evaluation. *See also* Self-evaluation
  approach behaviors and, 161
  compassion training and, 266–267
  shifting thinking styles and, 56–57, 183–184,
    218
Evidence supporting thoughts, 12, 37
Evidence-based treatment, 12–17, 306
Excuses, 37
Executive functioning, 8
Expectations
  therapy rationale and, 94
  treatment planning and, 168–169
Experiential evidence, 155
Experiential exercises. *See also* Behavioral exper-
  iments; Experiments; Imagery exercises
  absorption exercises and, 228–231, 232–234
  ACES (Active, Concrete, Experiential,
  Specific) rule and, 50–53

case examples, 280, 283–285
compassion training and, 242–248
components of RFCBT and, 39
group RFCBT and, 289*t*, 302, 303
homework and, 46–47
Internet-delivered RFCBT and, 306–307
rumination-focused cognitive-behavioral
  therapy and, 11
shifting thinking styles and, 56–57, 221–223
values and, 268–269
Experiments. *See also* Behavioral experiments;
  Experiential exercises
  components of RFCBT and, 39
  difficulties in implementing plans, 174
  If–Then plans and, 151
  processing style and, 191–193
Exposure approaches. *See also* Behavioral
  experiments; Experiential exercises;
  Imagery exercises
  emotional exposure and, 45–46
  overview, 10
  visualizations and imagery techniques and,
    214–215
Expression, 29

F

Facial expressions, 57, 196, 204, 219, 221, 252,
  254, 257, 308, 320
Failure
  functions of rumination, 35–36
  rumination as a form of avoidance and,
    28–29
Feedback
  compassion training and, 267
  concreteness training and, 196–199, 201–202
  flow and, 225–226
  Internet-delivered RFCBT and, 305, 307
Feelings. *See also* Emotions
  antecedent–behavior–consequence analysis
    (ABC approach) and, 41–42
  compassion training and, 260–264
  functions of rumination, 36–37
  rumination as a form of avoidance and, 29
  shifting thinking styles and, 56–57
  therapy rationale and, 97
  thinking style and, 208
  visualizations and imagery techniques and,
    215–216
Flow, 223–228, 234. *See also* Absorption
  training
Focused attention, 224–225. *See also* Attention
Focus on nonspecific factors, 57
Focus on Nonspecific Factors (RFCBT Principle
  8), 57–58, 176, 177, 178, 179, 193,
  246, 246–247, 308. *See also* Nonspecific
  factors; Principles of RFCBT
Follow through, 27
Forms. *See* Handouts and forms
Formulation. *See also* Case formulation;
  Functional analysis (FA)
  case examples, 162–172, 278–280
  components of RFCBT and, 40
  functional analysis (FA) and, 175–179
  If–Then plans and, 154–156
  overview, 38